DYSLEXIA IN ADULTHOOD

This groundbreaking book provides a comprehensive international perspective on how dyslexia manifests across the lifespan, with a rare and valuable focus on adults. Each chapter meticulously examines research on critical aspects of dyslexia relevant to adult populations.

The book delivers an in-depth assessment of the dyslexic reader's neurocognitive profile—exploring language processing, memory systems, learning mechanisms, executive functions, and neurobiological foundations. Readers will find evidence-based approaches to screening, diagnosis, and intervention specifically tailored to adults with dyslexia.

The text addresses crucial questions about long-term cognitive risk factors while highlighting how adults with dyslexia develop resilience through effective compensatory strategies. By synthesizing diverse research into a single authoritative resource, this book serves as an essential reference for scholars, students, and professionals worldwide who seek to understand how dyslexia impacts training, education, and employment throughout adulthood.

Eddy Cavalli is an Associate Professor in Cognitive Sciences and Neuropsychology at Lyon 2 University, France, and a member of the Laboratory for the Study of Cognitive Mechanisms.

Pascale Colé is a Full Professor in Cognitive Psychology at Aix-Marseille University, France, and a member of the Research Center in Psychology and Neurosciences.

Lynne G. Duncan is a Reader in Developmental Psychology at the University of Dundee, Scotland, UK.

DYSLEXIA IN ADULTHOOD

A Research Perspective

Edited by Eddy Cavalli, Pascale Colé and
Lynne G. Duncan

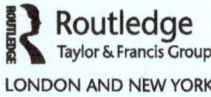

LONDON AND NEW YORK

Designed cover image: Getty Images

First published 2026
by Routledge
4 Park Square, Milton Park, Abingdon, Oxon OX14 4RN

and by Routledge
605 Third Avenue, New York, NY 10158

Routledge is an imprint of the Taylor & Francis Group, an informa business

© 2026 selection and editorial matter, Eddy Cavalli, Pascale Cole and Lynne G. Duncan; individual chapters, the contributors

The right of Eddy Cavalli, Pascale Colé and Lynne G. Duncan to be identified as the author[/s] of the editorial material, and of the authors for their individual chapters, has been asserted in accordance with sections 77 and 78 of the Copyright, Designs and Patents Act 1988.

All rights reserved. No part of this book may be reprinted or reproduced or utilised in any form or by any electronic, mechanical, or other means, now known or hereafter invented, including photocopying and recording, or in any information storage or retrieval system, without permission in writing from the publishers.

For Product Safety Concerns and Information please contact our EU representative GPSR@taylorandfrancis.com. Taylor & Francis Verlag GmbH, Kaufingerstraße 24, 80331 München, Germany.

Trademark notice: Product or corporate names may be trademarks or registered trademarks, and are used only for identification and explanation without intent to infringe.

British Library Cataloguing-in-Publication Data
A catalogue record for this book is available from the British Library

Library of Congress Cataloging-in-Publication Data
Names: Cavalli, Eddy editor | Cole, Pascale, 1960- editor | Duncan, Lynne G. editor
Title: Dyslexia in adulthood : a research perspective / edited by Eddy Cavalli, Pascale Cole and Lynne G. Duncan.
Description: Abingdon, Oxon ; New York, NY : Routledge, 2026. | Includes bibliographical references and index. |
Identifiers: LCCN 2025039987 (print) | LCCN 2025039988 (ebook) | ISBN 9781032792330 hbk | ISBN 9781032792323 pbk | ISBN 9781003491125 ebk
Subjects: LCSH: Dyslexia--Research | Dyslexics--Research
Classification: LCC RC394.W6 D976 2026 (print) | LCC RC394.W6 (ebook)
LC record available at https://lccn.loc.gov/2025039987
LC ebook record available at https://lccn.loc.gov/2025039988

ISBN: 978-1-032-79233-0 (hbk)
ISBN: 978-1-032-79232-3 (pbk)
ISBN: 978-1-003-49112-5 (ebk)

DOI: 10.4324/9781003491125

Typeset in Times New Roman
by SPi Technologies India Pvt Ltd (Straive)

CONTENTS

List of Contributors vii
Acknowledgements ix

Introduction: Understanding Adult Dyslexia—
Definitions, Challenges and Research Perspectives 1
Eddy Cavalli, Pascale Colé and Lynne G. Duncan

1 Adults with Learning Disorders in Reading: A Selective
Review of the Literature 22
H. Lee Swanson

2 Phonological Processing Skills in Adults with Dyslexia 41
*Kirsten Schraeyen, Jolijn Vanderauwera and
Maaike Vandermosten*

3 Oral Language Skills and Reading in Adults with Dyslexia 65
Jeremy M. Law and Eddy Cavalli

4 Visuo-orthographic Processing in Dyslexic Adults 105
Nadège Doignon-Camus and Anne Bonnefond

5 Executive Functions in Adults with Dyslexia 129
   James H. Smith-Spark

6 Memory in Adults with Dyslexia 153
   James H. Smith-Spark and Rebecca Gordon

7 Neurological Function in Adult Dyslexia 179
   Fabio Richlan

8 Screening and Diagnosis of Dyslexia in Higher Education 205
   Wim Tops and Marc Brysbaert

9 Learning Strategies and Metacognition in Adults with Dyslexia 219
   Rauno Parrila, Bradley W. Bergey and S. Helene Deacon

10 Cognitive Remediation and Neural Changes in Adults with Dyslexia 243
    Floriana Costanzo, Stefano Vicari and Deny Menghini

11 The Definition of Dyslexia, Still Debated After All These Years 287
    Franck Ramus

12 Compensatory Mechanisms in University Students with Dyslexia 298
    Pascale Colé, Lynne G. Duncan and Eddy Cavalli

13 Supporting Students with Dyslexia in Higher Education: Predictors of Success and Inclusive Adjustments 337
    Émilie Collette, Mariane Frenay and Marie-Anne Schelstraete

Index 372

CONTRIBUTORS

Bradley W. Bergey
Queens College
City University of New York
USA

Anne Bonnefond
University of Strasbourg
France

Marc Brysbaert
Ghent University
Belgium

Eddy Cavalli
Lyon 2 University
France

Pascale Colé
Aix-Marseille University
France

Émilie Collette
Université Catholique de Louvain
UCLouvain, Belgium

Floriana Costanzo
Sapienza University of Rome
Italy

S. Helene Deacon
Dalhousie University
Canada

Nadège Doignon-Camus
University of Strasbourg
France

Lynne G. Duncan
Dundee University
Scotland, UK

Mariane Frenay
Université Catholique de Louvain
UCLouvain, Belgium

Rebecca Gordon
University College London
UK

Jeremy M. Law
University of Glasgow
UK

Deny Menghini
Bambino Gesù Children's Hospital
Rome, Italy

Rauno Parrila
Australian Catholic University
Australia

Franck Ramus
CNRS
Ecole Normale Supérieure de Paris
Paris, France

Fabio Richlan
University of Salzburg
Austria

Marie-Anne Schelstraete
Université Catholique de Louvain
UCLouvain, Belgium

Kirsten Schraeyen
KU Leuven
Belgium

James H. Smith-Spark
London South Bank University
UK

H. Lee Swanson
University of California-Riverside
USA

Wim Tops
Hasselt University
Belgium

Jolijn Vanderauwera
Université Catholique de Louvain
UCLouvain, Belgium

Maaike Vandermosten
KU Leuven
Belgium

Stefano Vicari
University of Genova
Italy

ACKNOWLEDGEMENTS

This research was supported by funding from the Institute of Convergence ILCB (France 2030, ANR-16-CONV-0002), the Excellence Initiative of Aix-Marseille University A*MIDEX (ANR-11-IDEX-0001-02), the LABEX CORTEX (ANR-11-LABX-0042), the Excellence Initiative of the University of Lyon (ANR-11-IDEX-0007), and by the research grant "DYSsuccess" awarded to EC (ANR-18-CE28-0006).

INTRODUCTION

Understanding Adult Dyslexia—Definitions, Challenges and Research Perspectives

Eddy Cavalli, Pascale Colé and Lynne G. Duncan

0.1 Defining Developmental Dyslexia: Theories and Criteria

Formulating a definition of developmental dyslexia continues to prove challenging for researchers despite the existence of a wide-ranging literature on this neurodevelopmental disorder. A number of factors have complicated the definition process, including changing ideas about how to conceptualise the reading difficulty in dyslexia, shifting attitudes towards co-occurrence with other neurodevelopmental disorders, ongoing debates surrounding exclusionary criteria and the prevalence of popular myths about dyslexia.

Scientific studies and professional associations (e.g., International Dyslexia Association (IDA), 2002; British Dyslexia Association (BDA), 2010; European Dyslexia Association (Mather, White, & Youman, 2020)) propose definitions that outline specific criteria for characterising dyslexia. The IDA definition is representative of this approach:

> Dyslexia is a specific learning disability that is neurobiological in origin. It is characterised by difficulties with accurate and/or fluent word recognition and by poor spelling and decoding abilities. These difficulties typically result from a deficit in the phonological component of language that is often unexpected in relation to other cognitive abilities and the provision of effective classroom instruction.
>
> *(IDA Board of Directors, 2002)*

While the IDA definition offers a phonological explanation of reading difficulties in dyslexia, substantial disagreement exists over the aetiology of individual cases of dyslexia. Indeed, four main hypotheses are currently proposed as causal explanations of dyslexia, namely the auditory, visual, cerebellar and phonological hypotheses. These hypotheses are summarised briefly below and will be referenced throughout this book.

According to the **auditory hypothesis** (Tallal, 1980), the origin of dyslexia is related to an impairment in the rapid auditory processing necessary for the perception of the duration of certain sounds (verbal or non-verbal) or for the reproduction of a rhythm in a synchronous fashion (Wolff, 2002). Expressed more generally, dyslexia is a consequence of impairments to the perceptual organisation of the acoustic structure of speech sounds (Goswami et al., 2014), leading to the phonological difficulties suffered by individuals with dyslexia.

Among the **visual hypotheses**, a magnocellular deficit (Livingstone et al., 1991; Stein & Walsh, 1997) and a reduction in visuo-attentional span (Lobier et al., 2011) are the most influential. According to the latter, dyslexic deficits are linked to a reduced visuo-attentional span, which corresponds to the number of visual elements that can be processed in parallel after a brief exposure. This reduced span affects the capacity of individuals with dyslexia to perform accurate orthographic processing of written words.

The first two hypotheses, auditory and visual, have been brought together in a unifying theory known as the **magnocellular deficit theory** (Stein & Walsh, 1997), which postulates that the magnocellular deficit is generalisable across all perceptual modalities, especially visual and auditory perception (Ramus, 2003a).

The **motor or cerebellar hypothesis** was formulated in response to reports that a significant proportion of individuals with dyslexia exhibit difficulties in sequential and temporal processing, as well as in motor coordination and balance. Fawcett and Nicolson (1999) proposed that a cerebellar dysfunction is implicated in these difficulties, which impedes the normal formation of the perceptual (auditory and visual) and articulatory skills necessary for setting up the phonological system and for the recognition of written words. Such a deficit would subsequently interfere with the automatisation of the orthographic and phonological reading procedures, and with reading and writing activities more generally (Nicolson & Fawcett, 1990, 1999; Nicolson et al., 2001).

Finally, the hypothesis that attracts the most consensus is that a majority of individuals with dyslexia present with an oral language problem underpinned primarily by a phonological processing impairment, which leads to difficulties in the processing of written language (Peterson & Pennington, 2015). This **phonological hypothesis** receives support from a large body of data, documenting significant dyslexic difficulties in phonological tasks, of which the most important are word and pseudoword reading, phonological awareness and verbal short-term memory (Ramus, 2008). Such difficulties are observed among children with dyslexia and even before reading is acquired among children classified as being at risk of developing dyslexia (Law et al., 2017). The phonological deficit impairs the learning of grapheme–phoneme correspondences and thus interferes with the word decoding procedures that utilise this information during reading acquisition in alphabetic orthographies (Norton et al., 2014; Snowling, 1981; Ziegler & Goswami, 2006).

In 2010, Tunmer and Greaney proposed that research evidence about the causes of dyslexia should provide the basis for *inclusionary criteria* in developing any definition of dyslexia, although they were careful to emphasise that the inclusionary criteria might change as the field developed. Tunmer and Greaney followed the IDA in using *"a general deficit in phonological processing skills"* as their inclusionary criteria due to the extent of research support for the phonological hypothesis. This was one of four sets of criteria they identified as central to defining dyslexia, with the other three listed below:

- *Persistence of the symptoms linked to dyslexia throughout life*, especially in the accuracy of written word recognition, spelling and phonological decoding.
- *Adequate exposure to evidence-based instruction and education*, to rule out reading difficulties arising from inadequate educational experiences, which respond well to intervention (Fuchs & Fuchs, 2006; Vellutino et al., 1996; Vellutino et al., 2006).
- *Exclusionary criteria*, considered essential for precision in diagnosis. The principal exclusionary criteria are defined in terms of the absence of disorders of the following types: attentional, visual, auditory, mental, communication, emotional, behavioural, intellectual, neurological, developmental (e.g., autistic spectrum disorders and childhood psychotic disorders) and finally, general health (chronic or acute problems).

Exclusionary criteria have also proved controversial in defining dyslexia. For example, although intellectual impairment is often part of the exclusionary criteria, there is little research evidence to suggest that below-average IQ within the typical range excludes dyslexia (Stanovich & Siegel, 1994; Stuebing et al., 2002), and this is a key argument in the "Dyslexia Debate" (see Chapter 11). Furthermore, in the majority of the studies underpinning the different explanations of dyslexia presented earlier, a single hypothesis was tested without considering any alternative hypotheses, and it has been usual for data only to be reported at the group level rather than at the individual level. These design features may have led to instances of co-occurrence or individual variation in deficits being overlooked, leading to a lack of sensitivity in diagnosis due to the use of exclusionary criteria that were too broad.

To address these limitations, several studies have employed a multiple-case study design to examine the different explanatory hypotheses for dyslexia. Ramus (2003b) investigated university students with dyslexia, while White et al. (2006) and Saksida et al. (2016) studied children with dyslexia. Generally, the results from these studies confirmed the prevalence of phonological impairments, although a greater diversity in problems was apparent among children than adults. Indeed, in Ramus's (2003b) study, all the adults with dyslexia displayed a phonological impairment compared to a smaller percentage of children – 52% and 79% in the studies of White et al. (2006) and Saksida et al. (2016), respectively. It is, however, important to note that the very high prevalence of phonological impairments observed among the adults in Ramus's study could be due to the participant selection process, as all of the participants with dyslexia were university students. It is possible that these students with dyslexia manage to pursue academic study because they have few or no associated difficulties, thus constituting "pure" cases of dyslexia (Ramus, 2003b, but see Marchetti et al., 2023). Nevertheless, the deficits shown by these adults with dyslexia are *persistent* in terms of Tunmer and Greaney's (2010) criteria and hence, such deficits can be considered as behavioural markers of dyslexia.

The diversity of the symptoms with which dyslexia is commonly associated during development (Saksida et al., 2016; White et al., 2006) has gained increasing recognition in the research literature. Furthermore, dyslexia has greater-than-chance comorbidity links with other neurodevelopmental disorders such as developmental language disorder, dyscalculia and attention deficit hyperactivity disorder (ADHD) (McGrath et al., 2011; Snowling & Hulme, 2020). Recognition of the varied symptoms and high levels of comorbidity has resulted in several new approaches to the definition of dyslexia. The high co-occurrence rates prompted the *Diagnostic and Statistical Manual of Mental Disorders (5th Edition*; DSM-5; American Psychiatric Society, 2013) to define dyslexia as a particular case of specific learning disorder, which comprises a wide spectrum of disorders considered to be neurodevelopmental in nature that an individual can present throughout their life. Within this framework, dyslexia manifests primarily as persistent difficulties in recognising written words, slowed reading fluency and weak spelling performance; additional difficulties in reading comprehension may also be observed (DSM-5; APS, 2013). Nonetheless, the diagnostic criteria that have been established for dyslexia in DSM-5 are somewhat general and offer few explanations about the causes and nature of the observed difficulties in this disability.

Another approach to defining dyslexia has been to reject the idea of a single deficit in favour of multiple cognitive deficits as inclusionary criteria (Pennington, 2006). According to McGrath et al. (2020), there are numerous potential risk factors that relate to neurodevelopmental disorders in a probabilistic, rather than deterministic, manner. Where comorbidity occurs, shared risk factors can be identified, as in the case of processing speed deficits, which account for some of the co-occurrence between dyslexia, dyscalculia and ADHD (McGrath et al., 2011).

In line with this probabilistic perspective, a growing body of research over the last decade has focused on multifactorial models that integrate both cognitive and environmental dimensions. In these models, dyslexia—and especially its severity—is conceptualised as resulting from the combination or interaction of multiple risk factors, such as phonological deficits, rapid automatised naming (RAN) impairments and oral language difficulties. These risk factors, like dyslexia itself, are dimensional in nature and vary in severity across individuals. Importantly, as Catts and Petscher (2022) have pointed out, the effects of these risk factors are further influenced by contextual variables such as the quality of instruction received, variation in language exposure, parental support and the individual's broader sociocultural background. In this light, dyslexia is not seen as an inevitable consequence of specific deficits, but as a probabilistic outcome shaped by the interaction of risk and protective factors. Additional risk factors for learning disabilities—including dyslexia—may include comorbid developmental language disorders, attentional or anxiety disorders (Nelson & Harwood, 2011), exposure to trauma (Duplechain et al., 2008), the internalisation of stigma related to reading difficulties (Daley & Rappolt-Schlichtmann, 2018) and misinterpretation of dialectal differences by teachers (Washington & Seidenberg, 2021). On the other hand, positive influences such as high-quality mentoring (Haft et al., 2019), interventions that boost intrinsic motivation (Lovett et al., 2021), emotional resilience (Goldberg et al., 2003; Zheng et al., 2014), growth mindsets (Andersen & Nielsen, 2016), family practices related to reading (Willingham, 2015) and rich conversational interactions at home (Romeo et al., 2018) have been shown to mitigate dyslexia symptomatology. These factors can support the development of the reading brain network and enhance students' attitudes towards reading, in some cases even independently of socioeconomic status. This broader perspective calls for an inclusive and dynamic definition of dyslexia that considers not only weaknesses but also protective factors, personal assets and compensatory mechanisms. Recent work has begun to explore this direction, suggesting the integration of individual strengths into theoretical models (e.g., Palser et al., 2021; Sturm et al., 2021). In other words, it is increasingly important to consider the dynamic role of changing environmental influences and social-emotional resources in shaping the expression of dyslexia across individuals and developmental contexts.

In view of the ongoing debate, two recent studies have systematically re-examined the components of the definition of dyslexia. The first by Carroll et al. (2024) is a Delphi study, which surveyed a panel of 58 members with a range of relevant expertise (e.g., education, psychology and occupational support) in an attempt to achieve consensus across research and practice. The second by Catts et al. (2024) is one of several articles in a special issue of the journal *Dyslexia*, which have revisited the content of the IDA definition (2002) to present a series of recommendations for updating the definition.

There is agreement across the two studies that dyslexia can be identified as *a problem with reading and spelling*, with Catts (2024) also mentioning weak decoding skills and Carroll et al. (2024) emphasising poor reading fluency as a reliable marker. These difficulties are noted as *persistent despite exposure to quality reading instruction*. Weak phonological processing skills are highlighted in both as the most common impairment; however, this is viewed as one of *multiple risk factors*, which cause dyslexia to occur at varying degrees of severity and frequently to co-occur with other neurodevelopmental disorders.

Some issues remained unresolved or were explored in only one of the studies. Differing opinions were noted across both studies around the use of exclusionary criteria based on IQ, as this was often perceived as a useful indicator of "unexpectedness" in practice or research contexts, even if research evidence shows that an IQ achievement discrepancy is neither necessary nor sufficient for diagnosis (Stuebing et al., 2002). An important contribution of the work by Carroll et al. (2024) was to make it explicit that dyslexia can be expressed differently according to the language being learned. Further, this study found agreement about factors, which, regardless of popular belief, did not warrant a place in the inclusionary criteria of any definition of dyslexia due to lack of research evidence, namely visual stress (Griffiths et al., 2016) and creativity (Erbeli et al., 2022). Catts et al. (2024) examined the critical issue of bias and discrimination in relation to the diagnosis of dyslexia, recommending that the inclusionary criteria should specify that dyslexia occurs across all languages, races, ethnicities and socioeconomic categories. Finally, the impact of a variety of secondary consequences of dyslexia was acknowledged across studies. Carroll et al. highlighted academic challenges in later achievement, and Catts et al. drew attention to non-academic challenges with self-esteem, anxiety and depression, although such challenges were not regarded as diagnostic criteria for dyslexia in either study.

0.2 A Special Case: The Adult with Dyslexia in Higher Education

Although research is mainly focused on the manifestation and causes of dyslexia among children and adolescents, French language surveys make it possible to estimate a prevalence for dyslexia among adults of between 6% and 8% (De La Haye et al., 2008; Jonas, 2012; Murat, 2005). However, we do not have epidemiological data at our disposal for many other writing systems, and where these data are available, there is very little information concerning adults. The general prevalence of dyslexia varies between 3% and 8% in Italy and between 5% and 12% in the United States; the figures obtained here are also a function of the particular definition of dyslexia in use (Katusic et al., 2001; Lindgren et al., 1985). Nevertheless, longitudinal studies (Shaywitz et al., 1998; Sprenger-Charolles et al., 2000) indicate that dyslexia persists with age and, hence, constitutes a non-transient developmental disorder, which makes it possible to apply the globally estimated prevalence rate of dyslexia at 10% to adulthood (Dyslexia International, 2014).

A sizeable proportion of individuals with reading difficulty do not progress beyond secondary school in education and follow a short professional training (e.g., 8 out of 10 young people with reading difficulty according to a French investigation conducted by De La Haye et al. (2008)) or when no longer in school, often find themselves unemployed (e.g., over 14% of 16- to 24-year-olds in England; *Public Health England*, 2013). However, a growing number of individuals with dyslexia pursue and succeed in post-secondary studies despite significant and persistent impairments in reading (approximately 1.4% of the student population in France according to data from *University Disability Services*; between 4% and 6.3% in the United Kingdom, *UK Higher Education Statistic Agency*; between 1.6% and 6.4% in Spain, López-Escribano et al., 2018; and between 1.5% and 4% in Sweden, Wolff & Lundberg, 2003). This suggests that this population is likely to have developed compensations or adaptations induced by continued exposure to writing, as well as by a strong motivation to learn (Lefly & Pennington, 2000). In this context, some studies show that students with dyslexia can sometimes attain a level of reading comprehension comparable to that of adults of the same age who read normally (Deacon et al., 2012; Parrila et al., 2007; Simmons & Singleton, 2000), despite persistent low-level processing deficits in reading (decoding and written word recognition; Bruck, 1990, 1992; Cavalli et al., 2018; Kemp et al., 2009; Martin et al., 2010; Pennington et al., 1986). Consequently, the reading of an adult with dyslexia at university level poses a genuine scientific challenge, as it is unclear how a reader whose basic reading skills remain deficient manages to deal with the intensive exposure to writing necessary for academic advancement and, later, for obtaining university qualifications. The further exploration of this question is one of the objectives of this book.

The large body of reading research has increasingly been applied to the reading of university students with dyslexia, partly due to the ease of accessing this particular population via university disability services (e.g., Callens et al., 2012; Warmington et al., 2013). These studies have led to recommendations both for screening and diagnosis, as well as for the management and academic support of these students. All of these results lead us to expect that adults with dyslexia at the university level may develop reading strategies most likely different from those of typical adult readers, especially when engaged in the activity of reading comprehension.

Epidemiological studies have shown that dyslexia is a persistent problem in adulthood and represents a significant impediment in the pursuit of higher education. For example, although numbers continue to rise, the proportion of UK university students who were dyslexic in 2013 was only 3.2%, increasing to 5% by 2016 (Ryder & Norwich, 2019; Warmington et al., 2013). Such low prevalence attests to the difficulty for individuals with dyslexia in pursuing and succeeding in secondary and post-secondary studies. Further, although the majority of students concerned will have already received a diagnosis of dyslexia during childhood, a substantial proportion (30–40%, according to Warmington et al., 2013) might not yet have received a diagnosis at entry to university.

Many universities around the world benefit from a disability support service. Although the precise nature of this service varies from country to country, the general aim is to increase the inclusiveness and accessibility of higher education by organising the welcome and support of students with disabilities. Common themes emerge in relation to the role that this service plays in supporting students: (1) advising and assisting students in their requests for support; (2) providing guidance about relevant academic aspects of these requests to the university (e.g., studies, exams, professional placements and access to the work environment); (3) making recommendations about appropriate academic adjustments for individuals with disabilities (e.g., assistive technology and extra time for assessed work); and (4) improving inclusiveness in all teaching and supervision (e.g., general use of accessible teaching methods). In certain countries (e.g., France and the United Kingdom), dyslexia is officially recognised as a disability in law, which mandates entitlement to equal treatment in terms of rights and opportunities within higher education. However, many university students with dyslexia around the world receive some form of educational support even in the absence of legislation of this type.

0.3 Research on Adult Dyslexia (2000–2024): Trends, Themes and Gaps

Generally, research studies about dyslexia are conducted less frequently with adults than with children. We have quantified the number of research studies on adults with dyslexia as a function of their main research theme. In order to do this, we used the international database "PubMed®" (https://pubmed.ncbi.nlm.nih.gov/) to access the highest-quality scientific studies published in international journals. The time period targeted was between 2000 and 2024.[1]

This search led to the selection of more than 2,100 studies likely to have been conducted on adults with dyslexia. After reading the abstracts (or the Method section where necessary), we identified 717 studies conducted specifically on adults with dyslexia. Over the past two decades, research on adult dyslexia has significantly expanded, moving beyond childhood-focused models to address the lifelong developmental trajectory of reading difficulties. From 2000 to 2024, the scientific literature on adult dyslexia can be broadly grouped into three major and complementary research categories: (1) clinical and socio-educational practice, (2) cognitive and experimental research and (3) neuroscience and brain mechanisms.

- **Clinical and Socio-Educational Practice**: This first category encompasses applied research aimed at identifying, supporting and accommodating adults with dyslexia across educational, clinical and workplace contexts. Studies in

this area focus on diagnostic procedures in adulthood, the development and evaluation of intervention programmes and the implementation of inclusive strategies in higher education and professional environments. This body of research also addresses broader psychosocial dimensions, such as self-esteem, identity, resilience and the lived experience of dyslexia in adulthood. Methodologies are diverse, often involving qualitative or mixed-method approaches, and the overarching goal is to translate scientific findings into actionable practices that promote access, autonomy and well-being.
- **Cognitive and Experimental Research**: The second category includes studies focused on the cognitive underpinnings of reading and language in adults with dyslexia. Research in this area typically employs controlled experimental paradigms to investigate processes such as phonological awareness, working memory, executive functions and visual-attentional mechanisms. These studies aim to refine theoretical models of reading by accounting for the persistent or evolving profiles observed in adults, as well as their compensatory strategies. Tasks may include lexical decision-making, naming, priming or reaction time measures. This line of research provides essential insights into the variability and specificity of cognitive functioning in adult dyslexia.
- **Neuroscience and Brain Mechanisms**: The third category focuses on the neural correlates of dyslexia in adulthood, using neuroimaging and electrophysiological methods such as functional and structural MRI, EEG and MEG. These studies investigate both persistent atypicalities in brain organisation and the adaptive neuroplastic changes that occur over time. Research has highlighted differences in the activation and connectivity of brain networks involved in reading and language, often compared to typically developing adults. By linking behavioural profiles to brain function, this category contributes to a deeper understanding of the neurobiological foundations of reading disorders in adults.

Together, these three research categories reflect the complexity and multidimensionality of dyslexia in adults. By integrating clinical relevance, cognitive theory and neuroscientific evidence, they contribute to a more comprehensive and realistic understanding of reading difficulties across the lifespan. This typology serves as a useful framework for mapping the evolution of the field and identifying promising directions for future research.

0.3.1 Proportional Distribution of Research on Adult Dyslexia Across Categories (2000–2024)

Figure 0.1 presents a horizontal bar chart illustrating the global distribution of publications (N = 717) from 2000 to 2024 across the three major research domains. The data reveal the dominance of cognitive and experimental research, which accounts for 50% of the total studies. Neuroscience and brain-based approaches represent 29%, while clinical and socio-educational research

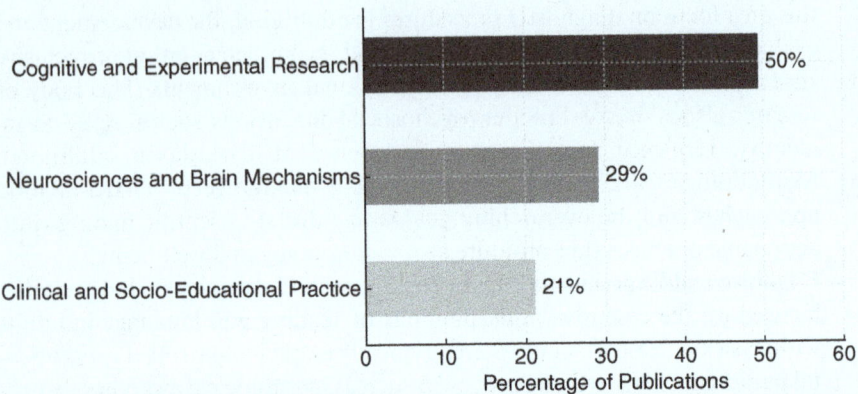

FIGURE 0.1 Proportional Distribution of Research on Adult Dyslexia Across Categories (2000–2024).

accounts for 21% of the total. However, this static picture does not illustrate the evolving dynamics of research in the field, which is investigated in the next section.

0.3.2 Annual Distribution of Research Categories on Adult Dyslexia (2000–2024)

Figure 0.2 presents a stacked bar chart illustrating the absolute number of studies published each year from 2000 to 2024 (N = 717), classified into the

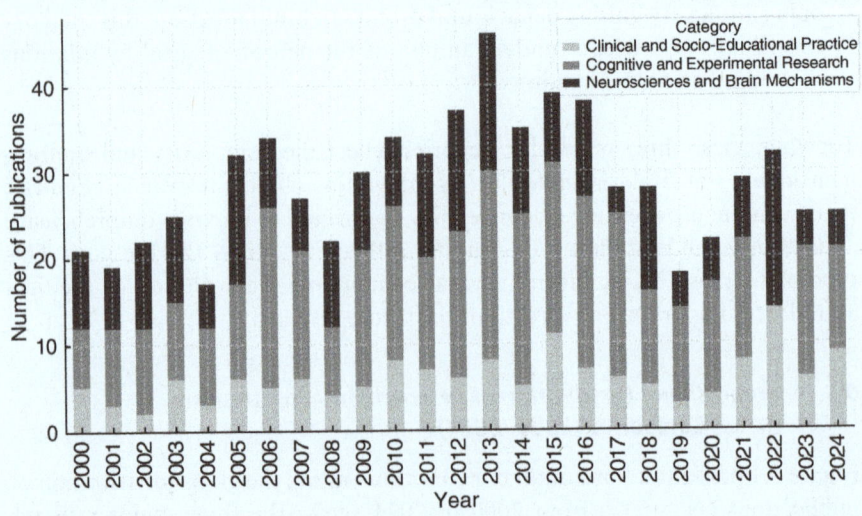

FIGURE 0.2 Annual Distribution of Research Categories on Adult Dyslexia (2000–2024).

three main research domains: *Clinical and Socio-Educational Practice, Cognitive and Experimental Research* and *Neurosciences and Brain Mechanisms*. The figure reveals a notable increase in research activity between 2005 and 2015, with a peak occurring around 2013–2015. During this period, cognitive research clearly dominated, followed by neuroscience. In contrast, the volume of neuroscience publications has remained relatively stable over time, generally ranging between 5 and 15 articles per year. This relative stagnation may be attributed to the complexity and resource intensiveness of neuroimaging studies, which often require specialised equipment, longer data acquisition times and advanced analytic techniques. Meanwhile, clinical and socio-educational studies, though less numerous overall, have shown steady growth in recent years, particularly between 2020 and 2024. This trend may reflect an increasing emphasis on applied research and the growing demand for practical interventions and inclusive support strategies for adults with dyslexia in higher education, the workplace and daily life.

0.3.3 Percentage of Scientific Studies (N = 717) on Adult Dyslexia by Research Subtheme (2000–2024)

Figure 0.3 presents a horizontal bar chart illustrating the distribution of subthemes across the 717 scientific studies on adults with dyslexia published between 2000 and 2024. Each study was classified into a thematic category based on the informed judgment of one of the authors of this book applying consistent criteria to ensure objective and coherent categorisation.

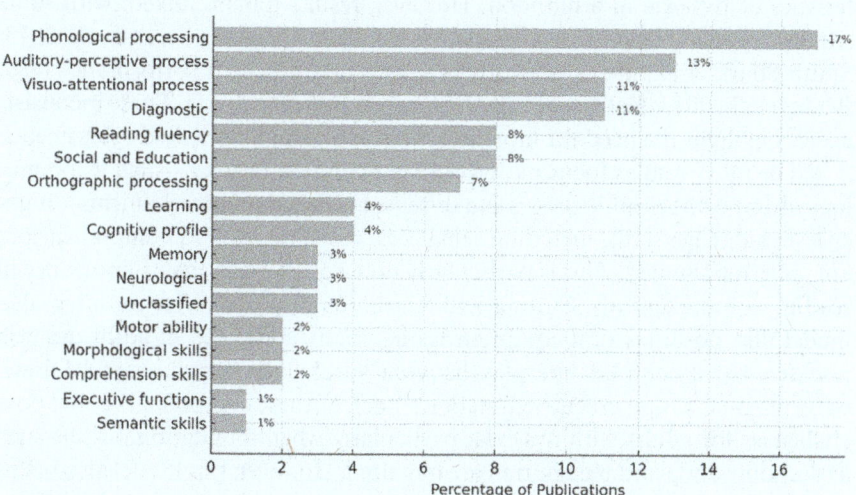

FIGURE 0.3 Percentage of Scientific Studies on Adult Dyslexia by Research Subtheme (2000–2024).

Unsurprisingly, phonological processing stands out as the most frequently investigated subtheme (17%), highlighting its central role in theoretical accounts of dyslexia. Research has also focused heavily on auditory-perceptive (13%) and visuo-attentional processes (11%), reflecting ongoing interest in sensory and attentional mechanisms. Other well-represented areas include diagnostic issues (11%), reading fluency (8%) and social and educational factors (8%). In contrast, topics such as semantic skills (1%), executive functions (1%) and morphological skills (2%) remain considerably underexplored.

Studies grouped under the "Social and Education" category account for a notable share of the literature (8%). These include investigations into psychosocial experiences—such as anxiety, identity development or social exclusion—as well as educational pathways and accommodations. This line of research emphasises the broader contextual and emotional factors influencing outcomes in adults with dyslexia and informs support strategies aimed at inclusion.

Although diagnostic issues appear in 11% of studies, only a small subset (~4%) focuses on comprehensive evaluation procedures. Few studies offer integrative assessments of reading-related skills (e.g., Callens et al., 2012; Warmington et al., 2013), and many lack a robust model of adult cognitive functioning. Furthermore, the predominance of English-language research limits cross-linguistic generalisability, although recent work in more transparent orthographies (e.g., Cavalli et al., 2018, in French; Tops et al., 2012, in Dutch; and Gagliano et al., 2015, in Spanish) has begun to address this gap.

Research on cognitive functioning—including learning (7%), memory (3%), executive functions (1%) and broader cognitive profiles (4%)—makes up about 17% of the literature. This body of work aims to clarify the cognitive characteristics of dyslexia in adulthood. However, results remain mixed, with some studies reporting deficits (e.g., Gabay et al., 2015; Martinez Perez et al., 2013; Smith-Spark et al., 2016), and others suggesting preserved performance (e.g., Beidas et al., 2013; Kelly et al., 2002; Shiran & Breznitz, 2011). These inconsistencies highlight the need for more nuanced, functionally oriented assessments.

While most studies focus on lower-level reading processes—such as phonological and orthographic processing or sensory-attentional mechanisms—higher-level language skills, including semantics, morphology and comprehension, are underrepresented. This is particularly noteworthy given their importance in reading comprehension. Cutting and Scarborough (2012) offer an integrated model that positions oral comprehension—rarely addressed in adult dyslexia research—as a complex interplay between vocabulary, syntax, world knowledge, pragmatics and executive functions. Each of these components could pose challenges for adults with dyslexia, particularly when foundational skills such as decoding and word recognition are impaired. However, this model also opens up the possibility that some individuals may rely on compensatory strengths—in oral language or higher-order cognition—to support comprehension.

This framework is especially relevant for understanding dyslexic adults pursuing higher education. Despite ongoing difficulties in word-level decoding and phonological processing, many of these individuals achieve reading comprehension levels comparable to their peers, particularly when time constraints are relaxed (Deacon et al., 2012; Parrila et al., 2007; Simmons & Singleton, 2000). Notably, only a few studies have directly examined the predictors of reading comprehension in this population (Brèthes et al., 2022; Ransby & Swanson, 2003). Their findings suggest that word recognition plays a relatively minor role, even among typical readers. In this context, the core deficits that define dyslexia in childhood appear to lose much of their explanatory power for reading comprehension in adulthood.

In sum, this distribution highlights the predominance of linguistic and low-level perceptual themes in adult dyslexia research, while revealing critical gaps in our understanding of higher-level language processes, reading comprehension and cognitive integration. These underexplored areas merit greater attention to develop a more complete understanding of dyslexia across the adult lifespan. This mapping of the research landscape provides essential context for understanding the structure of this book, which is designed to address both the most extensively studied domains and the key gaps identified.

0.4 Overview of the Book Structure and Content

This book brings together the expertise of internationally recognised specialists to provide a comprehensive and up-to-date perspective on adult dyslexia. While research in this field remains less extensive than that dedicated to children, a significant body of scientific knowledge is now available. This book offers a structured synthesis of that knowledge, combining theoretical insights with practical guidance for identifying, understanding and supporting adults with dyslexia. Each chapter highlights not only the latest scientific findings but also their practical implications for clinical practice, educational settings and everyday life.

The book is organised into three main sections that together provide a multidimensional view of adult dyslexia, integrating cognitive, clinical and educational perspectives. The first section explores in depth the cognitive and neurological functioning of adults with dyslexia, including the compensatory mechanisms they may develop. The second section focuses on screening, diagnosis and remediation, offering evidence-based approaches to assessment and intervention. The final section addresses current scientific debates and open questions related to dyslexia, with particular emphasis on the challenges and opportunities specific to the adult population.

0.4.1 Cognitive, Linguistic and Neurological Characteristics of Adults with Dyslexia

The first part of the book examines the cognitive, linguistic and neurological characteristics of adults with dyslexia, exploring both persistent difficulties and compensatory mechanisms. It opens with Chapter 1: *Adults with Learning*

Disorders in Reading: A Selective Review of the Literature (L. H. Swanson), which synthesises findings from 52 studies to map out the academic, cognitive and behavioural profiles of adults with dyslexia. This chapter highlights how difficulties in word recognition, spelling, naming speed and related cognitive processes often persist into adulthood, shaping their educational and professional trajectories.

Building on this foundation, Chapter 2: *Phonological Processing Skills in Adults with Dyslexia* (K. Schraeyen, J. Vanderauwera & M. Vandermosten) focuses on phonological deficits—consistently identified as central in dyslexia research—and examines how these difficulties endure even in adults who have developed effective reading strategies. This leads to Chapter 3: *Oral Language Skills and Reading in Adults with Dyslexia* (J. M. Law & E. Cavalli), where the role of semantics and morphology is explored, showing how certain oral language abilities may act as supports or compensatory strengths in reading comprehension.

The discussion then shifts to visual and attentional processes in Chapter 4: *Visuo-orthographic Processing in Dyslexic Adults* (N. Doignon-Camus & A. Bonnefond), which reviews evidence of difficulties in the allocation of visual attention and the processing of letter sequences. This chapter also considers how these challenges interact with phonological deficits. The cognitive exploration continues with Chapter 5: *Executive Functions in Adults with Dyslexia* (J. H. Smith-Spark), addressing how impairments in planning, inhibition and problem-solving can affect daily functioning and academic tasks, and how such difficulties might be mitigated.

Memory processes, essential for learning, are reviewed in Chapter 6: *Memory in Adults with Dyslexia* (J. H. Smith-Spark), which discusses how dyslexia affects short-term, working, long-term and prospective memory both in experimental settings and everyday contexts. The section closes with Chapter 7: *Neurological Function in Adult Dyslexia* (F. Richlan), offering an overview of neuroimaging research that reveals structural and functional brain differences associated with dyslexia and discusses the implications of these findings for understanding the disorder in adulthood.

0.4.2 Screening, Diagnosis and Remediation in Adults with Dyslexia

It is well established that the difficulties observed in children with dyslexia persist into adulthood. However, the cognitive profile of an adult can differ significantly from that of a child, particularly as a result of the cognitive adaptations and compensatory strategies that many adults develop in order to meet the demands of higher education and professional life. The second part of the book focuses on the assessment and intervention tools designed to address the specific needs of adults with dyslexia. Effective screening, diagnosis and remediation must take into account these distinctive features of adult cognitive functioning.

Chapter 8: *Screening and Diagnosis of Dyslexia in Higher Education* (W. Tops & M. Brysbaert) presents evidence-based approaches for identifying dyslexia in adults, demonstrating that a small, targeted battery of tests is sufficient for a reliable diagnosis. This streamlined approach facilitates the faster implementation of appropriate accommodations and support measures within university settings.

Building on this, Chapter 9: *Learning Strategies and Metacognition in Adults with Dyslexia* (R. Parrila, B. W. Bergey & H. S. Deacon) examines the role of study strategies and metacognitive skills in helping students with dyslexia manage their academic challenges. The chapter highlights both the compensatory strategies that students often develop spontaneously and the need for further research to optimise support in this area.

The section concludes with Chapter 10: *Cognitive Remediation and Neural Changes in Adults with Dyslexia* (F. Costanzo, S. Vicari & D. Menghini), which reviews the effectiveness of cognitive training and neurophysiological interventions aimed at improving reading skills in adults. The chapter underscores the potential of such interventions to promote neural plasticity and enhance reading performance, challenging the notion that remediation is less effective beyond childhood.

0.4.3 Current Debates and Perspectives on Adults with Dyslexia

The final section addresses broader conceptual and practical issues related to adult dyslexia. Chapter 11: *The Definition of Dyslexia, still debated after all these years* (F. Ramus) revisits the evolving debate around the definition of dyslexia, reflecting on Elliott and Grigorenko's (2024) updated position, which now accepts the term "dyslexia" but equates it with a broad notion of reading disability, without sufficient diagnostic criteria. The chapter provides a counterargument in Favor of a more rigorous and functional definition based on "harmful dysfunction" and response to intervention (RTI/MTSS), aligning with DSM-5 and promoting better-targeted support for struggling readers.

In Chapter 12: *Compensation Mechanisms in University Students with Dyslexia* (P. Colé, L. G. Duncan, & E. Cavalli), the concept of compensation is discussed through a review of genetic, cognitive, behavioural and neurological findings. The chapter reflects on how compensatory mechanisms may help explain the academic success of some adults with dyslexia and inform the development of more effective interventions.

The book concludes with Chapter 13: *How to Give the Best Support to Students with Dyslexia at University?* (E. Collette, M. Frenay & M-A. Schelstraete), which analyses the specific needs of students with dyslexia and the range of support strategies, aids and adjustments that can promote success. This discussion is framed within the broader context of inclusive pedagogy and factors contributing to academic achievement in higher education.

0.5 Conclusion

Taken together, the elements presented in this introductory chapter provide the conceptual, empirical and practical foundations necessary for approaching the chapters that follow. By combining theoretical models, research trends and an outline of the book's structure, this introduction aims to equip readers with a clear framework for understanding the complexity of dyslexia in adulthood. The subsequent contributions build on this foundation to offer in-depth analyses, evidence-based interventions and perspectives that address both scientific challenges and the real-world needs of adults with dyslexia. In this way, the book seeks not only to advance scientific understanding but also to inform practices that can meaningfully support adults with dyslexia in educational, professional and everyday contexts.

Note

1 Inclusion and exclusion criteria using PubMed Search: ((("dyslexia"[title] OR "dyslexic"[title] OR "adults with dyslexia"[All Fields] OR "dyslexic adults"[All Fields] OR "students with dyslexia"[All Fields] OR "high functioning adults with dyslexia"[All Fields] OR "reading disabilities"[All Fields] OR "reading disorders"[All Fields] OR "college students with dyslexia"[All Fields]) AND English[lang] AND ("2000/01/01"[Date - Publication] : "2024/12/31"[Date - Publication])) NOT ("children"[Title/Abstract] OR "adolescents"[Title/Abstract] OR "deep dyslexia"[Title/Abstract] OR "neglect dyslexia"[Title/Abstract] OR "animal"[Title/Abstract]).

References

American Psychiatric Society (2013) Diagnostic and statistical manual of mental disorders (DSM-5). www.dsm5.org/Pages/Default.aspx (accessed 10 July 2014).

Andersen, S. C., & Nielsen, H. S. (2016). Reading intervention with a growth mindset approach improves children's skills. *Proceedings of the National Academy of Sciences*, *113*(43), 12111–12113. https://doi.org/10.1073/pnas.1607946113

Beidas, H., Khateb, A., & Breznitz, Z. (2013). The cognitive profile of adult dyslexics and its relation to their reading abilities. *Reading and Writing*, *26*, 1487–1515.

Brèthes, H., Cavalli, E., Denis-Noël, A., Melmi, J. B., El Ahmadi, A., Bianco, M., & Colé, P. (2022). Text reading fluency and text reading comprehension do not rely on the same abilities in university students with and without dyslexia. *Frontiers in Psychology*, *13*, 866543.

British Dyslexia Association. (2010). *The dyslexia friendly quality mark*. British Dyslexia Association.

Bruck, M. (1990). Word-recognition skills of adults with childhood diagnoses of dyslexia. *Developmental Psychology*, *26*, 439–454.

Bruck, M. (1992). Persistence of dyslexics' phonological awareness deficits. *Developmental Psychology*, *28*, 874–886.

Callens, M., Tops, W., & Brysbaert, M. (2012). Cognitive profile of students who enter higher education with an indication of dyslexia. *PLoS One*, *7*.

Carroll, J., Holden, C., Kirby, P., Thompson, P. A., & Snowling, M. J. (2024, May 3). Towards a consensus on dyslexia: Findings from a Delphi study. https://doi.org/10.31219/osf.io/tb8mp

Catts, H. W., & Petscher, Y. (2022). A cumulative risk and protection model for reading disabilities. *Remedial and Special Education, 43*(4), 225–237.

Catts, H. W., Terry, N. P., Lonigan, C. J., et al. (2024). Revisiting the definition of dyslexia. *Annals of Dyslexia, 74*, 282–302. https://doi.org/10.1007/s11881-023-00295-3

Cavalli, E., Colé, P., Leloup, G., Poracchia-George, F., Sprenger-Charolles, L., & El Ahmadi, A. (2018). Screening for dyslexia in French-speaking university students: An evaluation of the detection accuracy of the Alouette test. *Journal of Learning Disabilities, 51*(3), 268–282.

Cutting, L. E., & Scarborough, H. S. (2012). Multiple bases for comprehension difficulties: The potential of cognitive and neurobiological profiling for validation of subtypes and development of assessments. In J. Sabatini, T. O'Reilly, & E. R. Albro (Eds.), *Reaching an understanding* (pp. 101–116). Lanham MD: Rowman & Littlefield Education.

Daley, S. G., & Rappolt-Schlichtmann, G. (2018). Stigma and reading disabilities: Exploring the interactions of context, culture, and identity. *Learning Disabilities Research & Practice, 33*(3), 155–166. https://doi.org/10.1111/ldrp.12173

De La Haye, F., Gombert, J. E., Riviere, J., & Rocher, T. (2008). Les evaluations en lecture dans le cadre de la journee d'appel de preparation a la defense, annee 2007. *Les notes 'information D.E.P.P.*

Deacon, S. H., Cook, K., & Parrila, R. (2012). Identifying high-functioning dyslexics: Is self-report of early reading problems enough? *Annals of Dyslexia, 62*(2), 120–134.

Duplechain, R., Reigner, R. C., & Packard, A. (2008). The impact of trauma on learning: A case for intervention. *Education, 128*(3), 446–453.

Elliott, J. G., & Grigorenko, E. L. (2024). *The dyslexia debate revisited*. Cambridge University Press.

Erbeli, F., Hart, S. A., & Taylor, J. (2022). Creativity and dyslexia: Disentangling myth from science. *Journal of Learning Disabilities, 55*(2), 123–135.

Fawcett, A. J., & Nicolson, R. I. (1999). Performance of dyslexic children on cerebellar and cognitive tests. *Journal of Motor Behavior, 31*, 68–78.

Fuchs, D., & Fuchs, L. S. (2006). Introduction to response to intervention: What, why, and how valid is it? *Reading Research Quarterly, 41*, 93–99.

Gabay, Y., Vakil, E., Schiff, R., & Holt, L. L. (2015). Probabilistic category learning in developmental dyslexia: Evidence from feedback and paired-associate weather prediction tasks. *Neuropsychology, 29*, 844–854.

Gagliano, A., Ciuffo, M., Ingrassia, M., Ghidoni, E., Angelini, D., Benedetto, L., & Stella, G. (2015). Silent reading fluency: Implications for the assessment of adults with developmental dyslexia. *Journal of Clinical and Experimental Neuropsychology, 37*, 972–980.

Goldberg, R. J., Higgins, E. L., Raskind, M. H., & Herman, K. L. (2003). Predicting academic achievement and grade retention with resilience and learning disabilities. *Learning Disability Quarterly, 26*(2), 58–70. https://doi.org/10.2307/1593594

Goswami, U., Power, A. J., Lallier, M., & Facoetti, A. (2014). Oscillatory "temporal sampling" and developmental dyslexia: Toward an over-arching theoretical framework. *Frontiers in Human Neuroscience, 8*, 904.

Griffiths, P. G., Taylor, R. H., Henderson, L. M., & Barrett, B. T. (2016). The effect of coloured overlays and lenses on reading: A systematic review of the literature. *Ophthalmic and Physiological Optics, 36*(5), 519–544. https://doi.org/10.1111/opo.12316

Haft, S. L., Myers, C. A., & Hoeft, F. (2019). Socio-emotional and cognitive resilience in children with reading disabilities. *Current Opinion in Behavioral Sciences, 25*, 109–116. https://doi.org/10.1016/j.cobeha.2018.10.003

International Dyslexia Association. (2002). *Definition of dyslexia*. Baltimore, MD: Author.

International Dyslexia Association. (2014). *Dyslexia in the classroom: What every teacher needs to know*. Baltimore, MD: Author.

Jonas, N. (2012). *Pour les générations les plus récentes, les difficultés des adultes diminuent à l'écrit, mais elles augmentent en calcul*. INSEE, 1426.

Katusic, S. K., Colligan, R. C., Barbaresi, W. J., Schaid, D. J., & Jacobsen, S. J. (2001). Incidence of reading disability in a population-based birth cohort, 1976–1982, Rochester. Minn. *Mayo Clinic Proceedings*, *76*(11), 1081–1092.

Kelly, S. W., Griffiths, S., & Frith, U. (2002). Evidence for implicit sequence learning in dyslexia. *Dyslexia*, *8*, 43–52.

Kemp, N., Parrila, R. K., & Kirby, J. R. (2009). Phonological and orthographic spelling in high-functioning adult dyslexics. *Dyslexia*, *128*, 105–128.

Law, J., Wouters, J., & Ghesquiere, P. (2017). The influences and outcomes of phonological awareness: A study of MA, PA and auditory processing in pre-readers with a family risk of dyslexia. *Developmental Science*, *20*(5), e12453.

Lefly, D. L., & Pennington, B. F. (2000). Reliability and validity of the adult reading history questionnaire. *Journal of Learning Disabilities*, *33*, 286–296.

Lindgren, S. D., De Renzi, E., & Richman, L. C. (1985). Cross-national comparisons of developmental dyslexia in Italy and the United States. *Child Development*, *56*, 1404–1417.

Livingstone, M. S., Rosen, G. D., Drislane, F. W., & Galaburda, A. M. (1991). Physiological and anatomical evidence for a magnocellular defect in develop- mental dyslexia. *Proceedings of the National Academy of Sciences, U.S.A*, *99*, 7943–7947.

Lobier, M., Zoubrinetzky, R., & Valdois, S. (2011). The visual attention span deficit in dyslexia is visual and not verbal. *Cortex*, *48*, 768–773.

López-Escribano, C., Elosúa, M. R., & García-Orza, J. (2018). Reading disabilities in Spanish: An overview of research findings. *Frontiers in Psychology*, *9*, 1406. https://doi.org/10.3389/fpsyg.2018.01406

Lovett, M. W., Frijters, J. C., Steinbach, K. A., & Wolf, M. (2021). Motivation-based interventions for struggling readers: Effects on engagement and achievement. *Reading and Writing*, *34*, 117–142.

Marchetti, R., Pinto, S., Spieser, L., Vaugoyeau, M., Cavalli, E., El Ahmadi, A., & Colé, P. (2023). Phoneme representation and articulatory impairment: Insights from adults with comorbid motor coordination disorder and dyslexia. *Brain Sciences*, *13*(2), 210.

Martin, J., Colé, P., Leuwers, C., Casalis, S., Zorman, M., & Sprenger-Charolles, L. (2010). Reading in French-speaking adults with dyslexia. *Annals of Dyslexia*, *60*, 238–264.

Martinez Perez, T., Majerus, S., & Poncelet, M. (2013). Impaired short-term memory for order in adults with dyslexia. *Research in Developmental Disabilities*, *34*, 2211–2223.

Mather, N., White, J., & Youman, M. (2020). Dyslexia debates: A comprehensive review of the history, evidence, and interpretations. *Annals of Dyslexia*, *70*(3), 298–327. https://doi.org/10.1007/s11881-020-00198-7

McGrath, L. M., Pennington, B. F., Shanahan, M. A., Santerre-Lemmon, L. E., Barnard, H. D., Willcutt, E. G., DeFries, J. C., & Olson, R. K. (2011). A multiple deficit model of reading disability and comorbid disorders: Implications for diagnosis and intervention. *Journal of Child Psychology and Psychiatry*, *52*(5), 547–557. https://doi.org/10.1111/j.1469-7610.2010.02346.x

McGrath, L. M., Peterson, R. L., & Pennington, B. F. (2020). The multiple deficit model: Progress, problems, and prospects. *Scientific Studies of Reading*, *24*(1), 7–13. https://doi.org/10.1080/10888438.2019.1706180

Murat, F. (2005). *Les competences des adultes a l'ecrit, en calcul et en comprehension orale*. Insee Première.

Nelson, J. M., & Harwood, H. R. (2011). Learning disabilities and anxiety: A meta-analysis. *Journal of Learning Disabilities, 44*(1), 3–17.

Nicolson, R. I., & Fawcett, A. J. (1990). Automaticity: A new framework for dyslexia research? *Cognition, 35*(2), 159–182. https://doi.org/10.1016/0010-0277(90)90013-A

Nicolson, R. I., & Fawcett, A. J. (1999). Developmental dyslexia: The role of the cerebellum. *Dyslexia, 5*(3), 155–177.

Nicolson, R. I., Fawcett, A. J., & Dean, P. (2001). Developmental dyslexia: The cerebellar deficit hypothesis. *Trends in Neurosciences, 24*, 508–511.

Norton, E. S., Beach, S. D., & Gabrieli, J. D. E. (2014). Neurobiology of dyslexia. *Current Opinion in Neurobiology, 30*, 73–78.

Palser, E. R., et al. (2021). From deficit to diversity: Developing a strengths-based approach to dyslexia. *Annals of Dyslexia, 71*, 217–239.

Parrila, R., Georgiou, G., & Corkett, J. (2007). University students with a significant history of reading difficulties: What is and is not compensated? *Exceptionality Education Canada, 17*, 195–220.

Pennington, B. E., McCabe, L. L., Smith, S. D., Lefly, D. L., Bookman, M. O., Kimberling, W. J., & Lubs, H. A. (1986). Spelling errors in adults with a form of familial dyslexia. *Child Development, 57*, 1001–1013.

Pennington, B. F. (2006). From single to multiple deficit models of developmental disorders. *Cognition, 101*(2), 385–413. https://doi.org/10.1016/j.cognition.2006.04.008

Peterson, R., & Pennington, B. F. (2015). Developmental dyslexia. *Annual Review of Clinical Psychology, 11*, 283–307.

Public Health England. (2013). Improving health and wellbeing through literacy and learning. Public Health England. https://www.gov.uk/government/publications/improving-health-and-wellbeing-through-literacy-and-learning

Ramus, F. (2003a). Developmental dyslexia: Specific phonological deficit or general sensorimotor dysfunction? *Current Opinion in Neurobiology, 13*, 212–218.

Ramus, F. (2003b). Theories of developmental dyslexia: Insights from a multiple case study of dyslexic adults. *Brain, 126*, 841–865.

Ramus, F. (2008). Genetique de la dyslexie. *Psychologie Schweizerische Zeitschrift Für Psychologie und Ihre Andwendungen, 67*(1), 9–14.

Ransby, M. J., & Swanson, H. L. (2003). Reading comprehension skills of young adults with childhood diagnoses of dyslexia. *Journal of Learning Disabilities, 36*, 538–555.

Romeo, R. R., Leonard, J. A., Robinson, S. T., West, M. R., Mackey, A. P., Rowe, M. L., & Gabrieli, J. D. (2018). Beyond the 30-million-word gap: Children's conversational exposure is associated with language-related brain function. *Psychological Science, 29*(5), 700–710. https://doi.org/10.1177/0956797617742725

Ryder, D., & Norwich, B. (2019). UK higher education lecturers' perspectives of dyslexia, dyslexic students and related disability provision. *Journal of Research in Special Educational Needs, 19*, 161–172.

Saksida, A., Iannuzzi, S., Bogliotti, C., Chaix, Y., Demonet, J. F., Bricout, L., & Ramus, F. (2016). Phonological skills, visual attention span, and visual stress in developmental dyslexia. *Developmental Psychology, 52*, 1503–1516.

Shaywitz, S. E., Shaywitz, B. A., Pugh, K. R., Fulbright, R. K., Constable, R. T., Mencl, W. E., & Gore, J. C. (1998). Functional disruption in the organisation of the brain for reading in dyslexia. *Proceedings of the National Academic of Science, USA, 95*, 2636–2641.

Shiran, A., & Breznitz, Z. (2011). The effect of cognitive training on recall range and speed of information processing in the working memory of dyslexic and skilled readers. *Journal of Neurolinguistics, 24*, 524–537.

Simmons, F., & Singleton, C. (2000). The reading comprehension abilities of dyslexic students in higher education. *Dyslexia, 6*, 178–192.

Smith-Spark, J. H., Henry, L. A., Messer, D. J., Edvardsdottir, E., & Zięcik, A. P. (2016). Executive functions in adults with developmental dyslexia. *Research in Developmental Disabilities, 53–54*, 323–341.

Snowling, M. (1981). Phonemic deficits in developmental dyslexia. *Psychological Research, 43*, 219–234.

Snowling, M. J., & Hulme, C. (2020). *The science of reading: A handbook* (2nd ed.). Wiley-Blackwell.

Sprenger-Charolles, L., Cole, P., Lacert, P., & Serniclaes, W. (2000). On subtypes of developmental dyslexia: Evidence from processing time and accuracy scores. *Canadian Journal of Experimental Psychology, 54*, 88–104.

Stanovich, K. E., & Siegel, L. (1994). Phenotypic performance profile for children with reading disabilities: A regression-based test of the phonological-core variable-difference model. *Journal of Educational Psychology, 86*, 1–30.

Stein, J., & Walsh, V. (1997). To see but not to read; the magnocellular theory of dyslexia. *Trends in Neurosciences, 20*, 147–152.

Stuebing, K. K., Fletcher, J. M., LeDoux, J. M., Lyon, G. R., Shaywitz, S. E., & Shaywitz, B. A. (2002). Validity of IQ-discrepancy classifications of reading disabilities: A meta-analysis. *American Educational Research Journal, 39*(2), 469–518. https://doi.org/10.3102/00028312039002469

Sturm, A., Moll, K., Kunze, S., & Landerl, K. (2021). Specific learning disorders across languages: Variability in reading, spelling, and arithmetic skills depends on orthographic consistency. *Frontiers in Psychology, 12*, 688901.

Tallal, P. (1980). Auditory temporal perception, phonics, and reading disabilities in children. *Brain and Language, 9*, 182–198.

Tops, W., Callens, M., Bijn, E., & Brysbaert, M. (2012). Spelling in adolescents with dyslexia: Errors and modes of assessment. *Journal of Learning Disabilities, 47*, 295–306.

Tunmer, W., & Greaney, K. (2010). Defining dyslexia. *Journal of Learning Disabilities, 43*, 229–243.

Vellutino, F. R., Scanlon, D. M., Sipay, E. R., Small, S. G., Pratt, A., Chen, R. S., & Denckla, M. B. (1996). Cognitive profiles of difficult- to- remediate and readily remediated poor readers: Early intervention as a vehicle for distinguishing between cognitive and experiential deficits as basic causes of specific reading disability. *Journal of Educational Psychology, 88*, 601–638.

Vellutino, F. R., Scanlon, D. M., Small, S., & Fanuele, D. P. (2006). Response to intervention as a vehicle for distinguishing between children with and without reading disabilities: Evidence for the role of kindergarten and first-grade interventions. *Journal of Learning Disabilities, 39*, 157–169.

Warmington, M., Stothard, S. E., & Snowling, M. J. (2013). Assessing dyslexia in higher education: The York adult assessment battery-revised. *Journal of Research in Special Educational Needs, 13*, 48–56.

Washington, J. A., & Seidenberg, M. S. (2021). Teaching reading to African American children: When home and school language differ. *Language, Speech, and Hearing Services in Schools, 52*(1), 1–15. https://doi.org/10.1044/2020_LSHSS-20-00067

White, S., Milne, E., Rosen, S., Hansen, P., Swettenham, J., Frith, U., & Ramus, F. (2006). The role of sensorimotor impairments in dyslexia: A multiple case study of dyslexic children. *Developmental Science, 9*, 237–255.

Willingham, D. T. (2015). *Raising kids who read: What parents and teachers can do.* Jossey-Bass.

Wolff, P. H. (2002). Timing precision and rhythm in developmental dyslexia. *Reading and Writing, 15*, 179–206.

Wolff, U., & Lundberg, I. (2003). A technique for group screening of dyslexia among adults. *Annals of Dyslexia, 53*, 324–339.

Zheng, Y., Plante, E., & Johnson, E. (2014). Life experiences, resilience, and risk factors among children with dyslexia. *Child and Adolescent Social Work Journal, 31*, 455–473. https://doi.org/10.1007/s10560-014-0334-8

Ziegler, J. C., & Goswami, U. (2006). Becoming literate in different languages: Similar problems, different solutions. *Developmental Science, 9*, 429–436.

1
ADULTS WITH LEARNING DISORDERS IN READING

A Selective Review of the Literature

H. Lee Swanson

1.1 Adults with Learning Disorders in Reading: A Selective Review of the Literature

Learning disorders is a general term that captures a number of specific areas of disability. The diagnosis of learning disorders in adults broadly reflects deficits in academic (i.e., reading, math, and writing), language (e.g., oral, expressive, and receptive), and motor skills (e.g., coordination) (e.g., see DSM-5; American Psychiatric Association, 2013; National Institute of Neurological Disorders and Stroke, 2010). One subgroup of learning disorder, learning disorders in reading (RD), refers to adults who experience problems isolated to deficits in reading achievement that fall substantially below what is expected given their age, intelligence, and education. Currently, adults classified with RD are those individuals of normal intelligence who have specific achievement deficits due to mental information processing difficulties. These individuals have **learning disorders** because their learning difficulties are caused by neurological inefficiencies that have a biological base, which in turn **disables** their performance on specific tasks such as reading, math, and related areas—hence the term RD. Neurological inefficiencies reflect differences in the process/organizing information as a function of brain anatomy and/or functionality. The purpose of this chapter is to review our previous syntheses of the experimental literature on the performance of adults with RD when compared to adults without RD. (In this chapter, the term RD is used interchangeably with the terms dyslexia, reading disabilities, learning disabilities in reading, and specific disabilities in reading.)

Although a critical focus of this chapter is on the identification of those constructs that separate the performance of adults with RD from those without RD, some discussion of the research with children is necessary. The majority of studies that synthesize the experimental work on children with RD focus on difficulties in phonological processes (see Zhang & Peng, 2022), as well as related problems in naming speed, orthography, morphology, and working memory (e.g., Araújo & Faísca, 2019; De Assis et al., 2023; Georgiou et al., 2023; Kudo et al., 2015; Melby-Lervåg et al., 2012; Peng et al., 2022). As a result, several measures of assessment within a theoretical framework that assumes a phonological core deficit have been developed for assessing childhood RD (i.e., dyslexia). In contrast, the literature on basic processing difficulties in adults with RD is less clear, and therefore, no research-based consensus has emerged as to the best assessment practices (e.g., Fletcher, 2010; Ottosen et al., 2022; Sadusky et al., 2022; Shuy, 2003).

Likewise, it is unclear how many adults suffer from RD. Although there has been no major epidemiological study focusing on RD among adults (Corley & Taymans, 2002; Gregg, 2011; Miller et al., 2010), the incidence of RD has been conservatively estimated at approximately 3–5% of the general population (National Adult Literacy Survey, 1992). Epidemiological data with children suggest that RD (i.e., dyslexia) fits a dimensional model in which proficient reading and RD occur along a continuum, with RD representing the lower tail of a normal distribution of reading ability (e.g., Fletcher et al., 1994; Grigorenko et al., 2019; cf. see Wagner et al., 2020, for review). Further, longitudinal studies indicate that RD is a persistent chronic condition across adulthood (e.g., Shaywitz et al., 1999). For example, in the U.S. Connecticut longitudinal project, approximately 70% of children identified with RD in grade 3 had RD as adults (e.g., Shaywitz & Shaywitz, 2005, 2013). Thus, over time and age, proficient readers and those with RD maintain their relative position among the spectrum of reading ability (Shaywitz & Shaywitz, 2013). Given these assumptions, we assume that approximately 5% of the adult population has RD. The literature characterizes the existence of RD as reflecting problems in accurate and fluent word recognition abilities. The literature also suggests that the difficulties experienced by these individuals are related to deficits within the phonological component of language, which is further unexpected relative to their other cognitive abilities.

Of course, a question emerges as to whether adults with RD can be distinguished from adults with general reading difficulties. Perhaps the most important distinction is that problems in reading for adults with RD (i.e., dyslexia) are attributed to neurological inefficiencies. This source of difficulty can be contrasted with adults who suffer from reading difficulties attributed to poor teaching, socioeconomic status, and/or comorbidity (e.g., attention deficit–hyperactivity disorder (ADHD) and specific language impairment (SLI)). More specifically, the American Psychiatric Association (2013) manual views a specific "learning disorder in reading" (i.e., dyslexia) as reflecting a neurodevelopmental disorder of biological origin. An example definition of dyslexia is provided by the National Institute of Neurological Disorders and Stroke (2010), which gives the following definition for dyslexia, implicating a biological origin:

> Dyslexia is a brain-based type of learning disability that specifically impairs a person's ability to read. These individuals typically read at levels significantly lower than expected despite having normal intelligence. Although the disorder varies from person to person, common characteristics among people with dyslexia are difficulty with spelling, phonological processing (the manipulation of sounds), and/or rapid visual-verbal responding. In adults, dyslexia usually occurs after a brain injury or in the context of dementia. It can also be inherited in some families and recent studies have identified a number of genes that may predispose an individual to developing dyslexia.

In terms of assessment, several researchers suggest that a focus on word identification or recognition measures is fundamental to evaluating adults with RD. This is because a cognitive process consistently implicated in RD is phonological awareness (e.g., Melby-Lervåg et al., 2012; Ottosen et al., 2022; Reis et al., 2020). Phonological awareness is "the ability to attend explicitly to the phonological structure of spoken words" (Scarborough, 1998, p. 95). Although several studies show that RD is related to phonological awareness (e.g., Melby-Lervåg et al., 2012; Ottosen et al., 2022), additional studies with adult samples suggest that other processes such as those related to rapid naming speed (e.g., Araújo et al., 2021; Ransby & Swanson, 2003), orthography (e.g., Collette et al., 2022; Purcell et al., 2014), morphology (e.g., Cheema et al., 2023), and working memory capacity (e.g., Schraeyen et al., 2019; Smith-Spark & Fisk, 2007) contribute statistically significant unique amounts of variance toward predicting adults classified as RD. Therefore, given the myriad cognitive problems reported in the literature for adults with RD, a brief review of outcomes related to a meta-analysis of the literature helps researchers as well as practitioners prioritize the academic and cognitive processes of importance that define such a disability.

Given this introduction, we review our findings, synthesizing the experimental literature on adults with RD. Because this chapter focuses on empirical comparative studies, a quantitative synthesis, referred to as a meta-analysis, will provide the basis of discussion. *Meta-analysis* is a statistical technique used to synthesize data from separate comparable studies to obtain a quantitative summary of research that addresses a common question (e.g., Hedges & Olkin, 1985). The *d-index* by Cohen (1988), commonly used to make comparisons, is a scale-free measure of the separation between two group means that is used when one variable in the comparison is dichotomous (e.g., adults with reading disabilities (RD) vs. without RD) and the other is continuous (e.g., vocabulary performance). To make d's interpretable, statisticians have adopted

Cohen's (1988) system for classifying *d*'s in terms of their size (i.e., .00–.19 is described as trivial; .20–.49, small; .50–.79, moderate; and .80 or higher, large).

1.2 Synthesis Questions

The most comprehensive synthesis to date on adults with RD was reported in Swanson (2012) and Swanson and Hsieh (2009). By admission, these meta-analytic findings appear dated. Although recent syntheses have focused on such areas as orthography (Carioti et al., 2021; Reis et al., 2020) and morphology (Georgiou et al., 2023), no published meta-analysis has covered the range of processes as the syntheses by Swanson (2012) and Swanson and Hsieh (2009). Thus, at a minimum, these syntheses serve as important "priors" for future meta-analyses (cf. Wagner et al., 2019). That is, this earlier work will supplement future comprehensive meta-analyses for a better understanding of adults with dyslexia. Given this context, this chapter will review some of their findings under the rubric of three questions that directed this work:

1 What domains of performance (i.e., intellectual, academic, cognitive, vocational, and life-adjustment) differentiate adults with RD from average-reading adults? The practical application is to show the similarities and differences between groups in terms of the magnitude of effect sizes (ESs) across an array of measures.
2 What performance similarities or differences among adults with and without RD are a function of variations in age, ethnicity, and gender? For example, it is of interest to determine if some of the same deficits (as reflected in the magnitude of ES) that emerge in studies that include older participants with RD also occur when the sample is of college age.
3 What performance differences emerge in adults with RD when compared to average reading adults as a function of the severity of the reading score? It is important to consider outcomes of studies as a function of the severity of the reading disability and the intelligence level.

1.3 Data Gathering

Several approaches were used to locate the relevant studies published in peer-reviewed journals. First, a computer search located studies comparing adults with reading disabilities and those without reading disabilities on psychological, occupational, and vocational variables using the PsycINFO, Medline, and ERIC databases. The computer search used the following terms: "adults, adult, students, college students," coupled with "dyslexia, learning disabilities, reading disabilities, reading disorders, specific reading disabilities, math disabilities, and dyscalculia." Entry of these terms yielded 9733 references. Because the computer search may have missed articles meeting selection criteria, a manual search was conducted of journals where the majority of articles were published (e.g., *Journal of Learning Disabilities, Learning Disabilities Research and Practice, Annals of Dyslexia*, and *Learning Disability Quarterly*).

1.4 Selection Criteria

Focusing on comparative studies (adults with RD vs. adults without RD) published in English-language journals narrowed the search down to 450 studies. The 450 "potential studies" were further evaluated according to the following criteria:

1 An adult group with RD (e.g., reading disabilities, dyslexia, and specific learning disabilities in reading) was compared to an adult group without RD (i.e., no indication of a learning or behavior deficit).
2 Within the RD groups, at least one RD subgroup has no reported comorbidities (e.g., math disabilities, ADHD, and SLI).
3 Each study reported a mean score on a standardized (norm-referenced) measure of intelligence for each comparison group (e.g., Wechsler tests or selected IQ subtests).
4 Each study reported a mean score from a standardized reading test for each comparison group.
5 The sample size of adults with RD in the study was greater than 9; this eliminated single-subject design studies and case studies.
6 Each study compared adults with RD and adults without RD on measures independent of the classification measures (i.e., reading).

Studies were excluded if: (a) they were not published in refereed journals, (b) they failed to provide enough quantitative data to calculate the ESs, (c) they failed to include a chronologically age-matched average achieving comparison group, and/or (d) they failed to provide information on ability group performance on a standardized (norm-referenced) reading and/or intelligence test.

1.5 Classification and Comparison Measures

Classification measures of adults with RD included measures of general intelligence (performance and nonverbal), word recognition, and reading comprehension.

Comparative measures (those not included as part of the classification criteria—i.e., general intelligence and reading scores) were organized into several categories: verbal intelligence, naming speed, phonological processing, word attack, math, vocabulary and language, spelling, writing, social skills, problem solving and reasoning, memory and cognitive monitoring, perceptual motor skills, visual perception skills, auditory perception skills, general information-facts, personality, and brain or neuropsychological measures (e.g., EEGs).

Thus, adults with RD were compared with their counterparts on measures related to the following categories:

Classification Measures

1 Real Word Reading. This category focused on the sight recognition of real words. Sample tasks include measures of irregular and regular words, experimental words, and real word identification.
2 Reading Comprehension. This category focused on measures of text or passage comprehension. The majority of dependent measures in this domain included reading comprehension and general reading measures.
3 General Intelligence. This category focused on standardized measures taken from tests of general intelligence.
4 Verbal Intelligence. This domain included general measures of verbal intelligence (e.g., composites of general information, word knowledge, and conceptual similarities).

Comparative Measures

1 Phonological Awareness. This category focused on oral tasks that required dividing spoken words into segments of sounds smaller than a syllable or learning about individual phonemes.
2 Naming Speed. This category focused on measures of speed (timed trials) related to the overt verbalizing of letters, sounds, words, objects, or colors.
3 Pseudo-Word Reading (Word Attack). This category focused on measures of word attack skills and was considered a separate entity of phonological processing.
4 Math. This category focused on measures related to calculation.
5 Vocabulary. This category focused on measures related to word meaning.
6 Spelling. This category focused on real-word spelling skills.
7 Writing. This category focused on written language and included measures of syntax and grammar.
8 Social Awareness. The category focused on measures of help-seeking, self-perception, perceived social support, and social competence.
9 Problem Solving/Reasoning. This category focused on general problem-solving on measures assumed to measure fluid intelligence.
10 Memory and Cognitive Monitoring. This category focused on span measures related to digits, words, sentences, and objects.

11 Perception and Motor Tasks. This category focused on measures of tactical performance balance.
12 Visual Perception. This category was visual–perceptual motor tasks.
13 Auditory Perception. This category was auditory–perceptual motor or listening tasks.
14 General Information. This category included measures that tapped previous knowledge or memory for general information.
15 External Criterion—School and Work. This domain included measures provided by professors, teachers (e.g., grades), and/or employers related to resource management and work performance.
16 Personality. This domain included measures of personality.
17 Brain and Neurological Measures. This domain primarily included measures of EEG function.

1.6 General Findings

The final synthesis included 52 articles with 776 ESs comparing adults with RD and adults without RD. The mean ES for the 52 studies across all measures was .72 (SD = .54), which placed differences between adults with RD and without RD according to Cohen's (1988) criteria in the moderate-to-high range. In terms of the reported study demographics, 74% of ESs came from the United States, 15% from the United Kingdom, 3% from Finland, 2% from France, 4% from Canada, and 2% from Australian samples. The total sample size across the 52 studies for adults with RD was 1793 (M = 31.73, SD = 28.01), and the total sample size for adults without RD was 1893 (M = 36.41, SD = 36.41). The age range for adults with RD varied from 18 to 42 years (M = 24.69, SD = 5.82), and adults without RD varied from 18 to 44 years (M = 23.93, SD = 5.95).

Thirty-nine studies provided data that allowed for the calculation of the ratio of males to females in participant selection. The gender ratio (number of males/total sample) in which the number of males and females was reported was .55 (SD = .17) for adults with RD. Ethnic background was reported in eight studies. The ethnic ratio (number of whites with RD/total sample of RD) was .83 (SD = .27). No study separated reading performance as a function of gender, ethnicity, or SES. Therefore, performance between adults with RD and without RD as a function of gender, ethnicity, and/or SES could not be compared across the studies.

The most common assessment measures (norm-referenced or experimental) by category were as follows: reading comprehension (e.g., Nelson–Denny, Woodcock–Johnson Psychoeducational Inventory, Woodcock Reading Mastery Test, and Gray Oral Reading Test), general intelligence (e.g., Wechsler Adult Intelligence Scale (WAIS)–Full Scale or Performance

Scale, and Raven's Standard Progressive Matrices), verbal intelligence (e.g., WAIS Verbal Scale, including composite scores of general information, similarities, and vocabulary), word recognition (e.g., WRAT, PIAT, and WRMT), naming speed (e.g., tasks related to the rapid naming of objects, colors, numbers and letters, WJPB-word fluency), phonological processing (e.g., experimental tasks related to phoneme deletion, nonword repetition, word comparisons), word attack (e.g., WRMT-word attack, WJPB-word attack, and experimental tasks), arithmetic (e.g., WJPB-math, WRAT-arithmetic, and PIAT-math), vocabulary (e.g., PPVT, WAIS-vocabulary, and TOAL), spelling (e.g., WRAT-spelling and PIAT-spelling), writing (e.g., TOAL and WJPB-written language), social skills (e.g., Harter tasks related to perceived support, self-perception profile, and help-seeking), problem-solving (e.g., WAIS tasks related to block design–comprehension, object assembly, and WJPB-cognitive and reasoning ability), verbal memory (e.g., WAIS-Digit Span and working memory tasks), visual–spatial memory (e.g., Corsi Block Span, VMS-visual index, and spatial working memory), cognitive monitoring (e.g., Trail Making, Token Test, and behavioral measure of attention), perceptual motor (e.g., balance measures and LNNB tactile), auditory perceptual (e.g., auditory-only Token Test and rhyming task), visual–perceptual (e.g., visual search, design recognition, perceptual (e.g., LNNB subtests and WAIS-visual matching), general information (e.g., WAIS-information, WJPB-knowledge aptitude), social expectations (e.g., GPA, organization, and manage time), personality (e.g., MMPI), and neurological (e.g., EEG).[1]

1.7 Characteristics of Sample on Classification Measures

Table 1.1 provides an overview of the reported norm-referenced psychometric information (e.g., intelligence and reading) for adult participants with and without RD. ESs on the norm-referenced measures are shown on the right side of Table 1.1. Positive ESs favored adults without RD. As shown, the aggregated mean standard scores for measures of word recognition, speed, phonological processing, word attack, and spelling were below the 25th percentile (< 90 standard score). For measures that included scale scores, verbal memory hovered around the 25th percentile (scale score of 8). As expected, ESs comparing adults with and without RD were large on measures of reading (i.e., comprehension and word recognition), naming speed, basic reading skills (e.g., phonological processing and word attack), and spelling. The category of measures that provided weak discrimination among readers was measures of general intelligence and problem-solving. Overall, the profiles for adults with RD were comparable to reported profiles of children with dyslexia (see Kudo et al., 2015; Peng et al., 2022).

TABLE 1.1 Psychological and Achievement Profiles on Standardized Normed Referenced Measures for Adult Participants with and without Reading Disabilities

	Average Adult Reader (N = 1162)		Adult with RD (N = 1719)		Effect Size	
	M	SD	M	SD	M	SD
Norm-Referenced						
Read. Comprehension[a]	109.87	11.29	93.05	12.29	1.25	.73
General Intelligence	110.55	6.89	104.64	11.62	.26	.67
Verbal Intelligence	110.60	9.00	101.36	12.63	.69	.61
Word Recognition	107.19	8.24	88.65	10.16	1.64	.79
Naming Speed	105.93	6.36	88.72	16.40	1.01	.65
Phonol. Processing	105.48	24.03	76.26	16.96	1.60	.68
Word Attack	105.82	8.23	87.17	11.88	1.68	.72
Math	106.23	8.71	93.64	10.31	.88	.82
Vocabulary	104.89	7.39	92.30	11.28	.88	.65
Spelling	107.89	7.02	87.62	9.88	1.77	.66
Writing	101.94	7.95	88.15	11.07	.81	1.10
Problem Solving/Reasoning[b]	11.94	1.88	11.32	1.70	.04	.30
Memory–Verbal[b]	9.99	3.38	8.13	2.21	.81	.80

Note. Positive effect size is in favor of average reading for adults.

[a] Reported as a standard score ($M = 100$, $SD = 15$).
[b] Reported as a scale score ($M = 10$, $SD = 3$).

1.8 Characteristics of Sample on Comparison Measures

Table 1.2 provides the mean ES (weighted by the reciprocal of the sampling variance) and standard errors, and a 95% confidence interval range. Using Cohen's criterion, high ESs (>.80) occurred across all areas of reading skills (i.e., reading comprehension, word recognition, speed of processing, phonological

TABLE 1.2 Effect Sizes, Standard Error, and Confidence Intervals of Categories for Comparisons between Adults with and without RD (Corrected for Outliers). Positive effect sizes favor adults without RD, and negative effect sizes favor the RD group.

Comparison	K	Effect Size	Standard Error	Lower	Upper
Total Across Categories	776	0.54	0.01	0.52	0.56
1. Reading Comprehension	53	1.20	0.04	1.12	1.28
2. General Intelligence	48	0.20	0.03	0.13	0.28
3. Verbal Intelligence	20	0.63	0.05	0.5	0.74
4. Word Recognition	43	1.37	0.04	1.28	1.44
5. Speed of Processing (e.g., Letter Naming, etc.)	56	0.96	0.03	0.88	1.04
6. Phonological Processing	42	0.87	0.05	0.77	0.98

(*Continued*)

TABLE 1.2 (Continued)

Comparison	K	Effect Size	Standard Error	Lower	Upper
7. Word Attack	55	1.33	0.03	1.25	1.41
8. Math	32	0.75	0.03	0.68	0.83
9. Vocabulary	29	0.71	0.04	0.62	0.8
10. Spelling	33	1.57	0.05	1.47	1.67
11. Writing	11	0.72	0.07	0.58	0.86
12. Social and Personal Skills	34	0.10	0.03	0.02	0.17
13. Problem Solving and Reasoning	38	0.11	0.04	0.03	0.20
14. Verbal Memory	44	0.62	0.04	0.53	0.71
15. Visual-Spatial Memory	6	−0.39	0.12	−0.63	−0.14
16. Cognitive Monitoring	19	0.27	0.06	0.15	0.39
17. Perceptual Motor Skills	66	−0.13	0.03	−0.19	−0.07
18. Auditory Perceptual	27	−0.18	0.06	−0.31	−0.06
19. Visual Perceptual	14	0.13	0.11	−0.09	0.35
20. General Information (LTM)	9	0.47	0.08	0.31	0.64
21. External Criterion	11	−0.23	0.05	−0.33	−0.12
22. Personality	16	0.28	0.04	0.19	0.37
23. Brain and Neuropsychological Areas (e.g., EEG)	57	−0.02	0.05	−0.12	0.07

Note. K = number of effects.
Sizes. Lower and upper = 95% level of confidence range.

processing, word attack, and spelling). Moderate ESs (.50 to .80) emerged across several categories, such as verbal IQ, math, vocabulary, writing, and verbal memory. Low ESs occurred for measures of personality, external criterion measures, visual and auditory perception, and problem-solving/reasoning measures.

1.9 Profile of High and Low IQ Studies

Although in the normal range, Table 1.3 shows *that* the intelligence scores of adults with RD varied across studies. To determine if the level of intelligence had some impact on the magnitude of ESs between RD and non-RD adults, studies were divided into those in which intelligence scores for adults with RD were above 100 and those in which intelligence scores for adults with RD were at or below 100. A profile of the scores as a function of studies that report high and relatively low IQs is shown in Table 1.3. As shown, the mean reading scores (i.e., word recognition and comprehension) were in the same range for studies with high IQ as those with relatively low IQs. Table 1.3 also shows that the studies with higher IQ had greater differences on phonological processing and memory measures with average achievers when compared to studies with RD samples that reported lower intelligence scores. The magnitude of ESs were also larger for the high IQ studies on measures of spelling ($M = .46$) and word attack ($M = .43$). Moderate ESs emerged in favor of low IQ studies (i.e., differences were greater between adults with and without RD) on measures of math

TABLE 1.3 Aggregated Means and Standard Deviations for the Classification and Comparison Categories as a Function of IQ

	High Intelligence Studies			Low Intelligence Studies			
Classification Measures	# Studies	Mean	SD	# Studies	Mean	SD	Effect Size[b]
Standard Scores							
General Intelligence	25	110.67	5.31	24	97.79	10.99	1.58
Verbal Intelligence	14	110.16	5.71	16	94.14	6.64	2.59
Read. Comprehension	12	90.03	12.81	16	93.46	6.54	−0.35
Word Recognition	18	94.38	7.1	16	86.85	10.22	0.86
Effect Sizes–Classification[a]		ES[a]	SD		ES[a]	SD	ES[c]
Read. Comprehension	10	1.25	0.62	15	1.27	0.63	−0.03
Gen. Intelligence	14	0.23	0.22	14	0.75	0.56	−1.33
Verbal Intelligence	10	0.57	0.49	8	0.94	0.76	−0.59
Word Recognition	14	1.72	0.66	14	1.69	0.92	0.03
Effect Sizes–Comparison[a]							
Measures							
Naming Speed	6	1.34	0.52	14	1.19	0.96	0.20
Phonological Processes	9	1.22	0.65	2	0.76	0.24	1.03
Word Attack	10	1.84	0.84	11	1.57	0.4	0.43
Math	8	0.65	0.68	6	1.01	0.69	−0.52
Vocabulary	4	0.72	0.76	13	0.87	0.63	−0.21
Spelling	12	2.02	0.61	8	1.68	0.85	0.46
Verbal Memory	12	1.36	0.54	8	0.69	0.44	3.90

Note. Only effect sizes (ESs) with > 3 studies were computed.

[a] Effect sizes between adults with and without RD.
[b] Effect sizes between studies with reported high and low intelligence scores.
[c] Effect sizes comparing the magnitude of ES differences between high and low intelligence studies.

($M = .43$). The analyses showed that adults with RD who have intelligence scores >100 are more likely to suffer greater deficits in phonological processing and verbal memory relative to their average reading peers than studies with IQ scores below 100.

1.10 Discussion

This chapter highlights some of the results of a quantitative synthesis of the published literature comparing adults with RD with chronologically age-matched average readers. Prior to reviewing our findings and making applications to the assessment, we address the three questions raised earlier in the chapter.

First, we sought to determine whether the deficits in adults with RD were distinct from their average-achieving counterparts. As expected, adults with RD varied substantially from adults without RD on the classification measures (i.e., $M = 1.20$ reading comprehension, $M = 1.37$ word recognition, and $M = .63$ verbal intelligence). More importantly, the results on the comparative measures (i.e., those not used as part of the classification criteria) yielded moderate to high (.50–1.33). ESs in favor of adults without RD on measures of phonological processes ($M = 1.60$), naming speed ($M = .96$), word attack (1.33), math ($M = .75$), vocabulary ($M = .71$), spelling ($M = 1.57$), writing ($M = .72$), general information ($M = .47$), and verbal memory ($M = .62$). Trivial-to-low ESs emerged on measures of general intelligence ($M = .20$), problem solving/reasoning ($M = .11$), visual memory ($M = -.39$), monitoring–executive processing ($M = .27$), perceptual skills ($M = -.13$), personality ($M = .28$), and neuropsychological indices ($M = -.02$). These findings coincide with a recent meta-analysis of children with RD (Kudo et al., 2015).

Second, the results support the notion that reading achievement and cognitive deficits in RD are persistent across age. As found with children, deficits in phonological processing, naming speed, and verbal memory continue to characterize RD even in adulthood. Performance on phonological processing measures was a clear discriminating variable between adults with RD and average adult readers. In fact, in terms of comparisons between children and adults, Miller-Shaul (2005) found that the differences between regular readers and adults with dyslexia were smaller in the adult group on orthographic tasks, but the difference increased substantially in adults on phonological tasks. This is not to suggest that adults do not become proficient in some areas of reading (as found in some studies), but the majority of studies found that adults with RD still exhibit poor phonological processing and reading relative to average-achieving readers. The results are consistent with more recent studies on adults with RD showing that the reading of familiar words is usually slow (Tighe & Schatschneider, 2016).

Finally, ESs varied as a function of severity in RD and intellectual level. The key finding on this issue was that variations in the level of intelligence significantly moderated the magnitude of ESs between adults with RD and without RD. Studies with low-IQ participants yielded *lower* ESs between adults with and without RD on measures of cognition and language than those with relatively high IQs. Thus, variations in IQ clearly moderated outcomes related to ESs.

1.11 Practical Application

Although the report meta-analysis synthesizes performance across a range of measures in adults with RD, the practical applications to assessment need to be highlighted. At a more general level, to assess adults with RD at the cognitive and behavioral level, it is assumed that systematic efforts are made to detect: (a) normal psychometric intelligence, (b) below normal achievement on standardized measures of achievement (e.g., word recognition) since childhood, (c) below normal performance on measures of specific cognitive processes (e.g., phonological awareness and working memory) since childhood, (d) that evidence-based instruction has been presented under optimal conditions over the individuals school experience, and there is (e) evidence that academic and/or cognitive processing deficits are not directly caused by environmental factors or contingencies (e.g., socioeconomic status [SES]). In essence, the identification of adults with RD is predicated on the assumption of documentation of normal intelligence (i.e., individuals do not suffer from intellectual disability) and deficient academic performance that persists after best instructional practices have been systematically provided throughout the individual's school experience.

Our synthesis of the literature did reveal a profile of adults with dyslexia with average normative scores on general and verbal intelligence tests (50th percentile range), low average scores in math and vocabulary (30th percentile range), but word recognition, word attack, fluency, spelling, and writing were below the 25th percentile (see Table 1.1). The average reported phonological processing skills for adults with dyslexia were below the 6th percentile, whereas paradoxically, the average reading comprehension scores were in the 30th percentile range. The largest differences between adults with dyslexia and those adults who were average readers were on measures of word recognition, word attack, reading comprehension, naming speed, phonological processing, and spelling.

The synthesis also revealed several frequently used instruments in defining the adult sample as RD. Tests such as the WAIS and the Woodcock–Johnson Tests of Cognitive Abilities were frequently used to evaluate overall cognitive skills. Academic achievement tests such as the Wechsler Individual Achievement Test, the Wide Range Achievement Tests, and the Woodcock–Johnson Test of Achievement frequently provided standardized methods for evaluating and documenting academic skills.

1.12 Implications

Besides the aforementioned descriptive findings, what are some of the nuances related to the assessment of adults with dyslexia commonly overlooked in the literature? There are at least three implications to diagnosing adults with RD that emerge from a meta-analysis of the literature.

1 *Processes related to rapid naming and verbal memory are just as important as the phonological process in defining RD.* Clear weaknesses in processing emerged on measures of rapid naming, phonological processing, and verbal

memory. It has generally been presumed that adults with RD experience difficulties in word recognition because they have a low degree of phonological awareness. This appears to be the case in the meta-analyses reviewed. However, other processes (e.g., rapid naming and verbal memory) were related to differences between adults with and without RD. Why is this the case? One possibility is that phonological skills are no more important in adult samples than other verbal processes. A similar observation has been made by Scarborough (1998) when they stated,

> what the adolescent and adult data indicate... is that phonemic awareness may not always be necessary for successful reading acquisition. Instead, some individuals may never come to appreciate the existence of phonemes and yet may attain high levels of achievement.
>
> *(p. 139)*

The results are consistent with those of Scarborough, suggesting that phonological awareness may be no more important than other processes in accounting for differences between adults with and without RD.

2 *Measures of Verbal intelligence should "not" be eliminated as part of the battery in defining adults with RD.* Several researchers have suggested eliminating IQ from the classification of RD (e.g., Fletcher et al., 1994; Francis et al., 2005; Stuebing et al., 2002). However, the Swanson and Hsieh (2009) synthesis supports the notion that verbal IQ should be included as part of the assessment process. Although not reported in this chapter, the original synthesis (Swanson & Hsieh, 2009) that included regression modeling showed that: (a) variations in reading did not partial out the influence of verbal IQ in predicting differences between adults with and without RD, and (b) variations in reading (whether word recognition or reading comprehension) did not eliminate the contribution of cognitive variables in accounting for ES differences between adults with and without RD. The results showed that the unique variables in the assessment process were measures of verbal IQ, reading (both word recognition and comprehension), phonological processing, naming speed, word attack, math, vocabulary, spelling, and verbal memory. These variables were significant moderators and independently contributed to discriminating the differences between adults with and without RD when the influence of all other variables was entered into the analysis (also see Swanson, 2012). Thus, the results are consistent with several assessment models (e.g., Carroll et al., 2016; Moll et al., 2016; Pourcin et al., 2016; Ramus et al., 2013; Re et al., 2011; Sadusky et al., 2022; Warmington et al., 2013), which emphasize that verbal IQ, word recognition, reading comprehension, math, spelling, and cognitive measures (e.g., phonological, naming speed, and verbal memory) should be included as part of the assessment battery for diagnosing individuals with RD.

3 The higher the IQ, the more severe the reading deficit. Paradoxically, adults with RD and relatively higher levels of IQ were worse off in terms of processing deficiencies than adults with RD and relatively lower IQs. Among studies with low composite reading scores (< 25th percentile), those that reported high IQ scores relative to their reading scores were "worse off" (i.e., higher ESs) on measures of cognition (verbal memory) and language (vocabulary) relative to adult readers in studies that reported IQ scores roughly in the same range as their reading scores. Thus, holding scores in reading below the 25th percentile constant, a critical factor related to assessing the severity of RD was that the higher the verbal IQ in adult samples with RD (IQs > 100), the poorer their performance was relative to adult skilled readers.

1.13 Summary

An analysis of ESs highlighted the primary areas to assess and diagnose adults suspected of having RD. It is important to note, however, that in contrast to current alternative assessment procedures suggested for children, such as response to instruction, dynamic testing, and progress monitoring, no empirical studies comparing adults with RD using these alternative models have been reported in the synthesis literature (cf. Fletcher et al., 2014). Thus, the literature reviewed included only studies that directly compared adults with RD and those without RD across a broad array of academic, cognitive, behavioral, vocational, and neuropsychological measures. However, the results are consistent with several earlier studies suggesting a phonological core deficit model (e.g., Snowling, 1998; Stanovich, 1998; Vellutino et al., 2004) where difficulties in phonological awareness and related phonological processes such as naming speed and verbal memory reflect a common construct.

The results indicate that specific cognitive and language processes of adults with RD with IQs greater than a standard score of 100 are clearly distinguishable from those of adult skilled readers, as well as adults with low IQ and reading scores. The results support the notion that the primary processes that underlie RD in children are the same as those in adults. For example, the results show that phonological processing deficits are related to RD in adults. However, the deficits in processing in adults with RD are much broader than a phonological core. Processes related to verbal memory and naming speed play just as important a role as phonological processes.

Note

1 Acronyms are as follows. WRAT = Wide Range Achievement Test, PIAT = Peabody individual achievement Test, WRMT = Woodcock Reading Mastery Test, WJPB = Woodcock–Johnson Psychoeducational Battery, PPVT = Peabody Picture vocabulary Test, TOAL = Test of Oral Language, WAIS = Wechsler Adult Intelligence Scale, LNNB = Lincoln Nebraska Neuropsychological Battery,

GPA = grade point average, MMPI = Minnesota Multiphasic Personality Inventory, EEG = Electroencephalogram.

The citations and description of each measure in terms of update and critique are found in the Nineteenth (2014) and Twentieth (2017) Mental Measurement Yearbook and Salvia et al. (2013).

References

American Psychiatric Association. (2013). *Diagnostic and statistical manual of mental disorders* (5th ed.). Washington, DC: American Psychiatric Association.

Araújo, S., & Faísca, L. (2019). A meta-analytic review of naming-speed deficits in developmental dyslexia. *Scientific Studies of Reading, 23*(5), 349–368. https://doi.org/10.1080/10888438.2019.1572758

Araújo, S., Huettig, F., & Meyer, A. S. (2021). What underlies the deficit in rapid automatized naming (RAN) in adults with dyslexia? Evidence from eye movements. *Scientific Studies of Reading, 25*(6), 534–549. https://doi.org/10.1080/10888438.2020.1867863

Carioti, D., Masia, M. F., Travellini, S., & Berlingeri, M. (2021). Orthographic depth and developmental dyslexia: A meta-analytic study. *Annals of Dyslexia, 71*(3), 399–438. https://doi.org/10.1007/s11881-021-00226-0

Carroll, J. M., Solity, J., & Shapiro, L. R. (2016). Predicting dyslexia using prereading skills: The role of sensorimotor and cognitive abilities. *Journal of Child Psychology and Psychiatry, 57*(6), 750–758. https://doi.org/10.1111/jcpp.12488

Cheema, K., Fleming, C., Craig, J., Hodgetts, W. E., & Cummine, J. (2023). Reading and spelling profiles of adult poor readers: Phonological, orthographic and morphological considerations. *Dyslexia: An International Journal of Research and Practice, 29*(2), 58–77. https://doi.org/10.1002/dys.1731

Cohen, J. (1988). *Statistical power analysis for the behavioral sciences* (2nd ed.). Hillsdale, NJ: Erlbaum.

Collette, E., Content, A., Schelstraete, M., & Chetail, F. (2022). The extraction of orthographic and phonological structure of printed words in adults with dyslexia. *Dyslexia: An International Journal of Research and Practice, 28*(1), 4–19. https://doi.org/10.1002/dys.1700

Corley, M., & Taymans, J. (2002). Adults with learning disabilities: A review of the literature. In J. Comings, B. Garner, & C. Smith (Eds.), *Annual review of adult learning and literacy, volume 3* (pp. 44–83). San Francisco, CA: Wiley & Sons, Inc.

de Assis, L., Sara, E. S., Lage, G. M., de Souza, R. P., Nogueira, d. H. M., Gardênia, N., & Pinheiro, Â. M. V. (2023). Working memory and manual dexterity in dyslexic children: A systematic review and meta-analysis. *Developmental Neuropsychology, 48*(1), 1–30. https://doi.org/10.1080/87565641.2022.2157833

Fletcher, J. M. (2010). Construct validity of reading measures in adults with significant reading difficulties. *Journal of Learning Disabilities, 43*(2), 166–168.

Fletcher, J. M., Shaywitz, S. E., Shankweiler, D. P., Katz, L., Liberman, I. Y., Stuebing, K. K., Francis, D. J., Fowler, A. E., & Shaywitz, B. A. (1994). Cognitive profiles of reading disability: Comparisons of discrepancy and low achievement definitions. *Journal of Educational Psychology, 86*, 6–23.

Fletcher, J. M., Stuebing, K. K., Morris, R. D., & Lyon, G. R. (2014). Classification and definition of learning disabilities: A hybrid model. In *Handbook of learning disabilities* (2nd ed., pp. 33–50). New York: Guilford Press.

Francis, D. J., Fletcher, J. M., Stuebing, K. K., Lyon, G. R., Shaywitz, B. A., & Shaywitz, S. E. (2005). Psychometric approaches to the identification of LD: IQ and achievement scores are not sufficient. *Journal of Learning Disabilities, 38*(2), 98–108. https://doi.org/10.1177/00222194050380020101

Georgiou, G. K., Vieira, A. P. A., Rothou, K. M., Kirby, J. R., Antoniuk, A., Martinez, D., & Guo, K. (2023). A meta-analysis of morphological awareness deficits in developmental dyslexia. *Scientific Studies of Reading, 27*(3), 253–271. https://doi.org/10.1080/10888438.2022.2155524

Gregg, N. (2011). Adults with learning disabilities: Barriers and progress. *Learning and Attention disorders in adolescence and adulthood: Assessment and treatment* (2nd ed., pp. 87–111). Hoboken, NJ: John Wiley & Sons Inc.

Grigorenko, E. L., Compton, D. L., Fuchs, L. S., Wagner, R. K., Willcutt, E. G., & Fletcher, J. M. (2019). Understanding, educating, and supporting children with specific learning disabilities: 50 years of science and practice. *American Psychologist.* https://doi.org/10.1037/amp0000452

Hedges, L. V., & Olkin, I. (1985). *Statistical methods for meta-analysis.* San Diego, CA: Academic Press.

Kudo, M. F., Lussier, C. M., & Swanson, H. L. (2015). Reading disabilities in children: A selective meta-analysis of the cognitive literature. *Research in Developmental Disabilities, 40,* 51–62. https://doi.org/10.1016/j.ridd.2015.01.002

Melby-Lervåg, M., Lyster, S. H., & Hulme, C. (2012). Phonological skills and their role in learning to read: A meta-analytic review. *Psychological Bulletin, 138*(2), 322–352. https://doi.org/10.1037/a0026744

Miller, B., McCardle, P., & Hernandez, R. (2010). Advances and remaining challenges in adult literacy research. *Journal of Learning Disabilities, 43,* 101–109.

Miller-Shaul, S. (2005). The characteristics of young and adult dyslexics readers on reading and reading related cognitive tasks as compared to normal readers. *Dyslexia: An International Journal of Research and Practice, 11*(2), 132–151. https://doi.org/10.1002/dys.290

Moll, K., Göbel, S. M., Gooch, D., Landerl, K., & Snowling, M. J. (2016). Cognitive risk factors for specific learning disorder: Processing speed, temporal processing, and working memory. *Journal of Learning Disabilities, 49*(3), 272–281. https://doi.org/10.1177/0022219414547221

National Adult Literacy Survey (1992). U.S. Department of Education, National Center for Education.

National Institute of Neurological Disorders and Stroke. (2010, May). Retrieved from: https://www.ninds.nih.gov/

Ottosen, H. F., Bønnerup, K. H., Weed, E., & Parrila, R. (2022). Identifying dyslexia at the university: Assessing phonological coding is not enough. *Annals of Dyslexia, 72*(1), 147–170. https://doi.org/10.1007/s11881-021-00247-9

Peng, P., Zhang, Z., Wang, W., Lee, K., Wang, T., Wang, C., & Lin, J. (2022). A meta-analytic review of cognition and reading difficulties: Individual differences, moderation, and language mediation mechanisms. *Psychological Bulletin, 148*(3–4), 227–272. https://doi.org/10.1037/bul0000361

Pourcin, L., Sprenger-Charolles, L., El Ahmadi, A., & Colé, P. (2016). Reading and related skills in grades 6, 7, 8 and 9: French normative data from EVALEC. *European Review of Applied Psychology/Revue Européenne De Psychologie Appliquée, 66*(1), 23–37. https://doi.org/10.1016/j.erap.2015.11.002

Purcell, J. J., Shea, J., & Rapp, B. (2014). Beyond the visual word form area: The orthography–semantics interface in spelling and reading. *Cognitive Neuropsychology, 31*(5–6), 482–510. https://doi.org/10.1080/02643294.2014.909399

Ramus, F., Marshall, C. R., Rosen, S., & van der Lely, H. K. (2013). Phonological deficits in specific language impairment and developmental dyslexia: Towards a multidimensional model. *Brain: A Journal of Neurology, 136*(2), 630–645. https://doi.org/10.1093/brain/aws356

Ransby, M. J., & Swanson, H. L. (2003). Reading comprehension skills of young adults with childhood diagnoses of dyslexia. *Journal of Learning Disabilities, 36*(6), 538–555. https://doi.org/10.1177/00222194030360060501

Re, A. M., Tressoldi, P. E., Cornoldi, C., & Lucangeli, D. (2011). Which tasks best discriminate between dyslexic university students and controls in a transparent language? *Dyslexia: An International Journal of Research and Practice, 17*(3), 227–241. https://doi.org/10.1002/dys.431

Reis, A., Araújo, S., Morais, I. S., & Faísca, L. (2020). Reading and reading-related skills in adults with dyslexia from different orthographic systems: A review and meta-analysis. *Annals of Dyslexia, 70*(3), 339–368. https://doi.org/10.1007/s11881-020-00205-x

Sadusky, A., Freeman, N. C., Berger, E., & Reupert, A. E. (2022). Psychologists' diagnostic assessments of adults with dyslexia: An Australian-based survey study. *The Educational and Developmental Psychologist, 39*(2), 151–160. https://doi.org/10.1080/20590776.2021.2011202

Salvia, J., Ysseldyke, J. E., & Bolt, S. (2013). *Assessment in special and inclusive education* (12th ed.). Belmont, CA: Wadsworth/Cencage Learning.

Scarborough, H. S. (1998). Early identification of children at risk for reading disabilities: Phonological awareness and some other promising predictors. In B. Shapiro, P. Accardo, & A. Capute (Eds.), *Specific reading disability: A view of the spectrum* (pp. 75–119). Timonium, MD: York Press.

Schraeyen, K., Van der Elst, W., Geudens, A., Ghesquière, P., & Sandra, D. (2019). Short-term memory problems for phonemes' serial order in adults with dyslexia: Evidence from a different analysis of the nonword repetition task. *Applied PsychoLinguistics, 40*(3), 613–644. https://doi.org/10.1017/S0142716418000759

Shaywitz, S. E., Fletcher, J. M., Holahan, J. M., Schneider, A. E., Marchione, K. E., Stuebing, K. K., Francis, D. J., & Shaywitz, B. A. (1999). Persistence of dyslexia: The Connecticut longitudinal study at adolescence. *Pediatrics, 104*, 1351–1359.

Shaywitz, S. E., & Shaywitz, B. A. (2005). Dyslexia (specific reading disability). *Biological Psychiatry, 57*, 1301–1309.

Shaywitz, S. E., & Shaywitz, B. A. (2013). Neurobiological indices of dyslexia. In H. L. Swanson, K. R. Harris, & S. Graham (Eds.), *Handbook of learning disabilities* (pp. 514–531). New York: Guilford Press.

Shuy, T. (2003). *Screening and measuring learning disabilities in adult education students*. Washington, DC: National Institute of Literacy.

Smith-Spark, J., & Fisk, J. E. (2007). Working memory functioning in developmental dyslexia. *Memory, 15*(1), 34–56. https://doi.org/10.1080/09658210601043384

Snowling, M. (1998). Dyslexia as a phonological deficit: Evidence and implications. *Child Psychology & Psychiatry Review, 3*(1), 4–11. https://doi.org/10.1017/S1360641797001366

Stanovich, K. E. (1998). Refining the phonological core deficit model. *Child Psychology & Psychiatry Review, 3*(1), 17–21. https://doi.org/10.1017/S136064179700138X

Stuebing, K. K., Fletcher, J. M., LeDoux, J. M., Lyon, G. R., Shaywitz, S. E., & Shaywitz, B. A. (2002). Validity of IQ-discrepancy classifications of reading disabilities: A meta analysis. *American Educational Research Journal, 39*, 469–518.

Swanson, H. L. (2012). Adults with reading disabilities: Converting a meta-analysis to practice. *Journal of Learning Disabilities, 45*(1), 17–30. https://doi.org/10.1177/0022219411426856

Swanson, H. L., & Hsieh, C. (2009). Reading disabilities in adults: A selective meta-analysis of the literature. *Review of Educational Research, 79*, 1362–1390.

The nineteenth mental measurements yearbook (2014). Lincoln, NE: The Buros Center for Testing. Retrieved from https://search.proquest.com/docview/1519510695?accountid=14521

The twentieth mental measurements yearbook (2017). Lincoln, NE: The Buros Center for Testing. Retrieved from https://search.proquest.com/docview/1946703224?accountid=14521

Tighe, E. L., & Schatschneider, C. (2016). Examining the relationships of component reading skills to reading comprehension in struggling adult readers: A meta-analysis. *Journal of Learning Disabilities*, *49*(4), 395–409. https://doi.org/10.1177/0022219414555415

Vellutino, F. R., Fletcher, J. M., Snowling, M. J., & Scanlon, D. M. (2004). Specific reading disability (dyslexia): What have we learned in the past four decades? *Journal of Child Psychology and Psychiatry*, *45*(1), 2–40. https://doi.org/10.1046/j.0021-9630.2003.00305.x

Wagner, R. K., Edwards, A. A., Malkowski, A., Schatschneider, C., Joyner, R. E., Wood, S., & Zirps, F. A. (2019). Combining old and new for better understanding and predicting dyslexia. *New Directions for Child and Adolescent Development*, *2019*(165), 11–23. https://doi.org/10.1002/cad.20289

Wagner, R. K., Zirps, F. A., Edwards, A. A., Wood, S. G., Joyner, R. E., Becker, B. J., & Beal, B. (2020). The prevalence of dyslexia: A new approach to its estimation. *Journal of Learning Disabilities*, *53*(5), 354–365. https://doi.org/10.1177/0022219420920377

Warmington, M., Stothard, S. E., & Snowling, M. J. (2013). Assessing dyslexia in higher education: The York adult assessment battery-revised. *Journal of Research in Special Educational Needs*, *13*(1), 48–56. https://doi.org/10.1111/j.1471-3802.2012.01264.x

Zhang, Z., & Peng, P. (2022). Reading real words versus pseudowords: A meta-analysis of research in developmental dyslexia. *Developmental Psychology*, *58*(6), 1035–1050. https://doi.org/10.1037/dev0001340

2
PHONOLOGICAL PROCESSING SKILLS IN ADULTS WITH DYSLEXIA

Kirsten Schraeyen, Jolijn Vanderauwera and Maaike Vandermosten

2.1 Content Chapter

Developmental dyslexia is a learning disorder defined in terms of persistent difficulties with reading and/or spelling (Siegel, 2006). More specifically, it is associated with reading decoding problems as well as slow and inaccurate word recognition (Gathercole, Frankish, Pickering, & Peaker, 1999; Ramus & Szenkovits, 2008). Although much research has been carried out in the field of dyslexia, there is still a continuous debate about the underlying cause(s) of developmental dyslexia (for a review, see Ramus & Ahissar, 2012; Elliott & Grigorenko, 2014; Peterson & Pennington, 2015; Snowling, Hulme, & Nation, 2020). In the past decades, however, a consensus has grown among researchers that phonological processing is important for reading (Share, 2021), and a consistent relation has been demonstrated between developmental dyslexia and deficient phonological processing skills (e.g., Lyon, 1995; Vellutino, Fletcher, Snowling, & Scanlon, 2004). Although phonological processing is not the only possible determinant of dyslexia (Pennington, 2006), the observed deficits in persons with dyslexia are larger than for other cognitive components. More specifically, meta-analyses have demonstrated effect sizes (representing the magnitude of the deficit), which are large for phonological processing ($d = 1.37$ in Melby-Lervåg, Lyster, & Hulme, 2012), whereas these are moderate for other frequently reported components such as oral language skills ($d = 0.82$ in Melby-Lervåg et al., 2012), speech sound identification and discrimination skills ($d = 0.86$ and $d = 0.66$ in Noordenbos & Serniclaes, 2015).

Phonological processing skills refer to a broad set of skills, such as phoneme identification (matching incoming speech sounds onto their corresponding phoneme, despite acoustic variation), phonological awareness

(awareness that words consist of individual syllables and phonemes and that these can be manipulated) and retrieval and short-term memory of phonological units (Snowling, 2000). These phonological skills are at the core of accurate written word recognition, reading comprehension and spelling (Liberman & Shankweiler, 1991; Rayner, Foorman, Perfetti, Pesetsky, & Seidenberg, 2002; Share & Stanovich, 1995; Share, 2023). Phonological processing skills are classically subdivided into three subdomains, i.e., phonological awareness, verbal short-term memory (VSTM) and lexical retrieval from long-term memory (LTM; Wagner & Torgesen, 1987). It is claimed that deviant phonological processing skills in individuals with dyslexia are exhibited in all three subdomains (e.g., Mann & Liberman, 1984; Ziegler & Goswami, 2005). Moreover, these phonological processing difficulties are not only shown in childhood (e.g., Ramus, 2003; Snowling, 2000) but also persist into adulthood (e.g., Elbro, Nielsen, & Petersen, 1994; Ramus et al., 2003; Reis, Araújo, Morais, & Faisca, 2020; Snowling, Nation, Moxham, Gallagher, & Frith, 1997), even in adolescents and adults who have achieved reading and writing skills within the normal range (e.g., Bruck, 1992; Paulesu et al., 1996; Snowling et al., 1997).

This chapter will explore these phonological processing skills in adults with dyslexia. Although this review is by no means exhaustive in terms of studies included, we hope to provide some key insights into this part of current dyslexia research.

2.2 Subdomains of Phonological Processing

2.2.1 Phonological Awareness

Phonological awareness refers to the metacognitive understanding that spoken words can be broken into smaller sound units such as syllables (syllable awareness), onsets and rimes (onset–rime awareness), body and codas (body–coda awareness) and phonemes (phonemic awareness) (Blachman, 1997; Liberman & Shankweiler, 1991; Share & Stanovich, 1995). It entails the ability to pay attention to these sound units and manipulate them. Phonological awareness is a dynamic construct that develops as a function of time (Anthony et al., 2002; Norris & Hoffman, 2002). During development, children start to understand that words can be divided into syllables, such as 'foot-ball' and, more complex, 'be-tter'. They gradually become aware that syllables can also be divided into smaller sound units, such as 'c-at' at the onset–rime level or 'ca-t' at the body–coda level to the smallest units of sounds, i.e., phonemes (Pennington & Lefly, 2001; Ziegler & Goswami, 2005). However, it is important to note that there is no such thing as a 'universal fixed' sequence of development. Based on a cross-linguistic study of six alphabetic writing systems, Duncan et al. (2013) clearly showed that phonological development – and, hence, the development of phonological awareness – is influenced by the native language, the instructional context and specific task demands.

In an alphabetic language, phonemes are the smallest unit of speech sounds that can change the meaning of a word (e.g., /cat/ that can be turned into /rat/ by replacing the speech sound /c/with/r/). In contrast to syllable awareness, phonemic awareness rarely emerges in the absence of explicit instruction (e.g., Huang & Hanley, 1995; Morais, Bertelson, Cary, & Alegria, 1986). Phonological awareness forms the basis for understanding the alphabetic principle, i.e., the realization that speech can be segmented into phonemes and that these phonemes are represented in printed forms (Blachman, 1997; Lyon, 1995).

Several tasks are available to measure individuals' phonological awareness at different representation levels (e.g., syllable level and phoneme level). Given that phonemic awareness is the most complicated stage of phonological awareness, most tasks for adults are situated at this level, albeit that performance on these tasks may vary according to their meta-cognitive demands and not just the unit of sound under study (see, for instance, Duncan et al., 2013). Before exploring different types of measures, it is important to understand that these phonological awareness tasks can be assessed based on both accuracy and reaction time. Accuracy is determined by the number of stimuli answered correctly, while reaction time refers to the time between stimulus presentation and an individual's response. While certain phonemic awareness tasks may be less demanding and could potentially lead to ceiling effects in accuracy, even among primary school children (e.g., Landerl & Wimmer, 2000), research consistently shows a measurable difference in reaction time between individuals with and without dyslexia (Callens, Tops, & Brysbaert, 2012). Given that these observed difficulties persist into adulthood and are particularly pronounced in speed measures, it is essential to incorporate speed measures when evaluating phonemic awareness in adults (see also Reis et al., 2020).

A first measure that has frequently been used is a *phoneme deletion task*. In this task, an individual is asked to delete a particular phoneme (the first or the last) from a word, mostly a non-existent word. For example, 'spoonk' without 'k' would be 'spoon'. Both accuracy and reaction time have been demonstrated to be hampered in adults with dyslexia (e.g., Beidas, Khateb, & Breznitz, 2013; De Smedt & Boets, 2010; Vandermosten et al., 2012). A similar task is a *phoneme substitution task*. In this task, an individual is asked to replace a particular phoneme in a word with a different phoneme. For example, replace 'n' of 'brain' with 'k'. For instance, Elbro and Jensen (2005) showed reduced performance in adolescents with dyslexia compared to younger reading-matched controls, indicating that there is a phoneme awareness *deficit* and not just a delay. Another task that is often used in adults because of a higher level of task complexity, and thus, a more sensitive measure, is the *spoonerisms task* (see de Jong & Van der Leij, 2003). In this task, an individual is requested to swap the initial phoneme of two (non)words [1]. For example, 'cal' and 'vook' become 'val' and 'cook'. This task is more difficult than the phoneme deletion task. Both accuracy and reaction time in this task have been demonstrated to be hampered in adults with dyslexia (e.g., Paulesu et al., 1996; Snowling et al., 1997; Ramus et al., 2003; Vandermosten et al., 2012). In addition, comparing adults with dyslexia and controls reveals that they perform less adequately on a *segmentation task*, in which an individual is asked to segment an auditorily presented nonword (e.g.,/spoors/) into its basic phonological sound units, i.e., phonemes, as rapidly as possible (e.g., Beidas et al., 2013). Another more complex task assessing phonological awareness is *a word reversal task*, in which an individual has to decide whether two spoken words are reversals or not (e.g., pen–nep). For instance, Tops, Callens, Lammertyn, Van Hees and Brysbaert (2012) used this task to compare first-year higher education students with and without dyslexia. Results revealed significant underperformance in adults with dyslexia, both in the level of accuracy and speed.

It is sometimes argued that these tasks in adults do not purely assess phonological awareness but also comprise, to some extent, a working memory component (e.g., in a spoonerism task, two words need to be remembered before they can be manipulated; e.g., Richardson et al., 2011) and an orthographic component (e.g., adults might visually imagine the written form of the auditory presented words; Landerl, Frith and Wimmer (1996) and also see Section 2.4 below for more information). Nevertheless, all tasks described above require individuals to reflect on the speech sounds and manipulate the sound structure of the word; hence, they involve phonological awareness, though potentially with influences of other cognitive components.

2.2.2 Verbal Short-term Memory

VSTM, a component of working memory (for details, see Baddeley, 2000, 2003), refers to a storage device in which phonological information can be maintained for a short period of time. Two essential features are necessary: a phonological storage that holds phonological information and a subvocal rehearsal mechanism that prevents decay of the stored information. VSTM tasks, therefore, typically require individuals to immediately recall a sequence of verbal items in the order they are presented. Different types of immediate serial recall tasks can be used to measure VSTM.

One such task is a *digit span task*. In a digit span task, individuals need to repeat progressively longer sequences of purely auditorily presented digits in direct order (digit span forward), e.g., an individual is asked to repeat the digit sequence /2–4/, /3–6–9/. The digit span is usually taken to be the number of sequences accurately recalled. Digit span backward, in which an individual is asked to repeat the reverse of the digit sequence /2–4/ (i.e., /4–2/) is less suited as a VSTM task, given that this task evaluates working memory capacity (presented digits need to be manipulated) and less VSTM (presented digits need to be remembered). There is evidence showing that children with dyslexia have poorer performance on digit span forward tasks compared to normal readers (e.g., Gallagher et al., 2000; Roodenrys, Koloski, & Grainger, 2001; Snowling, Muter, & Carroll, 2007), although this is not always confirmed (Dandache, Wouters, & Ghesquiére, 2014). The capacities of adults with dyslexia on those digit span forward tasks are also not that clear. Snowling et al. (1997) showed reduced performance on digit span forward in adults with dyslexia compared to skilled adult readers, although the effect disappeared when other metalinguistic skills were controlled for. Other studies, however, did find a difference. For instance, De Smedt and Boets (2010) showed an underperformance in adults with dyslexia on digit span forward as compared to adult skilled readers. Other studies showed similar results when comparing adult skilled readers and compensated[1] dyslexics (Brunswick, McCrory, Price, Frith, & Frith, 1999; Sela, Izzetoglu, Izzetoglu, & Onaral, 2012).

Another task that measures VSTM is (non)word span. In this task, individuals have to repeat a series of auditorily presented unrelated (non)words, e.g., recall of words 'blood-lamp-cool'. Differences have been shown between adults with dyslexia and controls, even after controlling for speech rate (Snowling et al., 1997), which is known to be an important determinant of VSTM (Hulme, Maughan, & Brown, 1991). One more prominent task that has been used is nonword repetition. In this task, individuals need to repeat auditorily presented nonwords[2] immediately from VSTM. Many studies revealed a reduced performance in adults with dyslexia compared to adult skilled readers (e.g., Dietrich & Brady, 2001; Ramus et al., 2003; Schraeyen, Van der Elst, Geudens, Ghesquière, & Sandra, 2019).

When considering tasks of VSTM, it is important to realize that the influence of LTM could not be ruled out (e.g., Schraeyen, Van der Elst, Geudens, Ghesquière, & Sandra, 2017). Indeed, many studies have shown that STM processing is influenced by long-term knowledge. For instance, a study showed that words are recalled better than nonwords (so-called lexicality effect, e.g., Gathercole, Pickering, Hall, & Peaker, 2001). Nonwords containing high phonotactic probabilities (i.e., the frequency with which phonological segments and sequences of phonological segments occur in words in a given language) are also shown to be easier to recall than nonwords containing low phonotactic probabilities (so-called word likeness effect, see Edwards, Beckman, & Munson, 2004).

2.2.3 Lexical Retrieval from LTM

Lexical retrieval refers to individuals' capacity to quickly retrieve stored phonological information from LTM. One of the most used measures to capture lexical retrieval is the rapid automatized naming (RAN) task. The RAN task consists of a strict set of high-frequency visually presented symbols, e.g., alphanumeric symbols (letters and digits) or non-alphanumeric symbols (objects and colors), that are repeated multiple times in a randomized order and that have to be named as quickly and accurately as possible. A wealth of evidence has been provided showing that RAN predicts later literacy performance in both transparent (e.g., de Jong & van der Leij, 2002; Lervag, Braten, & Hulme, 2009) and opaque orthographies (e.g., Georgiou, Parrila, Kirby, & Stephenson, 2008; Kirby, Parrila, & Pfeiffer, 2003). In addition, adults with dyslexia consistently underperform on such RAN tasks as compared to skilled readers (Bekebrede, Van der Leij, & Share, 2009; de Jong & Van der Leij, 2003; De Smedt & Boets, 2010; Jones, Branigan, & Kelly, 2009; Shaywitz & Shaywitz, 2005).

Although RAN has been conceptualized as a phonological processing (sub) skill for many years (e.g. Wagner & Torgesen, 1987), recent studies suggest that RAN should be considered as a separate and independent risk factor to reading development rather than a phonological subskill (Parrila & Protopapas, 2017; Rodríguez, van den Boer, Jiménez, & de Jong, 2015). This interpretation is based on the finding that RAN has been shown to account for variance in reading beyond the effects of phonological awareness (e.g., Parrila, Kirby, & McQuarrie, 2004) and phonological short-term memory (e.g., Bowers, Steffy, & Tate, 1988; Georgiou et al., 2008; Parrila et al., 2004).

2.3   Factors that Underpin Phonological Processing Difficulties

The fact that poor phonological awareness, reduced VSTM span and underperformance in rapid lexical retrieval in most individuals with dyslexia persist into adulthood calls for further understanding. Why is it so hard for these individuals to process the sound structure of a language? Many ideas have been suggested in the literature. Before elaborating on some of these ideas, it is crucial to understand that phonological awareness, VSTM and rapid lexical retrieval involve the storage and retrieval of phonological representations. Phonological representations refer to sound-based codes stored in the lexicon for each word (Anthony et al., 2010). Given that a phonological representation can be considered as a *sequence* of speech sounds, it comprises several phonemic representations. Hence, many researchers in the field of dyslexia believe that phonological processing problems are rooted in a basic problem with phonemic representations. One influencing idea is that sequences of phonemes are poorly specified (Elbro & Jensen, 2005), indistinct (Elbro, 1998), overspecified (Serniclaes, Van Heghe, Mousty, Carré, & Sprenger-Charolles, 2004) or less mature (Boada & Pennington, 2006). Here, it is important to note that, in contrast to the older view of Chomsky (Chomsky & Halle, 1968), converging evidence suggests that phonological representations are not innate but emerge gradually by natural language exposure. A child progressively learns to map the various sounds he is exposed to in his native language to specific phoneme categories, despite the acoustic variability in each of the sounds due to, for example, speaking rate, dialects, gender or co-articulation. Two mechanisms are important for learning to form robust representation of phonemes: (1) auditory processing abilities that enable a child to perceive the subtle acoustic cues (often within tens of milliseconds) that distinguish different speech sounds (such as formant transition to distinguish stop consonants); and (2) sensitivity to the statistical distribution of sounds in their native language, which allows them to define the phonemic structure of their language. Interestingly, impairments in each of these two mechanisms have been demonstrated in (at least some) dyslexic readers, thereby reinforcing the idea of impaired representations (for a review on auditory impairments, see Hämäläinen, Salminen, & Leppänen, 2012; for impairments in statistical learning of speech sounds, see Gabay & Holt, 2015; Vandermosten et al., 2020). In addition, dyslexic children perform more poorly on behavioral speech tasks such as categorical perception, lexical gating and priming experiments, which require no explicit attention to or metalinguistic manipulation of the speech sounds, thereby suggesting a deficit in the underlying phonological representations itself rather than problems in the metalinguistic processes computed on them (for a meta-analysis on categorical perception deficits, see Noordenbos & Serniclaes, 2015; for deficits in priming and lexical gating, see Boada & Pennington, 2006; Elbro, 2002; Metsala, 1997).

The strong emphasis on the quality of phonemic representations or speech sounds suggests a nearly restricted concentration on the representation of phonemes' identity. Given that a sequence of phonemic representations forms a phonological representation, phonemes' serial order may also be crucial in the representation/retrieval of phonological representations. Using a nonword repetition paradigm, recently some researchers showed a decreased retention for phonemes' serial order, both in young poor readers (Schraeyen, Geudens, Ghesquière, Van der Elst, & Sandra, 2017) and adults with dyslexia (Schraeyen et al., 2019). Therefore, serial order retention might also be a crucial factor to consider for understanding the processing of phonological information.

Based on experiments in adult university students, other researchers claimed that the basic problem might not be the nature of phonological representations but the access to these representations (i.e., the computational processes such as conscious awareness, manipulation and attention to the representations) (Dickie, Ota, & Clark, 2013; Ramus & Szenkovits, 2008). It should be acknowledged that all these cognitive experiments cannot purely measure either representation or access since the measured outcome is the result of the dynamic interplay between them. Therefore, Boets et al. (2013) used a specific brain imaging decoding technique that proved to be sensitive to measure the neural distinctiveness of phonemes, thereby providing a more direct index of phonemic representations. Yet when this technique was applied in university students with dyslexia, no evidence was found for less distinctive neural phonemic representations, although altered connectivity from the regions hosting these representations was found (Boets et al., 2013). This could mean that the neural systems supporting phonological representations operate properly, whereas the connections with other brain regions (those that take phonological representations as input) are disturbed, thereby supporting the idea of a deficit in access rather than in the representations themselves (Ramus, 2014). Remarkably, applying the same neuroimaging technique in beginning readers did display a neural representational deficit in dyslexic readers (Vandermosten, Wouters, Ghesquière, & Golestani, 2019). Language differences cannot explain the discrepant findings between these two studies since both were conducted in Dutch-speaking participants. Yet it might suggest, and this is convergent with the pattern observed in the behavioral studies, that a deficit in phonological representations is present in young children with dyslexia but resolves in older (compensated) adults with dyslexia. In the future, methodological advances to obtain more precise representational measures (e.g., Gwilliams, King, Marantz, et al., 2022) and their applications in infants and children prior to reading onset can shed more light on whether representational problems indeed explain the phonological processing deficits observed from kindergarten through adulthood.

Nonetheless, both ideas (nature of and access to phonological representations) emphasize the important role of phonemic representations in the reading process in children and adults, i.e., the capacity to fluently access these representations, and that such representations underlie high-quality phonological representations of words.

2.4 The Importance of Integrated Lexical Representations in Sight-Word Reading

Apart from the fact that phonological processing problems in individuals with dyslexia are able to explain reduced performance in decoding tasks, one might ask whether this basic phonological problem can also explain poor sight-word recognition, as often observed in adults with dyslexia.

In normal conditions, the link between oral word form (phonology) and word meaning (semantics) has already been established before actual reading development starts, namely, starting when a child learns to speak his or her first words by interacting with native-language speakers. However, when learning to read, children need to acquire the link between the written word form (orthography) and the oral word form (phonology). To this end, the acquisition of reading skills entails the insight that each grapheme corresponds to a phoneme. Thus, when an unfamiliar written word has to be read, a child needs to (1) break down the word into its constituent letters (graphemes) and (2) map these letters or letter strings onto their corresponding speech sounds (phonemes), i.e., the process of phonological decoding (Share, 1995, 1999, 2004). In turn, phonemic representations provide access to that word's phonological representation. After a reader has numerous opportunities to decode a new word multiple times, and a specific word has consequently been read sufficiently often, an orthographic representation in LTM will be formed and linked to the phonological representation and meaning in memory. Once the reader successfully anchors and connects knowledge about the orthography, phonology, morphology and meaning of a word in LTM, he no longer needs to decode the word letter by letter but possesses orthographic and word-specific knowledge (Van den Broeck & Geudens, 2016). This enables immediate word reading or sight-word reading the next time this word has to be read, as connections are made among the spelling, pronunciation and meaning of the word. In the literature, this process is referred to as orthographic mapping (Ehri, 2014). Through this process of orthographic learning, beginning readers progress to advanced and automated reading (Nation & Castles, 2017). With repeated practice, all words eventually become read automatically, which is the most efficient way to read words in a text (Ehri, 2017). According to the 'self-teaching' hypothesis (Share, 1995, 1999; Ziegler, Perry, & Zorzi, 2014), each successful attempt at decoding a word enables a beginning reader to store information about the word's orthography and meaning. In this view, efficient decoding skills – which rely on efficient phonological processing skills – thereby aid the storage of sight-words (Howland & Liederman, 2013). In addition, other studies concluded that phonological decoding is necessary, but not sufficient. Goulandris (2003), for instance, showed that individuals with dyslexia were inefficient in sight-word recognition, even though they managed to learn to phonologically decode words with sufficient accuracy. According to the lexical quality hypothesis (Perfetti, 2007; Perfetti & Hart, 2002), high-quality lexical representations, including detailed information about the word's orthography or spelling, phonology or pronunciation and semantics or meaning, are crucial for sight-word reading. For example, one must know the spelling of the word 'kitchen', the pronunciation /'kɪtʃɪn/ and the meaning (place to cook). Eventually, one integrated lexical representation (combining orthography, phonology and meaning) has to be established in a manner that activation of one element (e.g., when you see the word 'kitchen') immediately retrieves from memory both the pronunciation (/'kɪtʃɪn/) and meaning (place to cook) (Perfetti & Hart, 2001).

Adult studies including skilled and less-skilled/dyslexic readers provide evidence for the crucial role of fully integrated lexical representations by showing that less-skilled readers and adults with dyslexia were not able to form connections between phonology and orthography and, thus, were unable to build up fully integrated lexical representations during word learning (e.g., Di Betta & Romani, 2006; Howland & Liederman, 2013; Hulme, Goetz, Gooch, Adams, & Snowling, 2007; Perfetti, 2007; Perfetti, Wlotko, & Hart, 2005; Van den Broeck & Geudens, 2012).

The importance of fully integrated lexical representations, however, does not diminish the role of phonological processing skills. As elaborated above, phonological processing skills are crucial for phonological decoding and reading aloud in the early stages of reading, but also act as a feedback mechanism (at an implicit level) in sight-word reading (see de Jong & Share, 2007).

2.5 The Role of Orthographic Knowledge in Phonological Awareness

In the previous sections, we explained how phonological processing affects literacy. However, there is also a wealth of evidence showing the opposite impact, i.e., orthographic mediation in phonological tasks. Evidence comes from different types of studies, including different age groups using both metalinguistic phonological and more implicit speech recognition tasks. It has been shown that 9-year-old children tend to give orthographically based responses when they have to perform a phoneme deletion task (e.g., /baɪnd/ without /n/ is pronounced as /bɪd/ – orthographical response – instead of the phonological response /baɪd/), and more skilled spellers seem to do this even more frequently (Stuart, 1990). Ehri and Wilce (1980) showed that fourth graders tend to report the number of phonemes in a word based on its orthographic codes instead of its phonological codes (e.g., the word 'pitch' /pɪtʃ/ was judged as having more phonemes than the word 'rich' /rɪtʃ/, although both have the same number of sounds). Castles, Holmes, Neath and Kinoshita (2003) conducted a series of different experiments. In the first experiment, skilled adult readers performed a phoneme deletion and phoneme reversal task. Both tasks contained items with straightforward grapheme–phoneme correspondences (transparent items, e.g., dentist) and items that did not have straightforward grapheme–phoneme correspondences (opaque items, e.g., chemist). Results revealed that deletions and reversals were more accurate and faster in response to straightforward items. Based on a correlational analysis between participants' spelling ability and their performance on both tasks, they concluded that participants with stronger orthographic skills were relying more strongly on the orthographic word form, and therefore performed better than individuals with poorer orthographic skills in response to transparent but not opaque items. In a second experiment with a younger age group, the same results were obtained (Castles et al., 2003).

All conducted studies using auditory lexical decision tasks (e.g., Pattamadilok, Morais, & Kolinsky, 2011; Ventura, Morais, & Kolinsky, 2007; Ziegler & Ferrand, 1998) adhere to the idea that speech recognition is automatically shaped by orthographic knowledge, at least in skilled readers. Using a lexical decision task in which the density of phonological and orthographic neighbors was manipulated, Ziegler and Muneaux (2007) found an orthographic neighborhood effect in children with adequate reading skills, but not in children with dyslexia, while a phonological neighborhood effect was found in both groups.

Research with skilled and dyslexic adult readers, however, showed that individuals with dyslexia can make use of their orthographic knowledge and rely on this knowledge despite their assumed unbalanced or coarsely specified orthographic representations (Pattamadilok, Nelis, & Kolinsky, 2014). In line with this view, Miller-Shaul (2005) showed that compensated adults with dyslexia had persisting problems with the phonological channel, but not with the orthographic channel. Comparing young normal and dyslexic readers on the one hand, and normal and dyslexic adult readers, on the other, she found that differences in phonological processing (e.g., decoding single real words) between normal and dyslexic readers not only occurred in both age groups but also increased in the adult group. In contrast, differences in orthographic processing (using a recognition task in which participants had to recognize words from a meaningful context) significantly reduced with age. One possible explanation is that compensated dyslexic adults' years of exposure to print enable them to use meaningful context as a compensation tool. Most likely, they have created word patterns in their lexicon, which facilitates the recognition (but not the articulation) of real words, albeit that their performance and speed level still is not the same as that of adult skilled readers. In contrast, when they have to recognize nonwords, they cannot rely on these word patterns in their lexicon. Instead, they need to make use of their 'disrupted' phonological channel. For this reason, they (still) perform on the same level as young dyslexics (Miller-Shaul, 2005). In the same vein, many other researchers showed lower phonological ability in compensated dyslexic adults (e.g., Bruck, 1990, 1992; Yap & Van der Leij, 1993).

This discussion underscores the complex interplay between orthographic and phonological processing in reading. The ability to compensate for phonological difficulties by relying on orthographic knowledge further emphasizes the dynamic nature of reading acquisition and the various strategies employed by readers to overcome challenges in literacy. Nonetheless, there is evidence showing orthographic mediation when performing phonological tasks. For this reason, many phonological tasks that are employed in adults make use of nonwords to prevent LTM influence as much as possible.

2.6 The Universal Role of Phonological Processing Skills

Evidence for the crucial role of phonological processing skills in reading development primarily comes from studies focusing on alphabetic languages, both transparent and opaque writing systems. In transparent writing systems, almost every letter corresponds to one speech sound. Examples are the Greek, Finnish and Italian writing systems. In opaque writing systems, one specific letter can correspond to different speech sounds. Examples are the English and French writing systems. It has been claimed that the relevance of phonological processing skills to literacy might be different depending on the transparency of the writing system (Share, 2008). Support for this claim was found in studies in which languages with different degrees of transparency were contrasted. For instance, Ziegler et al. (2010) conducted a study in which Finnish (less opaque), Hungarian, Dutch, Portuguese and French (most opaque) were compared in a group of 1265 children from Grade 2. Although phonological awareness (and not rapid naming) turned out to be the main factor predicting reading performance (both accuracy and speed) in each language tested, its impact was stronger in more opaque languages (Ziegler et al., 2010). Similar results were found by Vaessen et al. (2010). Comparing performance in Grades 1 and 2 and in Grades 3 and 4, they showed that the association of phonological awareness with reading was modulated by the language transparency, while the association of RAN or VSTM was not. This finding was also confirmed by Furnes and Samuelsson (2011), who investigated 750 U.S./Australian children and 230 Scandinavian children longitudinally from kindergarten to Grade 2.

Hence, the development of phonological awareness seems to be dependent on specific patterns of the language the child speaks. Durgunogly and Öney (1999) showed that Turkish-speaking children from kindergarten and Grade 1 were able to manipulate syllables more accurately than English-speaking children of the same age, reflecting the more consistently defined syllable structure of the Turkish language. In addition, Moll et al. (2014) conducted a study comparing 1062 typically developing children beyond Grade 2, learning to read in Finnish, Hungarian, German, French and English. While phonological awareness and short-term memory significantly contributed to reading and spelling accuracy in all languages (however, most in English), RAN turned out to be the best predictor of reading fluency.

Landerl et al. (2013) conducted a large-scale European study in which the cognitive and literacy skills of 1000 eight- to 12-year-old children, with and without dyslexia, learning to read in Finnish, Hungarian, German, Dutch, French and English were tested. Results confirmed that both phonological awareness (phoneme deletion) and RAN strongly predicted developmental dyslexia in all languages tested. The role of both VSTM and general verbal abilities turned out to be minor, but still significant. Similar to the studies described above, the impact of phonological awareness and RAN was stronger in more opaque than in more transparent languages, while this was not found for VSTM.

All together, these studies provide evidence that the predictive power of phonological processing tasks increases with the degree of orthographic complexity of a language. For individuals with dyslexia, this means that reading is differently affected by phonological deficits, depending on the complexity of the writing system. Hence, phonological deficits cause larger problems for reading opaque orthographies such as English compared to more transparent orthographies such as Finnish. Important to note is that, next to orthographic complexity, psychometric qualities of tasks such as task difficulty (e.g., spoonerism being more difficult than segmentation; however, both measure phonological awareness) may be decisive in explaining the mixed results (Caravolas, Volín, & Hulme, 2005; de Jong & Van der Leij, 2003; Morfidi, Leij, Jong, Scheltinga, & Bekebrede, 2007).

An interesting question, however, is whether this association between phonological processing skills is specific and restricted to (both transparent and opaque) alphabetic writing systems or whether it also extends to logographic writing systems such as Chinese. This question is relevant given that alphabetic writing systems are based on phonology, while in logographic writing systems, the pronunciation of whole characters cannot systematically be retrieved, requiring readers to memorize the pronunciations of all characters (Chen & Shu, 2001; Tan, Spinks, Eden, Perfetti, & Siok, 2005). Although Tan et al. (2005) found a much weaker association between phonological awareness and Chinese reading, other studies did show a strong association. For instance, Hu and Catts (1998) showed that performance on the phonological tasks was related to performance on reading tasks and concluded that the relation between phonological processing skills and early reading ability is also present in non-alphabetic languages, and thus, not specific to reading an alphabetic orthography. Likewise, Chan and Siegel (2001) investigated 94 school-aged children and demonstrated that phonological processing plays a significant role in reading development in Chinese. A more recent study by Yang, Zheng and Liu (2023) focusing on the associations of phonological processing skills with reading ability in Chinese kindergartners, third graders and fifth graders revealed that phonological awareness and RAN showed stronger relations than phonological memory with reading across grades. Moreover, these researchers found that the associations of phonological awareness and RAN with reading were much stronger in kindergartners than in primary school children (Yang et al., 2023). Two other reviews focusing on Chinese individuals with dyslexia conclude that these individuals tend to have difficulties with one or more of the following constructs: phonological sensitivity (sensitivity to different levels of speech sounds, including tones), morphological awareness, visual-orthographic processing and fluency(McBride & Wang, 2015; McBride, Wang, & Cheang, 2018).

2.7 From Group Studies to Individual Care

Although valuable, group-level analyses as reported in the previous sections cannot disclose the proportion of adults with dyslexia who actually show a specific deviant performance on phonological processing measures. However, this is crucial information for a clinician. Therefore, examination of phonological performance at the *individual level* is relevant. A common method is to place a threshold at *n* standard deviations (SD) of the mean of the control group (Ramus et al., 2003). Although arbitrary, several studies used *n* = 1.65 SD as this corresponds to a scoring below percentile 5 and thus seems an acceptable threshold for deviance, i.e., a performance below the norm for a specific measure or task. Ramus et al. (2003) conducted a study in English-speaking adults with dyslexia, examining individual deviances for phonological processing as well as visual, auditory and motoric skills. They demonstrated that all dyslexic adults displayed a phonological deficit (based on a phonological composite score including phonological awareness, VSTM and RAN), whereas this was only 6% in typical readers. For comparison, for auditory, visual and motor tasks, respectively, 60%, 13% and 25% of the dyslexic adults failed, indicating the clinical importance of a phonological deficit for diagnosis relative to other contributing factors. Although this study suggests that every adult with dyslexia has a phonological deficit, other studies in English-speaking adults show lower deviance rates. For example, Hazan, Messaoud-Galusi, Rosen, Nouwens and Shakespeare (2009) conducted individual deviance analyses on a phonological compound factor, including phonological awareness (spoonerism) and VSTM (nonword repetition) measures. They found that around half of the dyslexic adults have a phonological deficit, versus 5% of the typical readers. Similarly, Law, Vandermosten, Ghesquière and Wouters (2014) reported on individual deviance analyses of phonological awareness, VSTM and rapid lexical retrieval in English-speaking adults with dyslexia, of whom some had compensated reading skills. They demonstrated that 72% of the dyslexic adults had a phonological awareness deficit and 53% showed a VSTM deficit, whereas 31% had a RAN deficit. In contrast, in typical readers, only 2% displayed a phonological awareness deficit, 4% showed a VSTM deficit and 6% a RAN deficit. Also, in other languages, the prevalence rates for a phonological deficit in dyslexia are high (but not 100%). Reid, Szczerbinski, Iskierka-Kasperek and Hansen (2007) examined deviance patterns for phonological fluency (including RAN and semantic/alliteration fluency) in Polish university students. They found that 60% of dyslexic students displayed a phonological fluency deficit, and 53% exhibited a phonological awareness deficit (spoonerism and phoneme deletion). Only 1% of the controls displayed a phonological fluency or phonological awareness deficit. Similar deviance rates for phonological processing have been found in school-aged dyslexic children, ranging from 92% in French-speaking children (Saksida et al., 2016) to 57% in English-speaking children (White et al., 2006).

Based on these studies, we can conclude that there seems to be a large variety in the proportion of persons with dyslexia who show deviant phonological processing. The variability in proportions could partially be due to the different methods and tests adopted for the diagnosis of adults with dyslexia. Nonetheless, the proportion of deviant phonological processing performance in adults with dyslexia is clearly higher than the proportion in control groups and than for other cognitive, perceptual or motoric measures.

2.8 Clinical Applications and Perspectives

To date, in most countries, the diagnosis of dyslexia is typically given based on clinical assessment of severe and persistent/resistant problems with accurate and/or fluent word recognition and poor spelling abilities. The reading and/or spelling abilities should be substantially and quantifiably below the performance level expected for the individual's chronological age (American Psychiatric Association, 2013). Fortunately, nowadays in many countries, most individuals with dyslexia receive a diagnosis before adulthood. For this diagnosis, generally, no assessment of the underlying cognitive profile of individuals with dyslexia is made. However, in some countries, like for example the Netherlands, the cognitive profile is required for reimbursement of therapy. The clinical diagnosis of adults with reading and spelling difficulties can be more difficult, as these adults have had years of reading and spelling experience, and might have developed some compensation strategies (e.g., Fitzgibbon & O'Connor, 2002). For these adults, it can be useful to include measurements of their cognitive profile, including important cognitive correlates of dyslexia such as phonological processing. A description of the cognitive profile has been suggested by the meta-analysis of Swanson and Hsieh (2009) and by Callens et al. (2012). Given the possible ceiling effects in accuracy, especially in transparent orthographies, it is important to include reaction time measurements for evaluating the adult's phonological abilities (see also Carioti, Masia, Travellini, & Berlingeri, 2021; Reis et al., 2020).

2.9 Conclusion

In this chapter, we outlined the role of phonological processing skills in reading performance and highlighted persistent problems among adult readers with dyslexia. In addition, we briefly explored the impact of language transparency on phonological processing.

Nonetheless, despite the persistent phonological processing problems in adults with dyslexia, we should note that a large group of these individuals successfully participate in academic education. This group is often referred to as 'high-functioning' adults with dyslexia (e.g., Deacon, Parrila, & Kirby, 2006). Indeed, they seem to be able to circumvent these problems using different compensatory or coping strategies (e.g., Beaton, McDougall, & Singleton, 1997; Fitzgibbon & O'Connor, 2002). Lexical cues such as the use of contextual information (Miller-Shaul, 2005; Nation & Hulme, 1998) or more general semantic support (Snowling, Bishop, & Stothard, 2000), as well as grammatical cues such as morphological knowledge (Elbro & Arnbak, 1996) and visual memory (Campbell & Butterworth, 1985), have proven to help to minimize the expression of reading difficulties in children, and seem also to play a role in adults with dyslexia (Cavalli, Duncan, Elbro, El Ahmadi, & Colé, 2017; Law, Wouters, & Ghesquière, 2015).

On the other hand, however, the presence and persistence of phonological processing problems seem not to explain all behavioral indicators that define dyslexia. This leads researchers to examine additional cognitive deficits to support the explanation of some behavioral symptoms that characterize dyslexia in adults (Pennington, 2006). These will be further elaborated in the next chapters.

Notes

1 In the literature, a distinction is made between 'non-compensated' dyslexics and 'compensated' dyslexics. While the former group's reading attainments remain low (thus, hampering academic education), the latter group's reading attainments are appropriate for academic education.
2 Even though two different terms are used in literature, i.e., 'nonwords' and 'pseudowords', in most tasks containing these words, pseudowords are used. Pseudowords comprise legal phoneme strings in the language tested (e.g., /adair/). For consistency, in this chapter we use the term 'nonword(s)'.

References

American Psychiatric Association. (2013). *Diagnostic and statistical manual of mental disorders* (5th ed.). Washington, DC: American Psychiatric Publishing.
Anthony, J., Williams, J., Aghara, R., Dunkelberger, M., Novak, M., & Mukherjee, A. (2010). Assessment of individual differences in phonological representation. *Reading and Writing, 23*, 969–994.
Anthony, J. L., Lonigan, C. J., Burgess, S. R., Driscoll, K., Phillips, B. M., & Cantor, B. G. (2002). Structure of preschool phonological sensitivity: Overlapping sensitivity to rhyme, words, syllables, and phonemes. *Journal of Experimental Child Psychology, 82*, 65–92.
Baddeley, A. (2003). Working memory: Looking back and looking forward. *Nature Reviews Neuroscience, 4*, 829–839.
Baddeley, A. D. (2000). The episodic buffer: A new component of working memory? *Trends in Cognitive Sciences, 4*, 417–423.
Beaton, A., McDougall, S., & Singleton, C. H. (Eds.) (1997). In *Dyslexia in literate adults*. Oxford: Blackwell.
Beidas, H., Khateb, A., & Breznitz, Z. (2013). The cognitive profile of adult dyslexics and its relation to their reading abilities. *Reading Writing, 26*, 1487–1515. https://doi.org/10.1007/s11145-013-9428-5
Bekebrede, J., van der Leij, A., & Share, D. L. (2009). Dutch dyslexic adolescents: Phonological-core variable-orthographic differences. *Reading Writing, 22*, 133–165. https://doi.org/10.1007/s11145-007-9105-7
Blachman, B. A. (Ed.) (1997). In *Foundations of reading acquisition and dyslexia*. Mahwah, NJ: Erlbaum.
Boada, R., & Pennington, B. (2006). Deficient implicit phonological representations in children with dyslexia. *Journal of Experimental Child Psychology, 95*, 153–193.

Boets, B., Op de Beeck, H. P., Vandermosten, M., Scott, S. K., Gillebert, C. R., Mantini, D., & Ghesquière, P. (2013). Intact but less accessible phonetic representations in adults with dyslexia. *Science*, *342*, 1251–1254. https://doi.org/10.1126/science.1244333

Bowers, P. G., Steffy, R., & Tate, E. (1988). Comparison of the effects of IQ control methods on memory and naming speed predictors of reading disability. *Reading Research Quarterly*, *23*, 304–309.

Bruck, M. (1990). Word recognition skills of adults with childhood diagnoses of dyslexia. *Developmental Psychology*, *26*, 439–454.

Bruck, M. (1992). Persistence of dyslexics' phonological awareness deficits. *Developmental Psychology*, *28*, 874–886.

Brunswick, N., McCrory, E., Price, C. J., Frith, C. D., & Frith, U. (1999). Explicit and implicit processing of words and pseudowords by adult developmental dyslexics: A search for Wernicke's Wortschatz? *Brain*, *122*, 1901–1917. https://doi.org/10.1093/brain/122.10.1901

Callens, M., Tops, W., & Brysbaert, M. (2012). Cognitive profile of students who enter higher education with an indication of dyslexia. *PlosOne*, *7*(6), e38081.

Campbell, R., & Butterworth, B. (1985). Phonological dyslexia and dysgraphia in a highly literate subject: A developmental case with associated deficits of phonemic processing and awareness. *The Quarterly Journal of Experimental Psychology*, *37*, 435–475.

Caravolas, M., Volín, J., & Hulme, C. (2005). Phoneme awareness is a key component of alphabetic literacy skills in consistent and inconsistent orthographies: Evidence from Czech and English children. *Journal of Experimental Child Psychology*, *92*, 107–139. https://doi.org/10.1016/j.jecp.2005.04.003

Carioti, D., Masia, M. F., Travellini, S., & Berlingeri, M. (2021). Orthographic depth and developmental dyslexia: A meta-analytic study. *Annals of Dyslexia*, *71*, 399–438. https://doi.org/10.1007/s11881-021-00226-0

Castles, A., Holmes, V. M., Neath, J., & Kinoshita, S. (2003). How does orthographic knowledge influence performance on phonological awareness tasks? *The Quarterly Journal of Experimental Psychology*, *56*, 445–467. https://doi.org/10.1080/02724980244000486

Cavalli, E., Duncan, L. G., Elbro, C., El Ahmadi, A., & Colé, P. (2017). Phonemic – Morphemic dissociations in university students with dyslexia: An index of reading compensation? *Annals of Dyslexia*, *67*, 63–84. https://doi.org/10.1007/s11881-016-0138-y

Chan, C. K. K., & Siegel, L. S. (2001). Phonological processing in Reading Chinese among normally achieving and poor readers. *Journal of Experimental Child Psychology*, *80*, 23–43.

Chen, H.-C., & Shu, H. (2001). Lexical activation during the recognition of Chinese characters: Evidence against early phonological activation. *Psychonomic Bulletin & Review*, *8*(3), 511–518. https://doi.org/10.3758/BF03196186

Chomsky, N. & Halle, M. (1968). *The sound pattern of English*. New York: Harper & Row.

Dandache, S., Wouters, J., & Ghesquière, P. (2014). Development of reading and phonological skills of children at family risk for dyslexia: A longitudinal analysis from kindergarten to sixth grade. *Dyslexia*, *20*, 305–329. https://doi.org/10.1002/dys.1482

de Jong, P. F., & Share, D. L. (2007). Orthographic learning during oral and silent reading. *Scientific Studies of Reading*, *11*, 55–71. https://doi.org/10.1080/10888430709336634

de Jong, P. F., & van der Leij, A. (2002). Effects of phonological abilities and linguistic comprehension on the development of Reading. *Scientific Studies of Reading*, *6*, 51–77. https://doi.org/10.1207/S1532799XSSR0601_03

de Jong, P. F., & van der Leij, A. (2003). Developmental changes in the manifestation of a phonological deficit in dyslexic children learning to read a regular orthography. *Journal of Educational Psychology*, *95*, 22–40. https://doi.org/10.1037/0022-0663.95.1.22

De Smedt, B., & Boets, B. (2010). Phonological processing and arithmetic fact retrieval: Evidence from developmental dyslexia. *Neuropsychologia*, *48*, 3973–3981.

Deacon, S. H., Parrila, R., & Kirby, J. R. (2006). Processing of derived forms in high-functioning dyslexics. *Annals of Dyslexia*, *56*, 103–128. https://doi.org/10.1007/s11881-006-0005-3

Di Betta, A. M., & Romani, C. (2006). Lexical learning and dysgraphia in a group of adults with developmental dyslexia. *Cognitive Neuropsychology*, *23*, 376–400. https://doi.org/10.1080/02643290442000545

Dickie, C., Ota, M., & Clark, A. (2013). Revisiting the phonological deficit in dyslexia: Are implicit nonorthographic representations impaired? *Applied PsychoLinguistics*, *34*, 649–672.

Dietrich, J. A., & Brady, S. A. (2001). Phonological representations of adult poor readers: An investigation of specificity and stability. *Applied PsychoLinguistics*, *22*, 383–418.

Duncan, L., Castro, S., Defior Seymour, P., Baillie, S., Leybaert, J., ... Serrano, F. (2013). Phonological development in relation to native language and literacy: Variations on a theme in six alphabetic orthographies. *Cognition*, *127*, 398–419. https://doi.org/10.1016/j.cognition.2013.02.009

Durgunoglu, A. Y., & Öney, B. (1999). A cross-linguistic comparison of phonological awareness and word recognition. *Reading and Writing*, *11*, 281–299.

Edwards, J., Beckman, M. E., & Munson, B. (2004). The interaction between vocabulary size and phonotactic probability effects on children's production accuracy and fluency in nonword repetition. *Journal of Speech, Language, and Hearing Research*, *47*, 421–436.

Ehri, L. (2014). Orthographic mapping in the Acquisition of Sight Word Reading, spelling memory, and vocabulary learning. *Scientific Studies of Reading*, *18*, 5–21. https://doi.org/10.1080/10888438.2013.819356

Ehri, L. (2017). Orthographic mapping and literacy development revisited. In K. Cain, D. L. Compton, & R. K. Parrila (Eds.), *Theories of reading development* (pp. 169–190). John Benjamins. https://doi.org/10.1075/swll.15.08ehr

Ehri, L. C., & Wilce, L. S. (1980). The influence of orthography on readers' conceptualisation of the phonemic structure of words. *Applied PsychoLinguistics*, *1*, 371–385.

Elbro, C. (1998). When reading is "readn" or somthn. Distinctiveness of phonological representations of lexical items in normal and disabled readers. *Scandinavian Journal of Psychology*, *39*, 149–153.

Elbro, C. (2002). Early linguistic abilities and reading development: A review and a hypothesis about distinctness of phonological representations. In L. Verhoeven, C. Elbro, & P. Reitsma (Eds.), *Precursors of functional literacy* (pp. 289–320). Amsterdam: John Benjamins.

Elbro, C., & Arnbak, E. (1996). The role of morpheme recognition and morphological awareness in dyslexia. *Annals of Dyslexia*, *46*, 209–240. https://doi.org/10.1007/BF02648177

Elbro, C., & Jensen, M. N. (2005). Quality of phonological representations, verbal learning, and phoneme awareness in dyslexic and normal readers. *Scandinavian Journal of Psychology*, *46*, 375–384. https://doi.org/10.1111/j.1467-9450.2005.00468.x

Elbro, C., Nielsen, I., & Petersen, D. K. (1994). Dyslexia in adults: Evidence for deficits in non-word reading and in the phonological representation of lexical items. *Annals of Dyslexia*, *44*, 205–226.

Elliott, J. G., & Grigorenko, E. L. (2014). *The dyslexia debate*. New York: Cambridge University Press.

Fitzgibbon, G., & O'Connor, B. (2002). *Adult dyslexia: A guide for the workplace*. London: Wiley.

Furnes, B., & Samuelsson, S. (2011). Phonological awareness and rapid automatized naming predicting early development in reading and spelling: Results from a cross-linguistic longitudinal study. *Learning and Individual Differences, 21*, 85–95.

Gabay, Y., & Holt, L. L. (2015). Incidental learning of sound categories is impaired in developmental dyslexia. *Cortex, 73*, 131–143.

Gallagher, H., Happé, F., Brunswick, N., Fletcher, P., Frith, U., & Frith, C. (2000). Reading the mind in cartoons and stories: An fMRI study of 'theory of mind' in verbal and nonverbal tasks. *Neuropsychologia, 38*, 11–21.

Gathercole, S., Frankish, C., Pickering, S., & Peaker, S. (1999). Phonotactic influences on short-term memory. *Journal of Experimental Psychology: Human Learning and Memory, 25*, 84–95.

Gathercole, S., Pickering, S., Hall, M., & Peaker, S. (2001). Dissociable lexical and phonological influences on serial recognition and serial recall. *Quarterly Journal of Experimental Psychology, 45A*, 1–30.

Georgiou, G., Parrila, R., Kirby, J. R., & Stephenson, K. (2008). Rapid naming components and their relationship with phonological awareness, orthographic knowledge, speed of processing, and different reading outcomes. *Scientific Studies of Reading, 12*, 325–350. https://doi.org/10.1080/10888430802378518

Goulandris, N. (2003). Introduction: Developmental dyslexia, language and orthographies. In N. Goulandris (Ed.), *Dyslexia in different languages: Cross-linguistic comparisons* (pp. 1–14). London: Whurr Publishers.

Gwilliams, L., King, J.R., Marantz, A. et al. (2022). Neural dynamics of phoneme sequences reveal position-invariant code for content and order. *Nature Communications, 13*, 6606. https://doi.org/10.1038/s41467-022-34326-1

Hämäläinen, J. A., Salminen, H. K., & Leppänen, P. H. T. (2012). Basic auditory processing deficits in dyslexia: Systematic review of the behavioral and event-related potential/ field evidence. *Journal of Learning Disabilities, 46*(5), 413–427.

Hazan, V., Messaoud-Galusi, S., Rosen, S., Nouwens, S., & Shakespeare, B. (2009). Speech perception abilities of adults with dyslexia: Is there any evidence for a true deficit? *Journal of Speech Language Hearing Research, 52*, 1510–1529. https://doi.org/10.1044/1092-4388(2009/08-0220)

Howland, K., & Liederman, J. (2013). Beyond decoding: Adults with dyslexia have trouble forming unified lexical representations across pseudoword learning episodes. *Journal of Speech, Language, and Hearing Research, 56*, 1009–1022. https://doi.org/10.1044/1092-4388(2012/11-0252)

Hu, C. F., & Catts, H. W. (1998). The role of phonological processing in early reading ability: What we can learn from Chinese. *Scientific Studies of Reading, 2*, 55–79.

Huang, H. S., & Hanley, J. R. (1995). Phonological awareness and visual skills in learning to read Chinese and English. *Cognition, 54*, 73–98.

Hulme, C., Goetz, K., Gooch, D., Adams, J., & Snowling, M. J. (2007). Paired-associate learning, phoneme awareness, and learning to read. *Journal of Experimental Child Psychology, 96*, 150–166. https://doi.org/10.1016/j.jecp.2006.09.002

Hulme, C., Maughan, S., & Brown, G. D. (1991). Memory for familiar and unfamiliar words: Evidence for a long-term memory contribution to short-term memory span. *Journal of Memory and Language, 30*, 685–701. https://doi.org/10.1016/0749-596X(91)90032-F

Jones, M. W., Branigan, H. P., & Kelly, M. L. (2009). Dyslexic and nondyslexic reading fluency: Rapid automatized naming and the importance of continuous lists. *Psychonomic Bulletin & Review, 16*, 567–572. https://doi.org/10.3758/PBR.16.3.567

Kirby, J. R., Parrila, R., & Pfeiffer, S.L. (2003). Naming speed and phonological awareness as predictors of reading development. *Journal of Educational Psychology*, *95*, 453–464.

Landerl, K., Frith, U., & Wimmer, H. (1996). Differences in phonological recoding fluency among German- and English-speaking children. *Scientific Studies of Reading*, *1*(2), 115–134.

Landerl, K., Ramus, F., Moll, K., Lyytinen, H., Leppänen, P. H. T., Lohvansuu, K., et al. (2013). Predictors of developmental dyslexia in European orthographies with varying complexity. *Journal of Child Psychology and Psychiatry*, *54*, 686–694. https://doi.org/10.1111/jcpp.12029

Landerl, K., & Wimmer, H. (2000). Deficits in phoneme segmentation are not the core problem of dyslexia: Evidence from German and English children. *Applied PsychoLinguistics*, *21*, 243–262. https://doi.org/10.1017/s0142716400002058

Law, J., Vandermosten, M., Ghesquière, P., & Wouters, J. (2014). The relationship of phonological ability, speech perception, and auditory perception in adults with dyslexia. *Frontiers in Human Neuroscience*, *8*, 1–12.

Law, J., Wouters, J., & Ghesquière, P. (2015). Morphological awareness and its role in compensation in adults with dyslexia. *Dyslexia*, *21*, 254–272. https://doi.org/10.1002/dys.1495

Lervag, A., Braten, I., & Hulme, C. (2009). The cognitive and linguistic foundations of early reading development: A Norwegian latent variable longitudinal study. *Developmental Psychology*, *45*, 764–781. https://doi.org/10.1037/A0014132

Liberman, I. Y., & Shankweiler, D. (1991). Phonology and the beginning reader: A tutorial. In L. Rieben & C. A. Perfetti (Eds.), *Learning to read: Basic research and its implications*. Hillsdale, NJ: Lawrence Erlbaum Associates.

Lyon, G. R. (1995). Toward a definition of dyslexia. *Annals of Dyslexia*, *45*, 3–27.

Mann, V. A., & Liberman, I. Y. (1984). Phonological awareness and verbal short-term memory. *Journal of Learning Disabilities*, *17*, 592–598.

McBride, C., & Wang, Y. (2015). Learning to read Chinese: Universal and unique cognitive cores. *Child Development Perspectives*, *9*(3), 196–200. https://doi.org/10.1111/cdep.12132

McBride, C., Wang, Y., & Cheang, L. M. L. (2018). Dyslexia in Chinese. *Current Developmental Disorders Reports*, *5*, 217–225. https://doi.org/10.1007/s40474-018-0149-y

Melby-Lervåg, M., Lyster, S.-A. H., & Hulme, C. (2012). Phonological skills and their role in learning to read: A metaanalytic review. *Psychological Bulletin*, *138*, 322–352. https://doi.org/10.1037/a0026744

Metsala, J. L. (1997). Spoken word recognition in reading disabled children. *Journal of Educational Psychology*, *89*, 159–169.

Miller-Shaul, S. (2005). The characteristics of young and adult dyslexics readers on reading and reading related cognitive tasks as compared to normal readers. *Dyslexia*, *11*(2), 132–151.

Moll, K., Ramus, F., Bartling, J., Bruder, J., Kunze, S., Neuhoff, N., & Landerl, K. (2014). Cognitive mechanisms underlying reading and spelling development in five European orthographies. *Learning and Instruction*, *29*, 65–77. https://doi.org/10.1016/j.learninstruc.2013.09.003

Morais, J., Bertelson, P., Cary, L., & Alegria, J. (1986). Literacy training and speech segmentation. *Cognition*, *24*, 45–64.

Morfidi, E., Leij, A., Jong, P. F., Scheltinga, F., & Bekebrede, J. (2007). Reading in two orthographies: A cross-linguistic study of Dutch average and poor readers who learn English as a second language. *Reading and Writing: An Interdisciplinary Journal*, *20*, 753–784. https://doi.org/10.1007/s11145-006-9035-9

Nation, K., & Castles, A. (2017). Putting the learning in orthographic learning. In K. Cain, D. Compton, & R. Parrila (Eds.), *Theories of reading development* (pp. 147–168). Amsterdam: John Benjamins.

Nation, K., & Hulme, C. (1998). The role of analogy in early spelling development. In *Reading and spelling: Development and disorder* (pp. 433–445). Mahwah, NJ: Routledge.

Noordenbos, M. W., & Serniclaes, W. (2015). The categorical perception deficit in dyslexia: A meta-analysis. *Scientific Studies of Reading, 19*(5), 340–359.

Norris, J. A., & Hoffman, P. R. (2002). Phonemic awareness: A complex developmental process. *Topics in Language Disorders, 22*, 1–34.

Parrila, R. K., Kirby, J. R., & McQuarrie, L. (2004). Articulation rate, naming speed, verbal short-term memory, and phonological awareness: Longitudinal predictors of early reading development? *Scientific Studies of Reading, 8*, 3–26.

Parrila, R. K., & Protopapas, A. (2017). Dyslexia and word reading problems. In K. Cain, D. Compton, & Parrila (Eds.), *Theories of reading development*. John Benjamins Publishing Company. https://doi.org/10.1075/swll.15

Pattamadilok, C., Morais, J., & Kolinsky, R. (2011). Naming in noise: The contribution of orthographic knowledge to speech repetition. *Frontiers in Psychology, 2*, 1–12. https://doi.org/10.3389/fpsyg.2011.00361

Pattamadilok, C., Nelis, A., & Kolinsky, R. (2014). How does reading performance modulate the impact of orthographic knowledge on speech processing? A comparison of normal readers and dyslexic adults. *Annals of Dyslexia, 64*, 57–76. https://doi.org/10.1007/s11881-013-0086-8

Paulesu, E., Frith, U., Snowling, M., Gallagher, A., Morton, J., Frackowiak, R. S. J., & Frith, C. D. (1996). Is developmental dyslexia a disconnection syndrome? Evidence from PET scanning. *Brain, 119*, 143–157. https://doi.org/10.1093/brain/119.1.143

Pennington, B., & Lefly, D. (2001). Early reading development in children at family risk for dyslexia. *Child Development, 72*, 816–833.

Pennington, B. F. (2006). From single to multiple deficit models of developmental disorders. *Cognition, 101*(2), 385–413.

Perfetti, C. (2007). Reading ability: Lexical quality to comprehension. *Scientific Studies of Reading, 11*, 357–383. https://doi.org/10.1080/10888430701530730

Perfetti, C., & Hart, L. (2002). The lexical quality hypothesis. In L. Verhoeven, C. Elbro, & P. Reitsma (Eds.), *Precursors of functional literacy* (pp. 189–213). Amsterdam: John Benjamin.

Perfetti, C., Wlotko, E., & Hart, L. (2005). Word learning and individual differences in word learning reflected through event-related potentials. *Journal of Experimental Psychology, 31*, 1281–1292. https://doi.org/10.1037/0278-7393.31.6.1281

Perfetti, C. A., & Hart, L. (2001). The lexical basis of comprehension skill. In D. S. Gorfein (Ed.), *On the consequences of meaning selection: Perspectives on resolving lexical ambiguity* (pp. 67–86). Washington, DC: American Psychological Association. https://doi.org/10.1037/10459-000

Peterson, R., & Pennington, B. (2015). Developmental dyslexia. *Annual Review of Clinical Psychology, 11*, 283–307. https://doi.org/10.1146/annurev-clinpsy-032814-112842

Ramus, F. (2003). Developmental dyslexia: Specific phonological deficit or general sensorimotor dysfunction? *Current Opinion in Neurobioly, 13*, 212–218. https://doi.org/10.1016/S0959-4388(03)00035-7

Ramus, F. (2014). Neuroimaging sheds new light on the phonological deficit in dyslexia. *Trends in Cognitive Sciences, 18*, 274–275. https://doi.org/10.1016/j.tics.2014.01.009

Ramus, F., & Ahissar, M. (2012). Developmental dyslexia: The difficulties of interpreting poor performance, and the importance of normal performance. *Cognitive Neuropsychology, 29*, 104–122.

Ramus, F., Rosen, S., Dakin, S., Day, B., Castellote, J., White, S., & Frith, U. (2003). Theories of developmental dyslexia: Insights from a multiple case study of dyslexic adults. *Brain, 126*, 841–865.

Ramus, F., & Szenkovits, G. (2008). What phonological deficit? *The Quarterly Journal Experimental Psychology, 61*, 129–141. https://doi.org/10.1080/17470210701508822

Rayner, K., Foorman, B., Perfetti, C. A., Pesetsky, D., & Seidenberg, M. S. (2002). How should reading be taught? *Scientific American, 286*, 84–91. https://doi.org/10.1038/scientificamerican0302-84

Reid, A. A., Szczerbinski, M., Iskierka-Kasperek, E., & Hansen, P. (2007). Cognitive profiles of adult developmental dyslexics: Theoretical implications. *Dyslexia, 13*, 1–24. https://doi.org/10.1002/dys.321

Reis, A., Araújo, S., Morais, I. S., & Faisca, L. (2020). Reading and reading-related skills in adults with dyslexia from different orthographic systems: A review and meta-analysis. *Annals of Dyslexia, 70*, 339–368. https://doi.org/10.1007/s11881-020-00205-x

Richardson, U., Thomson, J. M., Scott, S. K., & Goswami, U. (2011). Auditory processing skills and phonological representation in dyslexic children. *Dyslexia, 17*(1), 30–48.

Rodríguez, G., van den Boer, M., Jiménez, J. E., & de Jong, P. F. (2015). Developmental changes in the relations between RAN, phonological awareness, and reading in Spanish children. *Scientific Studies of Reading, 19*, 273–288. https://doi.org/10.1080/10888438.2015.1025271

Roodenrys, S., Koloski, N., & Grainger, J. (2001). Working memory function in attention deficit hyperactivity disordered and reading disabled children. *British Journal of Developmental Psychology, 19*, 325–337.

Saksida, A., Iannuzzi, S., Bogliotti, C., Chaix, Y., Démonet, J. F., Bricout, L., & Ramus, F. (2016). Phonological skills, visual attention span, and visual stress in developmental dyslexia. *Developmental Psychology, 52*(10), 1503–1516.

Schraeyen, K., Geudens, A., Ghesquière, P., Van der Elst, W., & Sandra, D. (2017). Poor performance on the retention of phonemes' serial order in short-term memory reflects young children's poor reading skills. *The Mental Lexicon, 12*, 129–158. https://doi.org/10.1075/ML.12.1.06SCH

Schraeyen, K., Van der Elst, W., Geudens, A., Ghesquière, P., & Sandra, D. (2017). Beyond global differences between monolingual and bilingual children on the nonword repetition task: Retention skills for phonemes' identity and serial order. *Bilingualism: Language and Cognition*, 1–16. https://doi.org/10.1017/S1366728917000244

Schraeyen, K., Van der Elst, W., Geudens, A., Ghesquière, P., & Sandra, D. (2019). Short-term memory problems for phonemes' serial order in adults with dyslexia: Evidence from a different analysis of the nonword repetition task. *Applied PsychoLinguistics, 40*(3), 613–644. https://doi.org/10.1017/S0142716418000759

Sela, I., Izzetoglu, M., Izzetoglu, K., & Onaral, B. (2012). A working memory deficit among dyslexic readers with no phonological impairment as measured using the n-back task: An fNIR study. *PLoS One, 7*, e46527. https://doi.org/10.1371/journal.pone.0046527

Serniclaes, W., Van Heghe, S., Mousty, P., Carré, R., & Sprenger-Charolles, L. (2004). Allophonic mode of speech perception in dyslexia. *Journal of Experimental Child Psychology, 87*, 336–361. https://doi.org/10.1016/j.jecp.2004.02.001

Share, D., & Stanovich, K. E. (1995). Cognitive processes in early reading development: Accommodating individual differences into a model of acquisition. In J. S. Carlson (Ed.), *Issues in education: Contributions from psychology* (pp. 1–57). Greenwich, CT: JAI.

Share, D. L. (1995). Phonological recoding and self-teaching: Sine qua non of reading acquisition. *Cognition, 55*, 151–218.

Share, D. L. (1999). Phonological recoding and orthographic learning: A direct test of the self-teaching hypothesis. *Journal of Experimental Child Psychology, 72*, 95–129.

Share, D. L. (2004). Orthographic learning at a glance: On the time course and developmental onset of self-teaching. *Journal of Experimental Child Psychology, 87*, 267–298. https://doi.org/10.1016/j.jecp.2004.01.001

Share, D. L. (2008). On the Anglocentricities of current reading research and practice: The perils of overreliance on an "outlier" orthography. *Psychological Bulletin, 134*, 584–615.

Share, D. L. (2021). Common misconceptions about the phonological deficit theory of dyslexia. *Brain Sciences, 11*(11). https://doi.org/10.3390/brainsci11111510

Share, D. L. (2023). Common cause and multiple deficit models of reading disability: Time for reconciliation. *Scientific Studies of Reading, 27*(3), 173–185.

Shaywitz, S. E., & Shaywitz, B. A. (2005). Dyslexia. *Biological Psychiatry, 57*, 1301–1309.

Siegel, L. S. (2006). Perspectives on dyslexia. *Paediatrics & Child Health, 11*, 581–587.

Snowling, M. (2000). *Dyslexia* (2nd ed.). Oxford: Blackwell.

Snowling, M., Bishop, D., & Stothard, S. (2000). Is preschool language impairment a risk factor for dyslexia in adolescence. *Journal of Child Psychology and Psychiatry, 41*, 587–600. https://doi.org/10.1111/1469-7610.00651

Snowling, M., Muter, V., & Carroll, J. (2007). Children at family risk of dyslexia: A follow-up in early adolescence. *Journal of Child Psychology & Psychiatry, 48*, 609–618.

Snowling, M., Nation, K., Moxham, P., Gallagher, A., & Frith, U. (1997). Phonological processing deficits in dyslexic students: A preliminary account. *Journal of Research in Reading, 20*, 31–34. https://doi.org/10.1111/1467-9817.00018

Snowling, M. J., Hulme, C., & Nation, K. (2020). Defining and understanding dyslexia: Past, present and future. *Oxford Review of Education, 46*(4), 501–513. https://doi.org/10.1080/03054985.2020.1765756

Stuart, M. (1990). Processing strategies in a phoneme deletion task. *The Quarterly Journal of Experimental Psychology, 42*, 305–327.

Swanson, H. L., & Hsieh, C. J. (2009). Reading disabilities in adults: A selective meta-analysis of the literature. *Review of Educational Research, 79*(4), 1362–1390.

Tan, L. H., Spinks, J. A., Eden, G., Perfetti, C. A., & Siok, W. T. (2005). Reading depends on writing, in Chinese. *Proceedings of the National Academy of Science, USA, 102*, 8781–8785.

Tops, W., Callens, M., Lammertyn, J., Van Hees, V., & Brysbaert, M. (2012). Identifying students with dyslexia in higher education. *Annals of Dyslexia, 62*, 186–203. https://doi.org/10.1007/s11881-012-0072-6

Vaessen, A., Bertrand, D., Tóth, D., Csépe, V., Faísca, L., Reis, A., & Blomert, L. (2010). Cognitive development of fluent word reading does not qualitatively differ between transparent and opaque orthographies. *Journal of Educational Psychology, 102*, 827–842.

Van den Broeck, W., & Geudens, A. (2012). Old and new ways to study characteristics of reading disability: The case of the nonword-reading deficit. *Cognitive Psychology, 65*, 414–456.

Van den Broeck, W., & Geudens, A. (2016). De rol van alfabetische en woord-specifieke kennis in didactiek en interventie van technisch lezen. In W. Van den Broeck (Ed.), *Handboek dyslexieonderzoek. Wetenschappelijke inzichten in diagnostiek, oorzaken, preventie en behandeling van dyslexie* (pp. 127–152). Leuven, Belgium: Acco.

Vandermosten, M., Boets, B., Poelmans, H., Sunaert, S., Wouters, J., & Ghesquière, P. (2012). A tractography study in dyslexia: Neuroanatomic correlates of orthographic, phonological and speech processing. *Brain, 135*, 935–948. https://doi.org/10.1093/brain/awr363

Vandermosten, M., Correia, J., Vanderauwera, J., Wouters, J., Ghesquière, P., & Bonte, M. (2020). Brain activity patterns of phonemic representations are atypical in beginning readers with family risk for dyslexia. *Developmental Science, 23*(1). https://doi.org/10.1111/desc.12857

Vandermosten, M., Wouters, J., Ghesquière, P., & Golestani, N. (2019). Statistical learning of speech sounds in dyslexic and typical Reading children. *Scientific Studies of Reading, 23*(1), 116–127. https://doi.org/10.1080/10888438.2018.1473404

Vellutino, F. R., Fletcher, J. M., Snowling, M. J., & Scanlon, D. M. (2004). Specific reading disability (dyslexia): What have we learned in the past four decades? *Journal of Child Psychology and Psychiatry, 45*, 2–40. https://doi.org/10.1046/j.0021-9630.2003.00305.x

Ventura, P., Morais, J., & Kolinsky, R. (2007). The development of the orthographic consistency effect in speech recognition: From sublexical to lexical involvement. *Cognition, 105*, 547–576.

Wagner, R., & Torgesen, J. (1987). The nature of phonological processing and its causal role in the acquisition of reading skills. *Psychological Bulletin, 101*, 192–212.

White, S., Milne, E., Rosen, S., Hansen, P., Swettenham, J., Frith, U., & Ramus, F. (2006). The role of sensorimotor impairments in dyslexia: A multiple case study of dyslexic children. *Developmental Science, 9*(3), 237–255.

Yang, X., Zheng, M., & Liu, K. (2023). Developmental changes in the contributions of phonological processing skills to Chinese character reading and arithmetic. *Learning and Instruction, 84*. https://doi.org/10.1016/j.learninstruc.2022.101730

Yap, R., & van der Leij, A. (1993). Word processing in dyslexics: An automatic decoding deficit? *Reading and Writing: An Interdisciplinary Journal, 5*, 261–279.

Ziegler, J. C., Bertrand, D., Tóth, D., Csépe, V., Reis, A., Faísca, L., & Blomert, L. (2010). Orthographic depth and its impact on universal predictors of reading: A cross-language investigation. *Psychological Science, 21*, 551–559.

Ziegler, J. C., & Ferrand, L. (1998). Orthography shapes the perception of speech: The consistency effect in auditory word recognition. *Psychonomic Bulletin and Review, 5*, 683–689.

Ziegler, J. C., & Goswami, U. (2005). Reading acquisition, developmental dyslexia and skilled reading across languages: A psycholinguistic grain size theory. *Psychological Bulletin, 13*, 3–29.

Ziegler, J. C., & Muneaux, M. (2007). Orthographic facilitation and phonological inhibition in spoken word recognition: A developmental study. *Psychonomic Bulletin & Review, 14*, 75–80. https://doi.org/10.3758/BF03194031

Ziegler, J. C., Perry, C., & Zorzi, M. (2014). Modelling reading development through phonological decoding and self-teaching: Implications for dyslexia. *Philosophical Transactions of the Royal Society B, 369*, 20120397.

3

ORAL LANGUAGE SKILLS AND READING IN ADULTS WITH DYSLEXIA

Jeremy M. Law and Eddy Cavalli

3.1 Introduction

Unlike reading, which requires explicit instruction over several years, oral language develops naturally as a result of biological and evolutionary processes, without the need for formal teaching. It is a complex cognitive system with specific structural properties that enables individuals to convey and receive verbal information. In the early years of life, children acquire oral language skills through listening and interaction, not only learning words used by adults around them but also understanding how these words function within communication. Through exposure to linguistic input, children internalize language rules from their environment well before encountering print-based instruction, such as sound-symbol correspondence and decoding.

Traditionally, oral language is viewed as consisting of five primary components, which interact dynamically and are organized hierarchically: phonology, semantics, morphology, syntax, and pragmatics (see Table 3.1 for a detailed overview of each component).

Research has consistently demonstrated that the quality of early oral language skills plays a crucial role in later reading achievement, as reading and oral language share many cognitive and linguistic processes (Hulme & Snowling, 2013; Metsala & Walley, 1998). According to the Simple View of Reading (SVR) (Gough & Tunmer, 1986; Hoover & Gough, 1990; for extensions, see Tunmer & Chapman, 2012b; Cutting & Scarborough, 2012; Hoover, 2023), reading is composed of two fundamental components: word recognition and reading comprehension. Word recognition refers to the ability to accurately and effortlessly identify printed words, enabling access to their stored representations in the mental lexicon. Reading comprehension, on the

TABLE 3.1 Five Primary Components of the Oral Language System

	Definition	Example	Method of Assessment
Phonology	Deals with the rules governing the structure and sequence of the sound patterns of language	In English, the final "s" sounds follow a phonological rule. If the word ends in an unvoiced consonant, it takes an /s/ sound as in cats. Yet if a word ends in a voiced consonant, it takes a /z/ sound, as in dogs	• Spoonerism (see Law, Wouters, & Ghesquière, 2015) • Phoneme blending and substitution (see Law & Ghesquière, 2017)
Semantics	Deals with the aspect of language that governs the meaning of words and word combinations, whether that be *intensional meaning* (the defining characteristics or critical features of a word) or *extensional meaning* (the set of objects, or events to which a word might apply in the world)	• Intensional meaning: a duck is a duck because it has a flat bill, feathers, wings, likes water, and quacks • Extensional meaning: involves related activities such as feeding bread to ducks in a pond, thus becoming an extension of the target word "duck"	• Semantic judgment tasks, Semantic memory, and Semantic interference (see Nation 2005). • Word-level semantics: vocabulary
Syntax	Refers to the rule system and principles that govern the combination of words and phrases into sentences and paragraphs to convey complex ideas and intentions. The primary function of syntax is to specify word order, sentence organization, and the relationship between words and word clauses	Consider: "Kyle chased the horse" and "the horse chased Kyle" Both sentences share the same words and word meaning; however, the interpretation of who the subject is within each sentence, or "who is doing the chasing and who is being chased," differs because of the syntax	• Grammatical judgments • Repetition of orally presented sentences with increasingly complex grammatical structures. (see Semel, Wiig, & Secord, 2003)

(*Continued*)

TABLE 3.1 (Continued)

	Definition	Example	Method of Assessment
Morphology	It is concerned with the use of morphemes, the smallest linguistic units of meaning, to form more complex words. Morphologically complex words convey subtle meaning and serve specific grammatical and pragmatic functions.	• Jumping can be broken down into two base morphemes: "jump" and "ing" Consider the sentences: "Kyle is riding a horse"; "Kyle rides a horse." The first sentence describes an action currently in progress, while the last sentence describes a routine event, resulting from a one-morpheme change	• Sentence completion tasks (see Carlisle, 2000). • Suffixation decision tasks (see Martin et al., 2013) • Lexical decision tasks in a visual priming paradigm (see Law, Wouters, & Ghesquière, 2017)
Pragmatics	Involves the rules that guide how language is used in context, such as sharing information, greeting, inquiring, or addressing questions that occur in a variety of differing contexts	Different kinds of discourse contexts (such as conversational, classroom, or narrative) may dictate differences in the set of rules that govern a topic's selection, formality, and required level of conveyed knowledge (Lund & Duchan, 1993)	Participants are asked to choose an address form appropriate for the orally presented social situations (e.g., setting, age, and familiarity) (see Kinginger & Farrell, 2004)

other hand, involves interpreting words, sentences, and discourse in a meaningful way, a process deeply rooted in oral language abilities (Gough & Tunmer, 1986). The development of these complex skills requires explicit instruction over several years, making it essential to explore the interactions between oral language and reading to fully understand how individuals acquire literacy. More importantly, for the objectives of this chapter, understanding how oral language—particularly semantics—interacts with word recognition and comprehension is essential for examining its role in the reading abilities of adults with dyslexia. This chapter will first explore the relationship between oral language and reading, focusing on visual word recognition and reading comprehension in typical readers. It will then provide an in-depth review of morphology and semantics in adults with dyslexia, analyzing how these linguistic skills may either support or hinder reading success in this population.

3.2 Oral Language and Word Recognition Skills

To examine the role of oral language in the reading abilities of adults with dyslexia, it is essential to first understand how typical readers process written words and how oral language skills contribute to this process.

3.2.1 The Role of Non-Phonological Oral Language Skills in Word Recognition

An understanding of the role of oral language in reading development has been formalized through two influential models of word reading: the dual-route cascade model (DRC), an extension of the original dual-route model (DRM) by Coltheart, Rastle, Perry, Langdon, and Ziegler (2001), and the connectionist triangle model proposed by Seidenberg and McClelland (1989) (see also Welbourne, Woollams, Crisp, & Ralph, 2011). Over time, these models have evolved to incorporate new behavioral and neuroimaging data, reflecting advancements in the study of word reading.

The DRM of reading focuses on the pronunciation of printed words and posits two distinct pathways for visual word recognition. The direct lexical route allows for immediate recognition of words by accessing their stored representations in the mental lexicon, irrespective of their regularity. In contrast, the indirect sub-lexical route relies on phoneme–grapheme correspondence rules to assemble word pronunciations before linking them to phonological and semantic representations. A notable extension of this model by Grainger and Ziegler (2011) incorporates morphemes, the smallest units of meaning, into the lexical route. This adaptation is particularly relevant for individuals with dyslexia, who face phonological processing difficulties and may rely more heavily on a morphological pathway for word recognition.

The triangle model of reading provides a framework for understanding how the brain learns and represents information during reading acquisition (Seidenberg, 2006). It conceptualizes reading as an interaction between orthographic, phonological, and semantic representations, with two key processing pathways. The phonological pathway (O → P) maps orthographic input directly onto phonological representations, while the semantic pathway (O → S → P) mediates this process through meaning. According to Woollams et al. (2010), reading development involves a shift from a reliance on phonological decoding to an increasing dependence on semantic processing, particularly for irregular or partially decoded words (see Cavalli & Colé, 2018, for a review).

This perspective suggests that semantic knowledge may play a compensatory role in individuals with dyslexia, supporting word recognition despite phonological deficits.

Despite the inclusion of a dedicated semantic pathway in many conceptions of the triangle model, semantics is often overlooked in empirical studies of word reading development and reading disorders. Similarly, although morphology has been shown to make an independent contribution to early visual word recognition across multiple languages—Dutch (Diependaele, Sandra, & Grainger, 2009; Law, Veispak, Vanderauwera, & Ghesquière, 2018), English (Marslen-Wilson, Bozic, & Randall, 2008; Rastle, Davis, & New, 2004), French (Cavalli et al., 2016b; Lefèvre, Law, Quémart, Anders, & Cavalli, 2022), Italian (Burani, Marcolini, De Luca, & Zoccolotti, 2008), and Spanish (Duñabeitia, Perea, & Carreiras, 2007)—morphology is frequently excluded from traditional reading models. With the exception of Grainger and Ziegler (2011) and the recently proposed Morphological Pathways Framework (Levesque, Breadmore, & Deacon, 2021), morphology is often treated as a subset of orthographic or semantic processing, rather than as a distinct linguistic system with its own influence on reading.

While there is no universal agreement on the precise role of oral language in early reading development, accumulating evidence suggests that broader oral language skills—including morphology, semantics, and syntax—contribute to reading attainment beyond phonological skills (Berninger et al., 2001; Catts et al., 1999; Colé et al., 2018; Dickinson et al., 2003; Law & Ghesquière, 2022; Lefèvre et al., 2022; Roth et al., 2002; Scarborough, 2005; Share & Leikin, 2004; Sénéchal et al., 2006). However, inconsistencies across studies have been noted, which may stem from differences in the assessment measures used to evaluate oral language abilities. Some studies rely on broad standardized assessments such as the *Clinical Evaluation of Language Fundamentals*, Fourth Edition (CELF-4) (Semel et al., 2003), which may obscure the specific contributions of morphology and semantics. This is particularly relevant in the context of dyslexia, where certain tasks may be more appropriate than others due to the inherent reading difficulties faced by this population. Consequently, future research should aim to refine oral language assessment tools and explore their clinical applications in reading intervention for individuals with dyslexia.

3.2.1.1 Semantics and Morphology in Word Recognition

The triangle model of reading highlights the crucial role of oral language skills and semantics in learning to decode print. However, how semantic representations influence word reading and its development over time remains insufficiently understood, particularly after children have grasped the alphabetic principle. Longitudinal studies examining the relationship between semantics and reading development suggest that the association between children's semantic knowledge—often assessed through oral vocabulary—and word reading ability strengthens with age (Nation & Snowling, 2004; Ricketts, Nation, & Bishop, 2007). For instance, a large-scale longitudinal study by Muter et al. (2004), conducted with native English-speaking children, found no significant predictive relationship between early receptive vocabulary skills (measured at school entry) and later decoding skills, assessed after one and two years of formal instruction. However, Nation and Snowling (2004), in their study of 8-year-old typically developing children, reported that expressive vocabulary and semantic skills, measured through word associations and synonym tasks, each explained a significant amount of variance in word recognition, even after controlling for age, nonverbal intelligence, and phonological skills. These findings suggest that semantic knowledge may become increasingly relevant in supporting word recognition as reading proficiency develops. Beyond behavioral studies, neuroimaging research provides additional support for the role of semantics in word reading. Studies comparing brain activation patterns during the reading of real words and pseudowords have identified the left angular gyrus and middle temporal gyrus as key regions involved in semantic processing (Taylor, et al., 2013). Moreover, research indicates that semantic activation occurs rapidly, emerging within the first 160–200 milliseconds of visual word presentation, and appears to be automatic during reading (Carreiras, Armstrong, Perea, & Frost, 2014). Further evidence comes from studies on neurologically impaired adults with semantic dementia, demonstrating a direct relationship between semantic knowledge and the ability to read low-frequency or irregular words (Funnell, 1996; Ralph, Patterson, Rogers & McClelland, 2004; Patterson & Hodges, 1992). These findings underscore the crucial role of semantics in word reading, particularly for words that do not conform to standard phoneme–grapheme correspondence rules.

Several theoretical accounts have been proposed to explain how semantic knowledge facilitates word reading. One widely supported hypothesis suggests that as children expand their semantic knowledge, they become more sensitive to sub-lexical detail, thereby enhancing phoneme awareness and facilitating reading development (Goswami, 2001; Metsala, 1999; Walley, Metsala, & Garlock, 2003). Another, not mutually exclusive, perspective posits that oral vocabulary knowledge assists in resolving partial decoding attempts and aids in reading irregularly spelled words (Share, 1995; Tunmer & Chapman, 2012a). According to Tunmer and Chapman (2012b), the process of identifying and assigning meaning to an unfamiliar printed word would be significantly hindered if its corresponding spoken form is absent from the reader's oral vocabulary. When encountering a novel word, children apply their developing grapheme–phoneme correspondences, producing a partially decoded form. If this approximate phonological representation sufficiently resembles a known word in the child's lexical memory, it facilitates correct word identification.

Recent research has increasingly recognized morphological knowledge as a critical factor in word recognition, independent of other psycholinguistic variables and reading-related skills (Carlisle, 2000; Deacon & Kirby, 2004; Catts, 2021; Lefèvre et al., 2022; Levesque & Deacon, 2022; Nagy, Berninger, & Abbott, 2006; Roman, Kirby, Parrila, Wade-Woolley, & Deacon, 2009; Tong, Deacon, Kirby, Cain, & Parrila, 2011). This shift in focus is largely due to the morpho-phonemic nature of the English language, which differentiates it from purely phonetic languages where letter-sound correspondences remain consistent. In English, morphological structure is embedded within the spelling system, preserving morpheme integrity even when pronunciation shifts. For example, the silent "g" in *sign* is retained to maintain its morphological link with *signature* and *signal*, illustrating how morphology influences spelling and connects related words.

Studies of pre-reading children have further demonstrated that morphological awareness—defined as the conscious understanding of a word's morphemic structure and the ability to recognize, comprehend, and manipulate morphemes in language processing (Carlisle & Feldman, 1995, p. 194)— emerges before the onset of formal reading instruction. Evidence from both English (Berko, 1958; Law et al., 2017) and French (Casalis & Louis-Alexandre, 2000) suggests that children develop an early sensitivity to morphological patterns, even in the absence of explicit teaching. This early acquisition highlights the fundamental role of morphology in language development and reading acquisition, reinforcing its importance in literacy instruction. However, previous studies have yielded contradictory findings regarding the role of morphological awareness in the early phases of word reading among typically developing English- and French-speaking children. Even in studies where a significant impact of morphological awareness on word reading has been observed, the interdependencies among morphological awareness, phoneme awareness, and vocabulary remain unclear. Among the rare studies conducted on the role of morphological awareness in the development of word reading, very few have explored the relationship between morphological skills, phonological awareness, and vocabulary, and how these skills interact in shaping early reading development. A recent study by Colé et al. (2018) investigated the role of morphological knowledge in the early stages of reading acquisition (decoding), before reading comprehension can be reliably assessed, among 703 French first-graders from low socioeconomic status (SES) backgrounds. Using a graphical modeling approach, they analyzed the network of oral language skills (vocabulary, listening comprehension, phoneme awareness, and morphological awareness) that influenced the acquisition of decoding and word recognition. This method revealed how these skills are interconnected and showed that morphological awareness and vocabulary have an indirect influence on word reading via both listening comprehension and phoneme awareness. This helps reconcile debates about whether semantic factors affect reading acquisition or word reading skills.

Morphological awareness refers to the ability to reflect on and manipulate morphemes, enabling individuals to construct words, understand word meanings, and recognize relationships between words, such as different derivations of a root word (e.g., *develop, developer, development*). However, early morphological awareness is often limited to inflectional morphology, including tense markers (*-ed*) and simple derivations that do not involve phonological shifts (e.g., *walk → walker*) (Berko, 1958; Law et al., 2017). While research has demonstrated developmental growth in derivational morphology—the ability to modify base words through prefixes and suffixes to create new words with distinct meanings or grammatical functions—this process evolves with age and reading experience (Nagy, Berninger, & Abbott, 1993; Carlisle & Fleming, 2003). For instance, Dawson, Rastle, and Ricketts (2017) investigated morphological decomposition in visual word recognition across different age groups, including children and adults. Using a timed lexical decision task, they found that older adolescents and adults were slower to reject pseudomorphemic nonwords (e.g., *cornment*), suggesting a greater sensitivity to morphological structure in word processing. This effect was absent in younger participants, indicating that morphological processing (MP) abilities continue to evolve throughout adolescence. Further studies have demonstrated that the independent contribution of morphological awareness to literacy outcomes strengthens over time (Deacon & Kirby, 2004; Singson et al., 2000). In a study examining predictors of reading development in English-speaking children, Roman et al. (2009) found that morphological awareness significantly predicted variations in word reading ability, even after controlling for age, phonological awareness, and naming speed.

Beyond explicit morphological awareness, research has also highlighted the role of MP—the implicit use of morphological structure during language processing—in literacy development. Studies employing priming paradigms with derived and inflected words suggest that MP enhances word recognition by facilitating lexical access and improving reading speed (Elbro, 1989; Diependaele, Sandra, & Grainger, 2005; Grainger & Beyersmann, 2017; Rastle, Davis, Marslen-Wilson, & Tyler, 2000; Rastle, Davis, & New, 2004; Raveh & Schiff, 2008). These findings indicate that as individuals develop reading expertise, they increasingly rely on morphological cues to decode complex words efficiently.

Research on skilled adult readers has provided additional evidence for the significant role of MP in word reading, revealing a distinct neural signature that goes beyond the combined activation of form and meaning (Beyersmann, Castles, & Coltheart, 2014; Rastle & Davis, 2008). Morphology-specific effects have been identified along the ventral stream and within a broadly distributed network, including the left inferior and superior temporal gyri, the left inferior frontal gyrus (IFG), and the left orbitofrontal gyrus (Cavalli et al., 2016b; Fruchter & Marantz, 2015; Whiting, Shtyrov, & Marslen-Wilson, 2015). In a recent magnetoencephalography (MEG) study employing a primed lexical decision task, Cavalli et al. (2016a) observed semantically driven morphological priming effects as early as 250 ms (M250) in the left superior temporal gyrus (STG). Around 350 ms (M350), orthographic and semantic contributions to morphological facilitation were detected along the ventral stream and in the left IFG. Furthermore, evidence for the recombination of morphemes and semantic unification emerged in the orbitofrontal cortex at 450–500 ms, further supporting the specialized role of morphology in reading and the unique and distributed neural basis of MP (see also Fruchter and Marantz, 2015).

The Morphological Pathways Framework (Levesque et al., 2021) provides a theoretical model to explain how morphological skills contribute to reading processes. This framework posits that morphological awareness influences reading through two distinct word-level mechanisms: morphological decoding and morphological analysis, both of which facilitate lexical access and have broader implications for reading comprehension (Deacon et al., 2017; Levesque et al., 2017; Levesque, Kieffer, & Deacon, 2019).

Morphological decoding refers to the process of using morphemes to read multimorphemic words (Deacon et al., 2017; Nagy et al., 2006; Carlisle & Stone, 2005). Through morphological decomposition, the constituent morphemes of complex words become recognizable units that assist in word identification and pronunciation. For example, when encountering the word *redevelopment*, a reader proficient in morphological decoding recognizes the boundary between morphemes (*re-* and *development*), rather than applying phonological rules that could lead to mispronunciations (e.g., *pronouncing "ed" as in "red"*). Studies have demonstrated that morphemic boundaries aid pronunciation in ways that phonics alone cannot explain (Nunes et al., 2012). Additionally, morphological decoding accounts for orthographic consistencies that phonics cannot, such as why *health* retains the spelling of *heal* rather than following phoneme–grapheme correspondence rules (Nunes, & Bryant, 2006). Thus, morphological decoding operates at the word form level, linking morphemic knowledge to the decomposition of complex words.

Morphological analysis, in contrast, functions at the word meaning level, utilizing syntactic and semantic cues from morphemes to support understanding of complex words within textual contexts (Baumann et al., 2002; Carlisle, 2007; Pacheco & Goodwin, 2013). This process plays a crucial role in vocabulary acquisition and sentence-level comprehension, as it enables readers to interpret the meanings and grammatical functions of words (Crosson & McKeown, 2016; Goodwin, Lipsky, & Ahn, 2012). For instance, when encountering the word *disagreement* in the sentence *"The meeting ended in disagreement about the budget,"* a reader employing morphological analysis would decompose the word into *dis-* (meaning "not" or "opposite of"), *agree* (to have the same opinion), and *-ment* (a suffix that turns a verb into a noun, indicating an action or result). By integrating these morphological cues, the reader infers that *disagreement* means *a state of not agreeing*, thus deriving meaning even without prior exposure to the word.

Empirical studies have confirmed the role of morphological-semantic and morphological-syntactic knowledge in vocabulary acquisition (Nagy et al., 2006; Singson, Mahony, & Mann, 2000; Sparks & Deacon, 2015) and reading comprehension in both children (Carlisle & Feldman, 1995; Deacon & Kirby, 2004) and adults (Nagy et al., 2006; Wilson-Fowler & Apel, 2015). These findings suggest that MP is not only central to word recognition but also plays a crucial role in higher-order reading skills.

3.3 Oral Language and Reading Comprehension Skills

Reading is fundamentally an act of extracting knowledge and meaning from text, making comprehension the ultimate goal of reading. This process requires the accurate decoding of individual words, as any failure in decoding can significantly alter the reader's interpretation of a sentence. For example, the sentences *"Kyle fell off the horse"* and *"Kyle fell off the house"* differ by only one letter, yet they convey entirely different meanings. This illustrates the necessity of precise word recognition for accurate comprehension.

However, while word reading accuracy and speed are essential, they do not fully account for reading comprehension. According to the SVR proposed by Gough and Tunmer (1986) and later tested by Hoover and Gough (1990), reading comprehension is not merely a function of word decoding but rather the combined product of decoding ability and oral language comprehension (see also Cutting & Scarborough, 2012; Hoover, 2023). A meta-analysis by Garcia and Cain (2014) provided strong empirical support for this model, showing that both decoding skills and oral language comprehension contribute significantly to reading comprehension. Furthermore, as decoding skills become more automatized, oral language comprehension plays an increasingly dominant role in determining reading comprehension outcomes (Foorman, Koon, Petscher, Mitchell, & Truckenmiller, 2015; Verhoeven & van Leeuwe, 2012).

For skilled adult readers, the primary challenge in reading is not decoding individual words but rather processing complex textual features, such as sophisticated vocabulary and intricate syntactic structures (Braze et al., 2007). As a result, skilled readers rely more heavily on oral language comprehension and associated linguistic skills, including morphology, syntax, and semantics (Lervag, Hulme, & Melby-Lervag, 2017). This is supported by findings from Ransby and Swanson (2003), who demonstrated that, among skilled adult readers, reading comprehension is predominantly explained by oral language comprehension rather than written word recognition. These results emphasize that, while decoding is a prerequisite for reading comprehension, the ability to extract and interpret meaning from text is primarily governed by higher-level language processing skills in proficient readers.

3.3.1 The Role of Non-Phonological Oral Language Skills in Reading Comprehension

Oral language comprehension, or listening comprehension, defined as *"the process by which, given lexical (i.e., word) information, sentences and discourses are interpreted"* (Gough & Tunmer, 1986, p. 7), has been shown to rely on the interaction and mastery of various component skills of oral language (e.g., morphology, syntax, and semantics (more specifically vocabulary)). Lervag, Hulme, and Melby-Lervag (2017) found that variations in oral language comprehension were nearly all explained by the variance shared by their collection of oral language measures containing syntax, semantics, and morphology. Additionally, it has been suggested that the oral language skills underlying listening comprehension may not only have an indirect effect on reading comprehension through oral language comprehension but, in addition, may have a direct effect (Adlof, Catts, & Lee, 2010; Geva & Farnia, 2012; Kirby & Savage, 2008; Silva & Cain, 2015). For instance, Perfetti and Stafura (2014) suggested that syntactic and semantic knowledge are not only fundamental for oral language comprehension but also directly influence reading comprehension, as together they constitute a lexicon or mental dictionary that is critical for comprehension to occur.

Additionally, basic syntactic, semantic, and morphological skills are essential to both reading and listening comprehension, as they both provide cues and information central to the understanding of the interrelationships of words within and between sentences (Kintsch & Kintsch, 2005); therefore they participate in the construction of a coherent representation of the text as a whole (also called the *Situation Model*; Kintsch, 1988). Moreover, evidence has been presented demonstrating that the underdevelopment of, or a deficit in, a reader's broad oral language skills may restrict higher-level comprehension processes, such as inference making and integration (Adlof et al., 2010; Nation, Cocksey, Taylor, & Bishop, 2010).

Oral language comprehension, also referred to as listening comprehension, is defined as *"the process by which, given lexical (i.e., word) information, sentences and discourses are interpreted"* (Gough & Tunmer, 1986, p. 7). It relies on the integration and mastery of multiple oral language components, including morphology, syntax, and semantics, particularly vocabulary. Research by Lervag, Hulme, and Melby-Lervag (2017) demonstrated that variations in oral language comprehension were almost entirely accounted for by shared variance among measures assessing syntax, semantics, and morphology. Beyond its established role in listening comprehension, oral language skills may contribute to reading comprehension both directly and indirectly. Studies have suggested that oral language skills influence reading comprehension indirectly via their impact on listening comprehension, but they may also exert a direct effect on reading comprehension (Adlof et al., 2010; Geva & Farnia, 2012; Kirby & Savage, 2008; Silva & Cain, 2015). For instance, Perfetti and Stafura (2014) posited that syntactic and semantic knowledge not only form the foundation of oral language comprehension but also play a direct role in reading comprehension, as they constitute the mental lexicon, a crucial component for understanding written text.

Fundamental syntactic, semantic, and morphological skills are integral to both reading and listening comprehension because they provide structural and relational cues that aid in interpreting the connections between words within and across sentences (Kintsch & Kintsch, 2005). These skills contribute to the construction of a coherent mental representation of the text, known as the Situation Model (Kintsch, 1988). Furthermore, research has demonstrated that deficits or underdeveloped oral language skills can limit higher-level comprehension processes, such as inference-making and text integration, ultimately impeding overall reading comprehension (Adlof et al., 2010; Nation et al., 2010).

3.3.1.1 *Semantics and Morphology in Reading Comprehension*

Recently, literature about the role of semantics in explaining reading performance has been increasingly emphasized in the body of reading research. A study of skilled adult readers by Guo, Roehrig, and Williams (2011) used structural equation modelling with a sample of 151 participants to demonstrate that reading comprehension was predicted directly by syntactic awareness and indirectly by vocabulary knowledge. Vocabulary knowledge, the most commonly utilized semantic assessment measure in reading research, made an independent contribution to reading comprehension above and beyond other oral language skills, such as syntactic and morphological awareness, thus highlighting the relevance of vocabulary measures in explaining individual differences in reading. This supports the view of vocabulary knowledge as an essential component of reading performance both in typically developing readers (Ouellette, 2006; Ouellette & Beers, 2010; Tunmer & Chapman, 2012b) and in skilled adult readers (Guo et al., 2011).

Compared to vocabulary and decoding skills, fewer studies have investigated the relationship between morphological knowledge and reading comprehension. However, research has consistently shown that morphological awareness is not only a strong predictor of reading comprehension later in life but also plays a role in early reading development (Levesque, Kieffer, & Deacon, 2017; Deacon & Kirby, 2004; Nagy et al., 2006). In a study of third-grade English-speaking children, Levesque et al. (2017) examined four potential intervening variables through which morphological awareness may contribute indirectly to reading comprehension. This study revealed evidence of two indirect relations and one direct relation between morphological awareness (as assessed through morphological decoding and morphological analysis tasks) and reading comprehension after controlling for phonological awareness and nonverbal ability. Levesque and colleagues noted that children with higher morphological awareness tend to have better reading comprehension skills.

In one of the few studies to examine this in an adult population, Guo et al. (2011) investigated the structural relationships among vocabulary knowledge, oral morphological awareness, syntactic awareness, and reading comprehension in English-speaking adults. After controlling for age, this study reported that morphological awareness directly influenced reading comprehension, thus supporting the view that morphological skills continue to contribute to reading comprehension across development into adulthood (also see Carlisle & Nomanbhoy, 1993; Mahony et al., 2000). Guo et al. (2011) argued that, for adult readers, the contribution of morphological skills to reading comprehension may be a function of increased accuracy and fluency in decoding words due to higher levels of morphological awareness, which would, in turn, affect reading comprehension. Similarly, in a recent study of 71 English-speaking undergraduate students, Kotzer, Kirby, and Heggie (2021) found that morphological awareness was a significant predictor of both reading speed and reading comprehension after controlling for all of the other predictors, such as vocabulary, phonological decoding, and memory. The results demonstrate that morphological awareness remains an important individual difference factor in reading proficiency among adults.

As discussed earlier in this chapter, the theoretical foundation for this contribution is supported by the Morphological Pathways Framework (Levesque et al., 2021). This framework emphasizes the role of morphological analysis skills, which utilize the syntactic and semantic information encoded in the morphemes of a target word. These skills aid in understanding complex words, their meanings, and grammatical functions within connected text, thereby enhancing word knowledge and contributing to improved reading comprehension.

3.3.1.2 *Syntax and Reading Comprehension*

The acquisition of basic syntax awareness, a meta-linguistic skill that reflects an individual's understanding of the rules for combining words into sentences, typically occurs by the age of five in typically developing children, with the exception of some complex word forms (Berman, 2007). Research has shown that syntax awareness plays a crucial role in both listening and reading comprehension from an early age (MacKay, Lynch, Duncan, & Deacon, 2021; Kim, 2016; Low & Siegel, 2005; Catts et al., 2002). This role evolves with development, as greater exposure to print and increasing text complexity enhances syntax awareness (Cain, Oakhill, & Bryant, 2004). A recent longitudinal study by Deacon and Kieffer (2018) involving 100 English-speaking children from Grades 3 to 4 showed that syntactic awareness uniquely contributed to reading comprehension but not to word reading skills. Additionally, syntactic awareness in Grade 3 predicted improvements in reading comprehension by Grade 4. Similarly, Brimo, Apel, and Fountain (2017), using path analysis, confirmed the significant effects of syntactic knowledge and syntactic awareness on reading comprehension among adolescent students, considering factors such as word-level reading, short-term memory, and vocabulary knowledge.

The mechanisms behind syntax's contribution to reading comprehension go beyond word order alone. As any Star Wars fan would attest: "Difficult to understand Yoda is." The predictability of a language's syntax and a reader's awareness of this structure aid in reading fluency and comprehension by assisting in the prediction of forthcoming words and word forms, thus reducing a reader's processing load. Tunmer (1989; Verhoeven & Perfetti, 2008) proposed that syntactic awareness provides a framework of syntactic and semantic context, enabling readers to accurately identify words and facilitating the comprehension of connected text. For example, in the sentence "Karen reads the s…," if a reader struggles to decode the final word, syntactic understanding can guide them to predict a noun, such as "sign" or "story," rather than a verb like "singing" or an adjective like "strong." This understanding enhances the activation of potential words within the reader's lexicon, helping to identify words that could appropriately complete the sentence.

Moreover, syntax plays a key role in accurately interpreting text. Consider the sentences (adapted from Cain, 2011, p. 48):

Max taught structural equation modelling to Kyle.
Max was taught structural equation modelling by Kyle.

Although the word order is preserved across both sentences, a shift from active to passive voice changes the meaning entirely. While studies have shown that readers may not retain exact word order in long-term memory (Sachs, 1967), syntactic awareness is essential during initial processing to extract meaning and ensure accurate comprehension.

3.4 Oral Language and Dyslexia

Individuals with developmental dyslexia have persistent difficulties with accurate or fluent word recognition and spelling despite receiving adequate instruction, having sufficient intelligence, and possessing intact sensory abilities (Carroll, Holden, Kirby, Thompson, & Snowling, 2024; Norton, Beach, & Gabrieli, 2014).

A recent study by Carroll et al. (2024) noted that the most common cognitive impairment observed among individuals with dyslexia is difficulty with phonological processing (such as phonological awareness, processing speed, or verbal short-term memory). However, phonological difficulties were noted to not fully explain the observed variability among this population. For instance, children and adolescents with dyslexia have been observed to possess oral language deficits beyond phonological processing. In a recent meta-analysis and review of oral language deficits in children at family risk of dyslexia, Snowling and Melby-Lervåg (2016) reported that as early as preschool, high-risk children demonstrate significant difficulties, not only in phonological processes but also with broader language skills. Snowling and Melby-Lervåg noted that within the longitudinal studies included in their review, the children at family risk who went on to be later diagnosed with dyslexia had more severe impairments in preschool language than those who were defined as normal readers. However, the broad oral language skill difficulties of children with dyslexia observed early in development were found to be nearly completely resolved within the first few years of primary education, with the notable exception of vocabulary and morphological knowledge, which have been observed to persist through adolescence (e.g., see Share & Silva, 1987). Further discussion of both morphology and semantics (vocabulary) deficits will be provided later in this chapter.

When oral language deficits persist, the direction of causation may be questioned, as such deficits in individuals with dyslexia could be attributed to limited print exposure, leading to delayed vocabulary, semantic, and morphological development. Recent studies have provided support for a bidirectional relationship between reading and morphological awareness (both oral and written). Morphological awareness was not only found to support later growth in reading, but reading skill was additionally found to influence later growth in morphological awareness ability (Deacon, Benere, & Pasquarella, 2013; Law & Ghesquière, 2017). As children encounter more complex and less phonologically transparent word derivations, explicit awareness of morphological structure and orthography becomes increasingly important. Law and Ghesquière (2017) argued that complex morphological representations and an understanding of many derivations may only become fully specified through repeated exposure to written language rather than spoken language, as morphemes are more consistently spelled than they are pronounced (e.g., Bowers & Kirby, 2010; Templeton & Scarborough-Franks, 1985). Additionally, vocabulary has been identified as a strong predictor of reading comprehension development, even several years later, after controlling for earlier word reading and reading comprehension. Conversely, reading comprehension has been found to account for the variance in vocabulary knowledge up to two years later, even after controlling for prior vocabulary knowledge (Seigneuric & Ehrlich, 2005).

3.4.1 Semantics and Morphology in Dyslexia

Research on semantic skills in dyslexia is highly underrepresented in the literature compared to other broad oral language skills, such as phonology or morphology. Of the studies that have examined semantic skills in dyslexia, the majority have focused on populations of children and adolescents. Results from this body of work, utilizing a range of methodologies, have suggested that children with dyslexia have impaired semantic skills in comparison to age-matched controls and that these deficits persist throughout the primary school years (Lyytinen et al., 2001; Torppa, Lyytinen, Erskine, Eklund, & Lyytinen, 2010; Vellutino, Scanlon, & Spearing, 1995). However, mixed results in studies comparing reading age-matched controls have raised questions about whether these semantic deficits are causal in the reading difficulties experienced by children with dyslexia (Betjemann & Keenan, 2008; Tsesmeli & Seymour, 2006). Despite challenges with reading fluency, some adolescents with dyslexia exhibit resilience, achieving adequate reading comprehension. Recent research highlights the potential role of semantic abilities in fostering this resilience (Lefèvre, Law, Prado, Anders, & Cavalli, 2025). However, the impact of semantic skills on reading comprehension appears to be indirectly shaped by SES, with SES having a particularly significant effect in individuals with dyslexia. These findings support the view that dyslexia primarily affects phonological processing and reading fluency. Semantic deficits, by contrast, are likely secondary and may stem from reduced reading exposure (Cain, Oakhill, & Bryant, 2004).

In adults, research is even scarcer, and among the few studies conducted examining the general semantic skills of adults with dyslexia, it has been reported that their semantic skills were comparable to those of typically developing adults (Elbro, Nielsen, & Petersen, 1994). In contrast, vocabulary skills of adults with dyslexia were reported to be significantly poorer when compared to normal reading controls, as shown by the meta-analysis of Swanson and Hsieh (2009). However, this review combined vocabulary breadth (i.e., number of words known) and depth (i.e., knowledge of word meanings), and the participants in the studies surveyed in this meta-analysis included both students and non-students with dyslexia, in addition to a more broadly defined group of adults with reading disabilities (not only dyslexia). In most studies involving adults with dyslexia, vocabulary is typically introduced as a control measure, with inconsistent or even contradictory results regarding both breadth and depth of vocabulary (Corkett & Parrila, 2008; Hatcher, Snowling, & Griffiths, 2002). These inconsistencies highlight the need for more focused and nuanced research on the vocabulary skills of adults with dyslexia. Specifically, a recent study by Cavalli et al. (2016b) distinguished between the evaluation of vocabulary breadth and depth, revealing group differences. Using a multiple-case study methodology, they reported no significant difference in the vocabulary breadth task between individuals with dyslexia and controls. However, university students with dyslexia outperformed their typically reading peers in the vocabulary depth task. Notably, using a logit Rasch scale (i.e., a scale that estimates person trait and item difficulty parameters on a common metric; Rasch, 1980), this study demonstrated that university students with dyslexia outperformed skilled adult readers on the most semantically complex items in the vocabulary depth task. Together, these findings support the hypothesis that strengths in vocabulary and semantics play an important role in reading compensation and strategies among university students with dyslexia.

Such behavioral evidence suggests that university students with dyslexia may develop compensatory mechanisms to support their reading process. Past research has suggested that adults with dyslexia may leverage relatively intact semantic skills as a compensatory strategy to help bootstrap the reading process. Consequently, this may lead to neural re-organization of the typical reading network, with lexical representations of words being (re)structured according to semantic rather than orthographic information (Cavalli et al., 2016b; Snowling, 2000; Stanovich, 1986). Consistent with this idea, some fMRI studies indeed reported overactivation of frontal areas during tasks of word and pseudoword reading that could potentially be associated with semantic processing (Brunswick et al., 1999; Salmelin et al., 1996; Shaywitz et al., 1998). However, over-activation in regions like the left IFG is more commonly interpreted as reflecting articulatory compensatory mechanisms or increased effort (Hancock et al., 2017; Richlan et al., 2011; Richlan et al., 2009). Additionally, neuroimaging studies specifically investigating semantic processing in dyslexia—such as sentence reading tasks manipulating semantic appropriateness (Helenius et al. 1999), pseudo-homophone reading tasks (Paz-Alonso et al., 2018), or semantic judgment tasks (Rüsseler et al., 2007)—generally found weaker activation in the left middle and superior temporal cortex, delayed N400 responses, or reduced hippocampal activation in individuals with dyslexia compared to controls. In summary, existing brain imaging studies provide little evidence for greater involvement of semantic brain areas or more efficient semantic processing, offering limited support for the hypothesis that semantics serves as a central compensatory mechanism in adults with dyslexia.

To further explore the question of compensatory reorganization of the reading network in adults with dyslexia, a recent fMRI study by Cavalli et al. (2024) employed multivariate representational similarity analyses (MVPA, RSA, Kriegeskorte et al., 2008) during an isolated word reading task (see also Tan et al., 2022). The goal was to identify regions of the reading network responsible for processing orthographic and semantic information and to examine differences between typical and dyslexic adult readers. Representational similarity analysis is based on the idea that words (or other representations), which are similar on a given dimension (e.g., semantics), should produce similar patterns of neural responses across voxels in a region that "cares" about that particular dimension. For example, in a semantic processing region, *shirt* and *dress* should produce more similar neural responses than *shirt* and *book*. In turn, in an orthographic processing region, *shirt* and *ship* should produce more similar neural responses than *shirt* and *book*. In accordance with the re-organization hypothesis, the authors predicted greater similarity between the neural representation of single words in adults with dyslexia than in typical readers (i.e., correlation of neural dissimilarity matrices between individual words) in regions associated with semantic processing and weaker similarity in regions associated with orthographic processing. However, the results did not confirm these predictions. They found sensitivity to semantic similarity in all three subparts of the fusiform gyrus (FG1, FG2, and FG3) bilaterally. Adults with dyslexia showed less (rather than more) sensitivity to semantic similarity in the posterior subpart of the fusiform gyrus (FG1) in the left hemisphere. Specifically, reading fluency (as a continuous variable) predicted the sensitivity of FG1 to semantic information/similarity (better readers show greater sensitivity to semantic information). In typical readers, sensitivity to orthographic information was not only found in the left fusiform gyrus (FG1, FG2, and FG3) but also in the left IFG. Adults with dyslexia, in contrast, did not show sensitivity to orthographic information in left IFG. However, they showed increased sensitivity to orthographic information in the right hemisphere FG1. Interestingly, reading fluency (as a continuous variable) was negatively related to the sensitivity to orthographic information/similarity in the right FG1, suggesting that poorer readers rely to a greater extent on orthographic processing in the right hemisphere homologue of FG1. Together, these results show atypical orthographic processing in left IFG and right FG1 and reduced semantic information in left FG1. While this study supports evidence for compensatory re-organization in adult dyslexia, the results do not support the hypothesis according to which adults with dyslexia rely more heavily on semantic information. Instead, they revealed atypical hemispheric organization of the reading network that is not restricted to the typical left language hemisphere, and more specifically, a lack of sharing semantic and orthographic information between key regions of the reading network that are more heavily dedicated to speech production (left IFG) and orthographic processing (left FG). These findings suggest that high-functioning adults with dyslexia seem to be less able to integrate semantic information during orthographic processes (left FG). They also seem to be impaired in processing orthographic similarity in left IFG, and the more severely impaired dyslexics (weaker reading fluency scores) seem to rely on right homologues of the FG to process orthographic information.

However, and interestingly, a recent fMRI study by Gavard et al. (2025) investigated the neural mechanisms underlying semantic and syntactic predictions in reading in adults with and without dyslexia during both a semantic and a syntactic predictive reading task, where participants had to read a final target word that was preceded by a semantically related context (e.g., orange – red – blue – purple – yellow) or a syntactically related context (the – big – carpet – is – yellow). The results support the dissociation between semantic and syntactic processes (Dapretto & Bookheimer, 1999) by revealing distinct neural networks for semantic prediction (i.e., activation in left frontal and temporal areas but also in the left angular gyrus and the left inferior occipital gyrus) and for syntactic prediction (i.e., activation in the left inferior frontal and temporal areas, in the left middle temporal gyrus and in the left superior frontal gyrus). Contrary to the initial hypothesis that university students with dyslexia would rely to a greater extent on context predictions than typical readers, the findings of this study revealed the opposite trend. While typical readers exhibited the expected facilitation effect of linguistic context, dyslexic readers showed no significant context effects. Nevertheless, the study demonstrated that dyslexic readers process predictive sentences and structured sequences more efficiently than scrambled or unrelated sequences, performing similarly to typical readers. fMRI data indicate that dyslexic readers engage in linguistic prediction, which likely supports reading comprehension. However, these predictive mechanisms do not improve word reading aloud, as bottom-up word identification remains significantly impaired in developmental dyslexia. This suggests that while neural compensation may support sentence-level comprehension, it does not extend to behavioral compensation in word reading.

Notably, compensatory mechanisms may only be present in dyslexic readers who have developed effective compensation strategies, which is not the case for all university students with dyslexia. Supporting this interpretation, Gavard et al. (2025) found a significant correlation between predictive reading and reading ability in dyslexic readers. Their results suggest that stronger readers (i.e., more compensated dyslexic readers) exhibit greater syntactic prediction effects, as indicated by faster reaction times for target words in syntactically correct sentences. This correlation implies that more compensated dyslexic readers might use linguistic context to facilitate word identification and reading aloud. Consistent with the findings of Cavalli et al. (2024), these results challenge the assumption that university students with dyslexia compensate for word reading deficits via increased reliance on semantic and syntactic predictions. Instead, compensation appears to occur primarily at the sentence level, enhancing reading comprehension rather than single-word recognition.

In summary, although some neural reorganization was observed in adults with dyslexia, the findings do not support the hypothesis that adults with dyslexia use higher-level semantic information more efficiently. In general, compensation at the neural level involves changes in neural activity or alternative neural pathways that support behavioral performance in individuals with dyslexia (Livingston & Happé, 2017; see also Chapter 12 of this book, which focused on compensatory mechanisms in adults with dyslexia). Given that individuals with dyslexia are frequently characterized by impaired access to phonological forms (Boets et al., 2013; Ramus & Szenkovits, 2008), strengths in semantic knowledge could theoretically support access to intact phonological forms. According to the triangle model of reading (Elbro & Arnbak, 1996; Elbro et al., 1994; Snowling, 2000), this process would facilitate lexical access by linking orthography to phonology through semantics (O → S → P).

To further understand why findings from existing brain imaging studies do not fully support the hypothesis that semantic processing plays a central compensatory role in adults with dyslexia, it is essential to consider alternative explanations that align with recent research on compensatory mechanisms in dyslexia. Building on this perspective, another compelling explanation is that adults with dyslexia may not primarily rely on broad semantic processing for compensation but rather on MP, which provides a more structured and direct link between form and meaning. Morphemes, the smallest units of meaning (e.g., *work-er*, *depart-ure*), inherently encode both form and meaning, reducing the arbitrariness of their association. Unlike single-word semantic processing, which requires more abstract inferencing, MP establishes systematic patterns that facilitate lexical access. For instance, morphologically related words (e.g., *work*, *worker*, and *working*) share both structural and semantic properties, making word recognition more predictable and efficient. This hypothesis aligns with findings suggesting that certain oral language skills, particularly vocabulary and morphological awareness, may serve as protective factors in dyslexia. University students with dyslexia who demonstrate stronger MP skills may be better equipped to compensate for phonological deficits, enabling more efficient word recognition and comprehension. These findings (for a review, see Haft, Myers, & Hoeft, 2016) further support the notion that compensation in dyslexia is not driven by enhanced reliance on broad semantic representations but rather by leveraging structured linguistic units—such as morphemes—to support word recognition and reading comprehension.

In line with this hypothesis, a key component of morphological knowledge is morphological awareness, which refers to the ability to recognize, manipulate, and analyze morphemes—the smallest units of meaning—within words (Carlisle & Feldman, 1995). This ability allows readers to break down complex words into their constituent parts, such as roots and affixes, facilitating more efficient lexical access and comprehension. Most studies examining the relationship between morphological awareness and dyslexia have focused primarily on children. Across various languages, research has constantly shown that children with dyslexia underperform on both written and oral morphological awareness tasks compared to their age-matched peers (Berthiaume & Daigle, 2014; Casalis, Dusautoir, Colé, & Ducrot, 2009; Fowler, Liberman, & Feldman, 1995; Law et al., 2017; Law et al., 2018; Tsesmeli & Seymour, 2006). However, when compared to younger children with similar reading abilities, those with dyslexia tend to perform at an equivalent or even superior level (Elbro, 1989; Fowler, Liberman, & Feldman, 1995; Tsesmeli & Seymour, 2006). This pattern of results suggests that morphological awareness deficits are not a primary cause of reading difficulties in dyslexia but rather a consequence of reduced reading experience or underlying phonological impairments. Supporting this view, research indicates that the ability of individuals with dyslexia to process morphological structures is highly dependent on the phonological demands of the task. For example, a study conducted in French by Casalis, Sopo, and Colé (2004) demonstrated that MP performance varies according to the phonological complexity of the task, highlighting the interdependence between phonological and morphological skills in dyslexia. These findings suggest that while morphological awareness may serve as a compensatory mechanism for some individuals with dyslexia, its effectiveness is constrained by the severity of phonological deficits.

Data on morphological skills in adults with dyslexia remain relatively scarce, despite the well-established role of morphological awareness in reading development and achievement, particularly among skilled adult readers (Guo et al., 2011). Although this skill has been extensively studied in children, research on morphological awareness in adults with dyslexia within alphabetic writing systems is still limited. Only a few studies have investigated this issue in English orthography (e.g., Farris, Cristan, Bernstein, et al., 2021; Law et al., 2015) and French orthography (e.g., Cavalli, Duncan, et al., 2017; Martin et al., 2013). Additionally, some research has examined Hebrew-speaking university students with dyslexia (e.g., Leikin & Zur Hagit, 2006; Schiff & Raveh, 2007).

Findings from studies conducted in Hebrew suggest that adults with dyslexia exhibit significant weaknesses in MP tasks. However, due to the unique structure of Hebrew morphology, these results cannot be easily generalized to Indo-European languages with alphabetic writing systems, such as English and French. In Hebrew, phonology and morphology are not dissociable, making it difficult to separate phonological deficits from MP challenges (see Leikin & Zur Hagit, 2006; Schiff & Raveh, 2007 for a detailed overview of Hebrew morphology). Given that phonological deficits are a well-documented characteristic of dyslexia, it is expected that Hebrew-speaking individuals with dyslexia would also exhibit difficulties in morphological awareness tasks, reinforcing the need for further cross-linguistic research on the relationship between MP and dyslexia across different orthographic systems.

However, in languages such as French, research by Cavalli, Duncan, et al. (2017) confirmed that university students with dyslexia retain intact MP abilities despite the presence of phonological deficits. This finding highlights a dissociation between phonological and morphological development, observed both at the individual and group levels. Moreover, the degree of this dissociation was correlated with reading ability, suggesting that university students with dyslexia may leverage their preserved MP skills to compensate for their reading difficulties. Specifically, these individuals may capitalize on the semantic dimension of morphology to acquire morphological knowledge and enhance reading comprehension.

Further supporting this idea, Law et al. (2015) found that when controlling for both vocabulary and phonological skills, compensated adults with dyslexia performed comparably to controls on measures of morphological awareness. However, when considering the dyslexic group as a whole, they underperformed compared to age-matched controls. One potential limitation of this study is that the written nature of the morphological awareness tasks (paper-and-pencil word and non-word sentence completion) made it difficult to determine whether the observed deficits in morphological awareness were due to difficulties in manipulating morphemes explicitly or simply a consequence of the participants' existing reading difficulties. Nevertheless, Law et al. (2015) demonstrated a stronger interaction between morphological awareness and word reading skills in adults with dyslexia compared to controls. Specifically, morphology accounted for 16.7% of the variance in word reading among dyslexic readers, whereas it did not significantly predict word reading ability in the control group. Similarly, a study by Farris et al. (2021) examined how morphological awareness and vocabulary knowledge contribute to reading resilience and comprehension in adults with dyslexia. Their findings indicated that both morphological awareness and vocabulary knowledge are significant predictors of reading resilience, further reinforcing the role of MP as a compensatory mechanism in dyslexia.

While much of the research has focused on morphological awareness in dyslexia, fewer studies have investigated MP in both children and adults with dyslexia. However, within this body of work, a growing consensus suggests that individuals with dyslexia retain the ability to rapidly process written morphology (Burani et al., 2008; Cavalli, Colé et al., 2017; Elbro & Arnbak, 1996; Quémart & Casalis, 2015; Law et al., 2018; Law & Ghesquière, 2022). However, some studies challenge this conclusion, suggesting possible deficits in MP in dyslexia (see Deacon, Kirby & Parrila, 2006; Lázaro et al., 2013). These mixed findings highlight the need for further research to clarify the extent to which MP can serve as a compensatory mechanism for individuals with dyslexia.

In a study of French-speaking adolescents, Quémart and Casalis (2015) provided evidence of intact MP skills in individuals with dyslexia using a masked priming paradigm. Their findings demonstrated significant morphological priming effects, indicating that individuals with dyslexia exhibit sensitivity to morphological structure and possess a degree of morphological organization within their lexicon. Moreover, dyslexic participants showed greater priming effects in derived word conditions compared to pseudo-derived conditions, a pattern not observed in controls. This suggests that individuals with dyslexia rely on the morpho-semantic properties of morphemes earlier during visual word recognition than typical readers.

Building on this research, Law et al. (2018) investigated the processing of derivational morphology and its relationship with literacy outcomes in Dutch-speaking adults with dyslexia, using a masked priming experiment embedded in a lexical decision task. This study specifically manipulated the semantic overlap between morphologically related word pairs to assess how dyslexic and typical readers process morphological information. Results showed a significant priming effect in the morphologically primed condition for both dyslexic and typical readers; however, adults with dyslexia exhibited significantly stronger priming effects compared to controls. Notably, although individuals with dyslexia showed significant priming effects in both derived and pseudo-derived conditions, the priming effect was significantly stronger for derived words, reinforcing the idea that they rely not only on the morpho-orthographic structure of morphemes but also on their morpho-semantic properties, a finding consistent with Quémart and Casalis (2015). Law and colleagues concluded that MP remains intact in adults with dyslexia and, in fact, appears to be a relative strength when compared to age- and reading comprehension-matched controls. These findings further support the hypothesis that morphological awareness serves as a compensatory mechanism in dyslexia, facilitating word recognition and reading comprehension.

A recent MEG study by Cavalli, Colé, et al. (2017) provided the first evidence of an earlier and stronger reliance on MP in high-achieving adults with dyslexia compared to typical readers. The study aimed to examine differences in morphological, orthographic, and semantic processing between high-achieving dyslexic adults and skilled readers using a primed lexical decision task. The results confirmed that dyslexic adults rely more on semantic rather than orthographic properties of morphemes, as indicated by greater morphological priming effects compared to controls. At the neural level, source-space analyses confirmed a spatiotemporal reorganization of the reading network in dyslexic readers, with earlier and stronger engagement of the left IFG. Notably, dyslexic readers exhibited a significant morpho-semantic priming effect in the left orbitofrontal gyrus between 45 and 170 ms, while in skilled readers, this effect only emerged later (435–500 ms, M350 time window). These findings challenge previous interpretations of frontal overactivation in dyslexic adults as mere compensatory phonological effort, instead suggesting a greater reliance on MP.

Another key finding was the difference in prelexical and lexico-semantic processing within the occipito-temporal cortex. Whereas typical readers showed early orthographic priming (~100 ms) in the left inferior temporal gyrus (ITG), dyslexic readers demonstrated morphological priming in the left anterior fusiform gyrus (100–200 ms) and lexico-semantic priming in the left middle fusiform gyrus (205–500 ms). In a later time window (385–500 ms), a global morphological priming effect emerged in the left middle fusiform gyrus, likely reflecting top-down feedback from frontal regions to the occipito-temporal cortex, facilitating lexical processing. These findings align with Stanovich's (1986) interactive compensatory hypothesis, which suggests that readers compensate for processing deficits by relying more on alternative linguistic cues. The earlier engagement of morpho-semantic processing in the left IFG appears to support morpho-orthographic processing in the occipito-temporal cortex, suggesting a functional interplay between these brain regions. A positive correlation between activity in the left IFG and the left middle fusiform gyrus further supports the hypothesis that top-down facilitation from frontal regions enhances word recognition in dyslexic readers. This mechanism is consistent with the predictive coding framework (Price & Devlin, 2011), which posits that higher-order cortical areas generate predictive models that shape lower-level sensory processing, allowing individuals with dyslexia to optimize reading strategies despite phonological decoding deficits (see Gavard et al., 2025).

The study by Cavalli, Colé, et al. (2017) provides strong evidence that high-achieving adults with dyslexia engage earlier and more strongly in MP than skilled readers, with an increased reliance on frontal regions to support morpho-semantic processing. These results highlight morphological awareness as a key compensatory mechanism in dyslexia, offering an alternative pathway to access meaning despite phonological difficulties. Further research should investigate the functional connectivity between the left IFG and the occipito-temporal cortex in high-achieving adults with dyslexia to directly test the interactive compensatory hypothesis within the predictive coding framework.

Cavalli and colleagues are not alone in highlighting the potential role of morphological knowledge in reading compensation for adults with dyslexia. Casalis et al. (2009) proposed that individuals with dyslexia differ from typical readers in the cognitive processes they engage during reading. Specifically, they may rely on morphological decomposition during initial visual word recognition, as opposed to phonological decoding. This reliance on morphology is thought to compensate for impaired grapheme–phoneme mapping, providing an alternative route for lexical access early in life. Similar findings have been reported across different languages, supporting the hypothesis that MP serves as a compensatory mechanism in dyslexia (see Law et al., 2015; Law & Ghesquière, 2022; Leikin & Zur Hagit, 2006; Tsesmeli & Seymour, 2006).

Recent theoretical perspectives on reading models provide further support for the role of morphological knowledge in compensatory mechanisms for dyslexia. A revised conceptualization of the DRM of reading (Coltheart et al., 2001) suggests that individuals with dyslexia, due to their phonological impairment, struggle to rely on the sub-lexical route, which involves decoding prior to lexical access. Consequently, they predominantly utilize the lexical route, which is hypothesized to encompass not only direct word recognition but also indirect access through complex graphemes and morphemes (Grainger & Ziegler, 2011). Empirical evidence supports this theoretical framework. A meta-analysis of neuroimaging studies by Jobard, Crivello, and Tzourio-Mazoyer (2003) validated the DRM at the neural level, demonstrating the existence of two distinct reading pathways: the ventral direct/lexical route, which involves the inferior occipito-temporo-frontal regions, and the dorsal indirect/sub-lexical route, which engages the superior parieto-temporo-frontal regions. Notably, recent tractography studies further corroborate the efficiency of the direct lexical route in adults with dyslexia. Vandermosten et al. (2012) found no difference between dyslexics and controls in fractional anisotropy of the left inferior fronto-occipital fasciculus, a critical tract supporting the ventral route. These findings align with the Grainger and Ziegler (2011) model, suggesting that the direct route linking the inferior frontal and occipito-temporal regions remains intact in adults with dyslexia and may serve as a compensatory mechanism for orthographic processing difficulties (Hoeft et al., 2011).

Beyond the studies highlighting relative strengths in morphological awareness and processing in adults with dyslexia, additional evidence supporting morphology's role in compensation comes from the pioneering work of Elbro and Arnbak (1996). Their research demonstrated that MP facilitates reading performance in dyslexic individuals, particularly through the use of semantically transparent morphemes. In their first study, dyslexic adolescents exhibited greater improvements in reading speed when processing words with clear morphological structures compared to matched control words. Notably, this increase in reading speed correlated with improvements in reading comprehension, a pattern that was not observed in non-dyslexic controls. A second study further confirmed this hypothesis. Dyslexic participants performed significantly better when reading texts segmented into morphemes compared to texts segmented into syllables, whereas reading-level-matched controls exhibited the opposite trend.

However, not all studies have provided consistent evidence supporting the compensatory role of MP in dyslexia. For instance, Deacon, Parrila, and Kirby (2006) found no evidence that adults with dyslexia benefit from morphological facilitation during a lexical decision task. Their results suggested that, unlike typical adult readers who demonstrate sensitivity to the derivational structure of written words, high-functioning dyslexic individuals do not exhibit the same advantage. Based on these findings, Deacon and colleagues concluded that MP may not universally serve as a compensatory mechanism in dyslexia, and its effectiveness may depend on individual differences or specific task demands.

3.4.2 Syntax in Dyslexia

Research on the syntactic abilities of individuals with dyslexia has consistently shown differences in syntactic processing compared to typical readers. Studies have reported deficits across various tasks, including sentence correction, grammatical acceptability, and sentence judgment (Badian, Duffy, Als, & McAnulty, 1991; Gottardo, Siegel, & Stanovich, 1997; Leikin & Assayag-Bouskila, 2004). Moreover, these deficits appear to persist across the lifespan, affecting both spoken and written modalities (Casalis, Leuwers, & Hilton, 2013; Leikin & Assayag-Bouskila, 2004; Wiseheart, Altmann, Park, & Lombardino, 2009; Nation & Snowling, 2000). A study by Wiseheart et al. (2009) examined the impact of syntactic complexity on written sentence comprehension in university students with dyslexia. Their findings confirmed the presence of syntactic processing difficulties even among high-achieving university students with dyslexia. However, they attributed these difficulties primarily to limitations in working memory and decoding rather than a fundamental syntactic impairment. Consistent with this, Robertson and Joanisse (2010) found that children with dyslexia comprehended sentences comparably to their non-dyslexic peers when working memory demands were controlled.

More recently, the study by Gavard et al. (2025), which we presented in the previous section, explored the neural mechanisms underlying semantic and syntactic prediction in reading and their potential link to domain-general statistical learning (SL) abilities. The study investigated whether individuals with dyslexia rely more heavily on semantic or syntactic prediction as a compensatory strategy during reading. Using fMRI, 50 university students (25 typical readers and 25 dyslexic readers) performed a predictive reading task in which target words appeared within semantically related or unrelated words or in syntactically correct or incorrect sentences. Additionally, participants completed a serial reaction time (SRT) task to assess SL abilities. The results revealed distinct neural networks for semantic and syntactic prediction, reinforcing prior research on their dissociation. Whole-brain and region-of-interest (ROI) analyses showed significant group differences in predictive reading, particularly in the left precentral gyrus and right anterior insula. Furthermore, in typical readers, predictive reading was linked to SL abilities in the left precentral gyrus, whereas dyslexic readers showed associations in multiple brain regions, including the left inferior frontal gyrus (BA47), right inferior frontal gyrus (BA44), left medial frontal gyrus, left fusiform gyrus, and left lingual gyrus. These findings suggest that dyslexic readers do not rely on predictive mechanisms to compensate for lower-level orthographic and articulatory deficits in single-word reading. However, their neural responses indicate that they process predictive sentences and sequences effectively, comparable to typical readers. This supports the idea that compensatory strategies in dyslexia function primarily at the sentence level rather than at the individual word level.

Despite extensive research on written syntactic skills in dyslexia, spoken language production remains relatively underexplored. Notably, a Dutch study by Tops, Callens, Bijn, and Brysbaert (2012) examined morpho-syntactic production using a dictation task in university students with dyslexia. The study found that while dyslexic students made fewer grammatical errors than their control peers, they produced more phonological and orthographic errors, suggesting that they capitalize on morpho-syntactic rules and leverage morphological knowledge in language production. These results align with the idea that dyslexic individuals develop compensatory language strategies to offset reading difficulties, relying on intact oral language skills. More recently, Wiseheart and Altmann (2017) investigated spoken sentence production in college students with dyslexia, assessing fluency, grammaticality, and completeness. Dyslexic students exhibited slower response times and reduced precision in sentence production compared to controls. The primary predictors of precision and efficiency were working memory, which differed between groups, and vocabulary, which did not. These results indicate that working memory deficits play a significant role in sentence formulation difficulties, but strong vocabulary skills may help mitigate some of these challenges. This aligns with findings suggesting that greater vocabulary knowledge is associated with enhanced lexical and grammatical competence (Bates et al., 1995). Moreover, Rose and Rouhani (2012) proposed that the relationship between vocabulary and working memory strengthens during adolescence, which may explain why some dyslexic individuals can partially compensate for working memory deficits through enhanced vocabulary knowledge. These findings suggest that vocabulary plays a crucial compensatory role, potentially counteracting verbal working memory limitations. From a clinical perspective, Wiseheart and Altmann (2017) recommended that interventions focusing on vocabulary development could improve spoken language fluency in individuals with dyslexia, providing an effective strategy to enhance communication skills despite underlying cognitive constraints.

3.5 Implications for Practice and Intervention

Although significant progress has been made in understanding oral language skills in adults with dyslexia, critical gaps remain, limiting both intervention strategies and assessment methods across different age and language groups. These limitations continue to impede the integration of oral language instruction into traditional remediation programs, restricting its potential to support reading and linguistic development in dyslexic individuals.

This chapter highlights the increasing body of evidence supporting morphology as a compensatory mechanism in adults with dyslexia. Research on MP and reading in dyslexic adults continues to provide valuable insights into how morphological awareness contributes to academic success. The benefits of morphological instruction have also been demonstrated in children, as evidenced by a meta-analysis conducted by Bowers, Kirby, and Deacon (2010). Their study examined the impact of morphological training on reading, spelling, vocabulary, and morphological skills in school-aged children, revealing significant improvements across all learners, with the greatest benefits observed in struggling readers. Although the review focused on children from preschool to Grade 8, the findings suggest that morphological instruction could be effective across all age groups, including adults.

More recently, Colenbrander et al. (2024) conducted a pre-registered meta-analysis assessing the effectiveness of morphology instruction on literacy outcomes in primary school children in English-speaking countries. Their study examined reading and spelling improvements while also exploring whether knowledge transferred to untrained words and broader reading comprehension. The analysis included twenty-eight studies with 177 effect sizes, applying robust variance estimation methods to account for data dependencies. Results indicated that morphology instruction had a small to moderate positive effect on reading and spelling, with greater benefits for explicitly taught words. While spelling improvements transferred to untrained words, such transfer was not observed for reading outcomes, suggesting that morphology instruction primarily enhances trained vocabulary rather than general reading skills. Moreover, no significant effects were found for reading comprehension, highlighting potential limitations in the broader application of morphological instruction.

A key challenge identified in the meta-analysis was the high level of heterogeneity and imprecision across studies due to variations in intervention content, dosage, outcome measures, and control group types. The authors emphasized the need for rigorously designed research to identify key components of effective morphology instruction and better understand knowledge transfer and retention patterns. They also stressed the importance of pre-registration, data transparency, and detailed reporting to improve the reliability of future research. While the meta-analysis supports morphology instruction as a tool to improve reading and spelling, further research is necessary to refine instructional methods, assess long-term effects, and clarify its role within broader literacy programs.

In a similar vein, Goodwin and Ahn (2010) conducted a meta-analysis of 17 studies on morphological intervention in children with literacy difficulties (kindergarten to ninth grade). Their findings demonstrated significant improvements in phonological and morphological awareness, vocabulary, reading comprehension, and spelling, though no effects were found for reading fluency or decoding. Interestingly, morphological instruction was particularly effective for children with reading, learning, and speech and language disabilities, reinforcing its potential for targeted intervention in dyslexic populations.

Despite these promising results, research on oral morphological training in dyslexic individuals remains scarce, particularly in adolescents and adults. To date, the only study explicitly targeting dyslexic participants was conducted by Arnbak and Elbro (2000), which examined the effects of oral morphological training on children with dyslexia (Grades 4 and 5). Their study found positive effects on morphological awareness, reading comprehension, word reading, and spelling accuracy, providing early evidence of the educational benefits of morphological instruction. However, the lack of research exploring these interventions in older populations highlights the need for further studies across different age groups, languages, and ability levels. Addressing these research gaps would provide a more comprehensive understanding of morphology's role in literacy development and help refine intervention strategies for individuals with dyslexia.

3.6 Conclusion

This review highlights the significant influence of early oral language skills on later word reading and reading comprehension development. Since reading and oral language share many cognitive and linguistic processes, understanding how broad oral language abilities contribute to reading acquisition is essential for the study, assessment, and intervention of reading disabilities. Despite this established relationship, research on semantic, morphological, and syntactic skills in adults with dyslexia remains limited, restricting our understanding of oral language's role in reading compensation in this population.

A major challenge in this area of research is the lack of well-validated oral language assessment tools, which limits their applicability in clinical and educational settings. Additionally, screening and diagnostic tests for oral language skills are scarce outside of English and Dutch, making cross-linguistic comparisons difficult. Another complication arises in the longitudinal assessment of oral language skills in adults, as standardized comprehension tests for this age group are largely absent. Moreover, existing assessments may measure abilities beyond oral language, such as executive functions, phonological processing, and memory, which are often impaired in individuals with dyslexia and may confound results.

Despite these challenges, emerging evidence suggests that vocabulary and MP strengths play a role in reading compensation among university students with dyslexia (e.g., Law et al., 2015; Cavalli et al., 2016b). These findings raise important questions about whether targeted oral language training could serve as an effective remediation strategy to support the reading development of dyslexic adults. While theoretically promising, future research is needed to systematically evaluate the impact of oral language interventions in mitigating reading difficulties and enhancing literacy outcomes for adults with dyslexia.

References

Adlof, S. M., Catts, H. W., & Lee, J. (2010). Kindergarten predictors of second versus eighth grade reading comprehension impairments. *Journal of Learning Disabilities*, *43*(4), 332–345.

Arnbak, E., & Elbro, C. (2000). The effects of morphological awareness training on the reading and spelling skills of young dyslexics. *Scandinavian Journal of Educational Research*, *44*, 229–251.

Badian, N. A., Duffy, F. H., Als, H., & McAnulty, G. B. (1991). Linguistic profiles of dyslexic and good readers. *Annals of Dyslexia*, *41*(1), 221–245.

Bates, E., Burani, C., D'Amico, S., & Barca, L. (1995). Word reading and picture naming in Italian. *Memory & Cognition, 23*(4), 451–461.

Baumann, J. F., Edwards, E. C., Boland, E. M., Olejnik, S., & Kame'enui, E. J. (2002). Vocabulary tricks: Effects of instruction in morphology and context on fifth-grade students' ability to derive and infer word meanings. *American Educational Research Journal, 39*(3), 447–478.

Berko, J. (1958). The child's learning of English morphology. *Word, 14*(2–3), 150–177.

Berman, R. A. (2007). Developing linguistic knowledge and language use across adolescence. In E. Hoff & M. Shatz (Eds.), *Blackwell handbook of language development* (pp. 347–367). Oxford: Blackwell.

Berninger, V. W., Abbott, R. D., Abbott, S. P., Graham, S., & Richards, T. (2001). Writing and reading: Connections between language by hand and language by eye. *Journal of Learning Disabilities, 34*(1), 39–58.

Berthiaume, R., & Daigle, D. (2014). Are dyslexic children sensitive to the morphological structure of words when they read? The case of dyslexic readers of French. *Dyslexia, 20*(3), 241–260.

Betjemann, R. S., & Keenan, J. M. (2008). Phonological and semantic priming in children with reading disability. *Child Development, 79*(4), 1086–1102.

Beyersmann, E., Castles, A., & Coltheart, M. (2014). Morphological processing during visual word identification: Evidence from masked priming. *Quarterly Journal of Experimental Psychology, 67*(4), 683–692.

Boets, B., de Beeck, H. P. O., Vandermosten, M., Scott, S. K., Gillebert, C. R., Mantini, D., & Ghesquière, P. (2013). Intact but less accessible phonetic representations in adults with dyslexia. *Science, 342*(6163), 1251–1254.

Bowers, P. N., & Kirby, J. R. (2010). Effects of morphological instruction on vocabulary acquisition. *Reading and Writing, 23*(5), 515–537.

Bowers, P., Kirby, J., & Deacon, H. (2010). The effects of morphological instruction on literacy skills: A systematic review of the literature. *Review of Educational Research, 80*, 144–179.

Braze, D., Tabor, W., Shankweiler, D. P., & Mencl, W. E. (2007). Speaking up for vocabulary: Reading skill differences in young adults. *Journal of Learning Disabilities, 40*(3), 226–243.

Brimo, D., Apel, K., & Fountain, T. (2017). Examining the contributions of syntactic awareness and syntactic knowledge to reading comprehension. *Journal of Research in Reading, 40*, 57–74. https://doi.org/10.1111/1467-9817.12050

Brunswick, N., McCrory, E., Price, C. J., Frith, C. D., & Frith, U. (1999). Explicit and implicit processing of words and pseudowords by adult developmental dyslexics: A search for Wernicke's Wortschatz? *Brain, 122*(10), 1901–1917. https://doi.org/10.1093/brain/122.10.1901

Burani, C., Marcolini, S., De Luca, M., & Zoccolotti, P. (2008). Morpheme-based reading aloud: Evidence from dyslexic and skilled Italian readers. *Cognition, 108*(1), 243–262.

Cain, K. (2011). *Reading development and difficulties*. Wiley-Blackwell.

Cain, K., Oakhill, J., & Bryant, P. (2004). Children's reading comprehension ability: Concurrent prediction by working memory, verbal ability, and component skills. *Journal of Educational Psychology, 96*(1), 31–42.

Carlisle, J. F. (2000). Awareness of the structure and meaning of morphologically complex words: Impact on reading. *Reading and Writing: An Interdisciplinary Journal, 12*(3), 169–190.

Carlisle, J. F. (2007). Fostering morphological processing, vocabulary development, and reading comprehension. In R. K. Wagner, A. E. Muse, & K. R. Tannenbaum (Eds.), *Vocabulary acquisition: Implications for reading comprehension* (pp. 78–103). New York, NY: Guilford Press.

Carlisle, J. F., & Feldman, L. B. (1995). Morphological awareness and early reading achievement. In L. B. Feldman (Ed.), *Morphological aspects of language processing* (pp. 189–209). Hillsdale, NJ: Lawrence Erlbaum Associates.

Carlisle, J. F., & Fleming, J. E. (2003). Lexical processing of morphologically complex words in the elementary years. *Scientific Studies of Reading*, 7(3), 239–253.

Carlisle, J. F., & Nomanbhoy, D. M. (1993). Phonological and morphological awareness in first graders. *Applied PsychoLinguistics*, 14(2), 177–195. https://doi.org/10.1017/S0142716400009541

Carlisle, J. F., & Stone, C. A. (2005). Exploring the role of morphemes in word reading. *Reading Research Quarterly*, 40(4), 428–449.

Carreiras, M., Armstrong, B. C., Perea, M., & Frost, R. (2014). The what, when, where, and how of visual word recognition. *Trends in Cognitive Sciences*, 18(2), 90–98.

Carroll, J., Holden, C., Kirby, P., Thompson, P. A., & Snowling, M. J. (2024). Towards a consensus on dyslexia: Findings from a Delphi study. OSF Preprints. https://osf.io/preprints/osf/tb8mp

Casalis, S., Dusautoir, M., Colé, P., & Ducrot, S. (2009). Morphological effects in children word reading: A priming study in fourth graders. *British Journal of Developmental Psychology*, 27(3), 761–766.

Casalis, S., Leuwers, C., & Hilton, H. (2013). Syntactic comprehension in reading and listening: A study with French children with dyslexia. *Journal of Learning Disabilities*, 46(3), 210–219.

Casalis, S., & Louis-Alexandre, M. F. (2000). Morphological analysis, phonological analysis, and learning to read French: A longitudinal study. *Reading and Writing: An Interdisciplinary Journal*, 12(3), 303–335.

Casalis, S., Sopo, D., & Colé, P. (2004). Morphological awareness in developmental dyslexia. *L'Année Psychologique*, 104(4), 469–487.

Catts, H. W. (2021). Commentary: The critical role of oral language deficits in reading disorders: Reflections on Snowling and Hulme (2021). *Journal of Child Psychology and Psychiatry*, 62(5), 654–656. https://doi.org/10.1111/JCPP.13389

Catts, H. W., Fey, M. E., Tomblin, J. B., & Zhang, X. (2002). A longitudinal investigation of reading outcomes in children with language impairments. *Journal of Speech, Language, and Hearing Research*, 45(6), 1142–1157.

Catts, H. W., Fey, M. E., Zhang, X., & Tomblin, J. B. (1999). Language basis of reading and reading disabilities: Evidence from a longitudinal investigation. *Scientific Studies of Reading*, 3(4), 331–361.

Cavalli, E., Chanoine, V., Anton, J.-L., Tan, Y., Ziegler, J. C., & et al. (2024). Atypical hemispheric re-organization of the reading network in high-functioning adults with dyslexia: Evidence from representational similarity analysis. *Imaging Neuroscience*. Advance online publication.

Cavalli, E., & Colé, P. (2018). Les dyslexies chez l'adulte. In S. Casalis (Ed.), *Les Dyslexies*. Elsevier Masson.

Cavalli, E., Colé, P., Badier, J.-M., Zielinski, C., Chanoine, V., & Ziegler, J. C. (2016a). Spatiotemporal dynamics of morphological processing in visual word recognition: An MEG study. *Cortex*, 74, 25–38.

Cavalli, E., Colé, P., Badier, J.-M., Zielinski, C., Chanoine, V., & Ziegler, J. C. (2016b). Spatiotemporal dynamics of morphological processing in visual word recognition: An MEG study. *Journal of Cognitive Neuroscience*, 28(8), 1228–1242.

Cavalli, E., Colé, P., Pattamadilok, C., Badier, J.-M., Zielinski, C., Chanoine, V., & Ziegler, J. C. (2017). Spatiotemporal reorganization of the reading network in adult dyslexia. *Cortex*, 92. https://doi.org/10.1016/j.cortex.2017.04.012

Cavalli, E., Duncan, L. G., Elbro, C., El Ahmadi, A., & Colé, P. (2017). Phonemic–morphological dissociation in university students with dyslexia: An index of reading compensation? *Annals of Dyslexia*, 67(1), 63–84. https://doi.org/10.1007/s11881-016-0138-y

Colé, P., Cavalli, E., Duncan, L. G., Theurel, A., Gentaz, E., Sprenger-Charolles, L., & Ahmadi, E. (2018). What is the influence of morphological knowledge in the early stages of reading acquisition among low SES children? A graphical modelling approach. *Frontiers in Psychology, 9*, 547.

Colenbrander, D., Anglim, J., Bellocchi, S., & Crewther, S. G. (2024). The effectiveness of morphology instruction for improving literacy outcomes: A pre-registered meta-analysis. *Reading Research Quarterly. Advance online publication.* https://doi.org/10.1002/rrq.599

Coltheart, M., Rastle, K., Perry, C., Langdon, R., & Ziegler, J. (2001). DRC: A dual route cascaded model of visual word recognition and reading aloud. *Psychological Review, 108*(1), 204.

Corkett, J. K., & Parrila, R. (2008). Use of context in the word recognition process by adults with a significant history of reading difficulties. *Annals of Dyslexia, 58*(2), 139–161.

Crosson, A. C., & McKeown, M. G. (2016). Morphological instruction in vocabulary learning: Development and examination of a pedagogical framework. *Contemporary Educational Psychology, 44–45*, 167–178. https://doi.org/10.1016/j.cedpsych.2016.02.003

Cutting, L. E., & Scarborough, H. S. (2012). Multiple bases for comprehension difficulties: The potential of cognitive and neurobiological profiling for validation of subtypes and development of assessments. In J. Sabatini, T. O'Reilly, & E. R. Albro (Eds.), *Reaching an understanding* (pp. 101–116). Lanham MD: Rowman & Littlefield Education.

Dapretto, M., & Bookheimer, S. Y. (1999). Form and content: Dissociating syntax and semantics in sentence comprehension. *Neuron, 24*(2), 427–432. 10.1016/S0896-6273(00)80855-7

Dawson, N., Rastle, K., & Ricketts, J. (2017). Morphological effects in visual word recognition: Children, adolescents, and adults. *Journal of Experimental Psychology: Learning, Memory, and Cognition, 44*(4), 645–654.

Deacon, S. H., Benere, J., & Pasquarella, A. (2013). Reciprocal relationship: Children's morphological awareness and their reading accuracy across grades 2 to 3. *Developmental Psychology, 49*(6), 1113.

Deacon, S. H., & Kieffer, M. J. (2018). Understanding how syntactic awareness contributes to reading comprehension: Evidence from a longitudinal study. *Journal of Educational Psychology, 110*(2), 240–256.

Deacon, S. H., Kieffer, M. J., & Laroche, A. (2017). The influence of morphological awareness on word reading and reading comprehension: A longitudinal examination of mediation. *Journal of Educational Psychology, 109*(5), 669–681.

Deacon, S. H., & Kirby, J. R. (2004). Morphological awareness: Just "more phonological"? The roles of morphological and phonological awareness in reading development. *Applied PsychoLinguistics, 25*(2), 223–238.

Deacon, S. H., Kirby, J. R., & Parrila, R. K. (2006). Decomposing the relationships between morphological awareness, vocabulary, and reading. *Canadian Journal of Behavioural Science / Revue canadienne des sciences du comportement, 38*(4), 271–284.

Deacon, S. H., Parrila, R., & Kirby, J. R. (2006). Processing of derived forms in high-functioning dyslexics. *Annals of Dyslexia, 56*(1), 103–128.

Dickinson, D. K., McCabe, A., Anastasopoulos, L., Peisner-Feinberg, E. S., & Poe, M. D. (2003). The comprehensive language approach to early literacy: The interrelationships among vocabulary, phonological sensitivity, and print knowledge among preschool-aged children. *Journal of Educational Psychology, 95*(3), 465–481.

Diependaele, K., Sandra, D., & Grainger, J. (2005). Masked cross-modal morphological priming: Evidence for morpho-orthographic decomposition in visual word recognition. *Journal of Memory and Language, 53*(2), 257–277.

Diependaele, K., Sandra, D., & Grainger, J. (2009). Semantic transparency and masked morphological priming: The case of prefixed words. *Memory & Cognition, 37*(6), 895–908.

Duñabeitia, J. A., Perea, M., & Carreiras, M. (2007). Do transposed-letter similarity effects occur at a morpheme level? *Evidence for morpho-orthographic decomposition. Cognition, 105*(3), 691–703.

Elbro, C. (1989). Morphological awareness in dyslexia. In *Brain and language* (pp. 279–291). Palgrave Macmillan.

Elbro, C., & Arnbak, E. (1996). The role of morpheme recognition and morphological awareness in dyslexia. *Annals of Dyslexia, 46*(1), 209–240.

Elbro, C., Nielsen, I., & Petersen, D. K. (1994). Dyslexia in adults: Evidence for deficits in non-word reading and the phonological representation of lexical items. *Annals of Dyslexia, 44*, 205–226.

Farris, E. A., Cristan, T., Bernstein, S. E., et al. (2021). Morphological awareness and vocabulary predict reading resilience in adults. *Annals of Dyslexia, 71*(3), 347–371. https://doi.org/10.1007/s11881-021-00236-y

Foorman, B. R., Koon, S., Petscher, Y., Mitchell, A., & Truckenmiller, A. (2015). Examining general and specific factors in the dimensionality of oral language and reading in 4th–10th grades. *Journal of Educational Psychology, 107*(3), 884.

Fowler, A. E., Liberman, I. Y., & Feldman, L. (1995). The role of phonology and orthography in morphological awareness. In *Morphological aspects of language processing* (pp. 157–188).Hillsdale, NJ: Lawrence Erlbaum Associates.

Fruchter, J., & Marantz, A. (2015). Decomposition, lookup, and recombination: MEG evidence for the full decomposition model of complex visual word recognition. *Brain and Language, 143*, 81–96.

Funnell, E. (1996). Response biases in oral reading: The effect of word frequency on oral reading errors in deep dyslexia. *Cognitive Neuropsychology, 13*(3), 401–422.

Garcia, J. R., & Cain, K. (2014). Decoding and reading comprehension: A meta-analysis to identify which reader and assessment characteristics influence the strength of the relationship in English. *Review of Educational Research, 84*(1), 74–111.

Gavard, E., Chanoine, V., Geringswald, F., Anton, J-L., Cavalli, E., & Ziegler, J. C. (2025) (accepted with minor reviews). Neural networks for semantic and syntactic prediction and visuo-motor statistical learning in adult readers with and without dyslexia. *Neurobiology of Language*, 1–34.

Geva, E., & Farnia, F. (2012). Developmental changes in the nature of language proficiency and reading fluency paint a more complex view of reading comprehension in ELL and EL1. *Reading and Writing, 25*(8), 1819–1845.

Goodwin, A. P., & Ahn, S. (2010). A meta-analysis of morphological interventions: Effects on literacy achievement of children with literacy difficulties. *Annals of Dyslexia, 60*(2), 183–208.

Goodwin, A. P., Lipsky, M., & Ahn, S. (2012). Word detectives: Using units of meaning to support literacy. *Reading Teacher, 65*(7), 461–470.

Goswami, U. (2001). Early phonological development and the acquisition of literacy. *Handbook of early literacy research* (Vol. 1, pp. 111–125). New York, NY: Guilford Press.

Gottardo, A., Siegel, L. S., & Stanovich, K. E. (1997). The assessment of adults with reading disabilities: What can we learn from experimental tasks? *Journal of Research in Reading, 20*(1), 42–54.

Gough, P. B., & Tunmer, W. E. (1986). Decoding, reading, and reading disability. *Remedial and Special Education, 7*(1), 6–10.

Grainger, J., & Beyersmann, E. (2017). Edge-aligned embedded word activation initiates morpho-orthographic segmentation. In B. Ross (Ed.), *Psychology of learning and motivation* (pp. 285–312). Cambridge: Academic Press.

Grainger, J., & Ziegler, J. C. (2011). A dual-route approach to orthographic processing. *Frontiers in Psychology*, *2*, 1–13.

Guo, Y., Roehrig, A. D., & Williams, R. S. (2011). The relation of morphological awareness and syntactic awareness to adults' Reading comprehension. *Journal of Literacy Research*, *43*(2), 159–183. https://doi.org/10.1177/1086296X11403086

Haft, S. L., Myers, C. A., & Hoeft, F. (2016). Socio-emotional and cognitive resilience in children with reading disabilities. *Current Opinion in Behavioral Sciences*, *10*, 133–141.

Hancock, R., Gabrieli, J. D. E., & Hoeft, F. (2017). Shared temporoparietal dysfunction in dyslexia and typical readers with discrepantly high IQ. *Trends in Neuroscience and Education*, *6*(3), 91–99. https://doi.org/10.1016/j.tine.2016.11.002

Hatcher, J., Snowling, M. J., & Griffiths, Y. M. (2002). Cognitive assessment of dyslexic students in higher education. *British Journal of Educational Psychology*, *72*(1), 119–133.

Helenius, P., Salmelin, R., Service, E., & Connolly, J. F. (1999). Semantic cortical activation in dyslexic readers. *Journal of Cognitive Neuroscience*, 11(5), 535–550. https://doi.org/10.1162/089892999563652

Hoeft, F., McCandliss, B. D., Black, J. M., Gantman, A., Zakerani, N., Hulme, C., et al. (2011). Neural systems predicting long-term outcome in dyslexia. *Proceedings of the National Academy of Sciences of the United States of America*, *108*, 361–366.

Hoover, W. A. (2023). The simple view of reading: Three decades later. *Reading and Writing*, *36*(2), 241–263.

Hoover, W. A., & Gough, P. B. (1990). The simple view of reading. *Reading and Writing: An Interdisciplinary Journal*, *2*, 127–160.

Hulme, C., & Snowling, M. J. (2013). Learning to read: What we know and what we need to understand better. *Child Development Perspectives*, *7*, 1–5.

Jobard, G., Crivello, F., & Tzourio-Mazoyer, N. (2003). Evaluation of the dual route theory of reading: A metanalysis of 35 neuroimaging studies. *NeuroImage*, *20*, 693e712.

Kim, Y. S. G. (2016). Direct and mediated effects of language and cognitive skills on comprehension of oral narrative texts (listening comprehension) for children. *Journal of Experimental Child Psychology*, *141*, 101–120.

Kinginger, C., & Farrell, K. (2004). Assessing development of meta-pragmatic awareness in study abroad. *Frontiers: The Interdisciplinary Journal of Study Abroad*, *10*, 19–42.

Kintsch, W. (1988). The role of knowledge in discourse comprehension: A construction integration model. *Psychological Review*, *95*, 163–182.

Kintsch & Kintch (2005). In S. G. Paris & S. A. Stahl (Eds.), *Children's reading comprehension and assessment*. Routledge.

Kirby, J. R., & Savage, R. S. (2008). Can the simple view deal with the complexities of reading? *Literacy*, *42*, 75–82.

Kotzer, M., Kirby, J. R., & Heggie, L. (2021). Morphological awareness, vocabulary, and reading comprehension in university students. *Reading and Writing*, *34*(8), 2029–2051.

Kriegeskorte, N., Mur, M., & Bandettini, P. A. (2008). Representational similarity analysis—Connecting the branches of systems neuroscience. *Frontiers in Systems Neuroscience*, *2*, Article 4. https://doi.org/10.3389/neuro.06.004.2008

Law, J. M., & Ghesquière, P. (2017). Early development and predictors of morphological awareness: Disentangling the impact of decoding skills and phonological awareness. *Research in Developmental Disabilities*, *67*, 47–59.

Law, J. M., & Ghesquière, P. (2022). Morphological processing in children with developmental dyslexia: A visual masked priming study. *Reading Research Quarterly*, *57*(3), 863–877.

Law, J. M., Veispak, A., Vanderauwera, J., & Ghesquière, P. (2018). Morphological awareness and visual processing of derivational morphology in high-functioning adults with dyslexia: An avenue to compensation? *Applied PsychoLinguistics*, *39*(3), 483–506.

Law, J. M., Wouters, J., & Ghesquière, P. (2015). Morphological awareness and its role in compensation in adults with dyslexia. *Dyslexia*, *21*(3), 254–272.

Law, J. M., Wouters, J., & Ghesquière, P. (2017). The influences and outcomes of phonological awareness: A study of MA, PA and auditory processing in pre-readers with a family risk of dyslexia. *Dyslexia*, *23*(3), 250–267.

Lázaro, M., García, N., & Defior, S. (2013). Morphological processing in Spanish-speaking children with dyslexia: The role of regularity and frequency. *Annals of Dyslexia*, *63*(2), 151–167.

Lefèvre, E., Law, J. M., Prado, J., Anders, R., & Cavalli, E. (2025). Reading comprehension resiliency in adolescents with and without dyslexia relates to vocabulary, listening comprehension and socioeconomic status. *Learning & Instruction.*, *96*, 102081. https://doi.org/10.1016/j.learninstruc.2025.102081

Lefèvre, E., Law, J. M., Quémart, P., Anders, R., & Cavalli, E. (2022). What's morphology got to do with it: Oral reading fluency in adolescents with dyslexia. *Journal of Experimental Psychology: Learning, Memory, and Cognition*, *49*(8), 1345–1360.

Leikin, M., & Assayag-Bouskila, O. (2004). Expression of syntactic complexity in sentence comprehension: A comparison between dyslexic and regular readers. *Reading and Writing*, *17*(7–8), 801–821.

Leikin, M., & Zur Hagit, E. (2006). Morphological processing in adult dyslexia. *Journal of Psycholinguistic Research*, *35*(6), 471–490.

Lervag, A., Hulme, C., & Melby-Lervag, M. (2017). Unpicking the developmental relationship between oral language skills and reading comprehension: It's simple, but complex. *Child Development*, *89*(5), 1821–1838.

Levesque, K. C., Breadmore, H. L., & Deacon, S. H. (2021). How morphology impacts reading and spelling: Advancing the role of morphology in models of literacy development. *Child Development*, *92*(3), 1048–1062.

Levesque, K. C., & Deacon, S. H. (2022). Clarifying links to literacy: How does morphological awareness support children's word reading development? *Applied PsychoLinguistics*, *43*(4), 921–943.

Levesque, K. C., Kieffer, M. J., & Deacon, S. H. (2017). Morphological awareness and reading comprehension: Examining mediating factors. *Journal of Experimental Child Psychology*, *160*, 1–20.

Levesque, K. C., Kieffer, M. J., & Deacon, S. H. (2019). Inferring meaning from meaningful parts: The contributions of morphological skills to reading comprehension. *Reading Research Quarterly*, *54*(1), 63–80.

Livingston, L. A., & Happé, F. (2017). Conceptualising compensation in neurodevelopmental disorders: Reflections from autism spectrum disorder. *Neuroscience & Biobehavioral Reviews*, *80*, 729–742. https://doi.org/10.1016/j.neubiorev.2017.06.005

Low, P. A., & Siegel, L. S. (2005). A comparison of the cognitive processes underlying reading comprehension in good and poor comprehenders. *Learning and Individual Differences*, *15*(3), 221–239.

Lund, N. J., & Duchan, J. F. (1993). *Assessing children's language in naturalistic contexts*. Prentice Hall.

Lyytinen, H., Ahonen, T., Eklund, K., Guttorm, T. K., Laakso, M. L., Leinonen, S., & Richardson, U. (2001). Developmental pathways of children with and without familial risk for dyslexia during the first years of life. *Developmental Neuropsychology*, *20*(2), 535–554.

MacKay, E., Lynch, E., Duncan, T. S., & Deacon, S. H. (2021). Informing the science of Reading: Students' awareness of sentence-level information is important for Reading comprehension. *Reading Research Quarterly*, *56*, S221–S230. https://doi.org/10.1002/rrq.397

Mahony, D., Singson, M., & Mann, V. (2000). Reading ability and sensitivity to morphological relations. *Reading and Writing*, *12*(3), 191–218.

Marslen-Wilson, W. D., Bozic, M., & Randall, B. (2008). Early decomposition in visual word recognition: Dissociating morphology, form, and meaning. *Language and Cognitive Processes*, *23*(3), 394–421.

Martin, J., Colé, P., Leuwers, C., Casalis, S., & Zorman, M. (2013). Reading in French-speaking adults with dyslexia. *Annals of Dyslexia*, *63*(1), 1–23.

Metsala, J. L. (1999). Young children's phonological awareness and nonword repetition as a function of vocabulary development. *Journal of Educational Psychology*, *91*(1), 3–19.

Metsala, J. L., & Walley, A. C. (1998). Spoken vocabulary growth and the segmental restructuring of lexical representations: Precursors to phonemic awareness and early reading ability. In J. L. Metsala & L. C. Ehri (Eds.), *Word recognition in beginning literacy* (pp. 89–120). Mahwah, NJ: Erlbaum.

Muter, V., Hulme, C., Snowling, M. J., & Stevenson, J. (2004). Phonemes, rimes, vocabulary, and grammatical skills as foundations of early reading development: Evidence from a longitudinal study. *Developmental Psychology*, *40*(5), 665–681.

Nagy, W. E., Berninger, V. W., & Abbott, R. D. (1993). Contributions of morphology beyond phonology to literacy outcomes of upper elementary and middle school students. *Journal of Educational Psychology*, *85*(4), 648–661.

Nagy, W. E., Berninger, V. W., & Abbott, R. D. (2006). Contributions of morphology beyond phonology to literacy outcomes of upper elementary and middle school students. *Journal of Educational Psychology*, *98*(1), 134–147.

Nation, K. (2005). Children's reading comprehension difficulties. In M. J. Snowling & C. Hulme (Eds.), *The science of reading: A handbook* (pp. 248–265). Oxford, UK: Blackwell Publishing.

Nation, K., Cocksey, J., Taylor, J. S., & Bishop, D. V. M. (2010). A longitudinal investigation of early reading and language skills in children with poor reading comprehension. *Journal of Child Psychology and Psychiatry and Allied Disciplines*, *51*(9), 1031–1039.

Nation, K., & Snowling, M. J. (2000). Factors influencing syntactic awareness skills in normal readers and poor comprehenders. *Applied PsychoLinguistics*, *21*(2), 229–241.

Nation, K., & Snowling, M. J. (2004). Beyond phonological skills: Broader language skills contribute to the development of reading. *Journal of Research in Reading*, *27*, 342–356.

Norton, E. S., Beach, S. D., & Gabrieli, J. D. E. (2014). Neurobiology of dyslexia. *Current Opinion in Neurobiology*, *30*, 73–78.

Nunes, T., & Bryant, P. (2006). *Improving literacy by teaching morphemes*. London, UK: Routledge.

Nunes, T., Bryant, P., & Olson, J. (2012). Learning morphological and phonological spelling rules: An intervention study. *Scientific Studies of Reading*, *7*(3), 289–307.

Ouellette, G. P. (2006). What's meaning got to do with it: The role of vocabulary in word reading and reading comprehension. *Journal of Educational Psychology*, *98*(3), 554.

Ouellette, G., & Beers, A. (2010). A not-so-simple view of reading: How oral vocabulary and visual-word recognition complicate the story. *Reading and Writing*, *23*(2), 189–208. https://doi.org/10.1007/s11145-008-9159-1

Pacheco, M. B., & Goodwin, A. P. (2013). Putting two and two together: Middle school students' morphological problem-solving strategies for unknown words. *Journal of Adolescent & Adult Literacy*, *56*(7), 541–553.

Patterson, K., & Hodges, J. R. (1992). Deterioration of word meaning: Implications for reading. *Neuropsychologia*, *30*(12), 1025–1040.

Paz-Alonso, P. M., Oliver, M., Lerma-Usabiaga, G., Caballero-Gaudes, C., Quinones, I., Suarez-Coalla, P., Duñabeitia, J. A., Cuetos, F., Carreiras, M., & Laka, I. (2018). Neural correlates of phonological, orthographic, and semantic reading processing in dyslexia. *NeuroImage: Clinical*, *20*, 433–447. https://doi.org/10.1016/j.nicl.2018.08.021

Perfetti, C., & Stafura, J. (2014). Word knowledge in a theory of reading comprehension. *Scientific Studies of Reading*, *18*(1), 22–37.

Price, C. J., & Devlin, J. T. (2011). The interactive account of ventral occipitotemporal contributions to reading. *Trends in Cognitive Sciences*, *15*(6), 246–253. https://doi.org/10.1016/j.tics.2011.04.001

Quémart, P., & Casalis, S. (2015). Sensitivity to morphological structure in children with developmental dyslexia: Evidence from masked priming. *Annals of Dyslexia*, *65*(1), 15–33.

Ralph, M. A. L., Patterson, K., Rogers, T. T., & McClelland, J. L. (2004). Semantic dementia and the distributed neural system for conceptual knowledge. *Philosophical Transactions of the Royal Society of London. Series B: Biological Sciences*, *359*(1451), 1207–1214.

Ramus, F., & Szenkovits, G. (2008). What phonological deficit? *The Quarterly Journal of Experimental Psychology*, *61*(1), 129–141.

Ransby, M. J., & Swanson, H. L. (2003). Reading comprehension skills of young adults with childhood diagnoses of dyslexia. *Journal of Learning Disabilities*, *36*(6), 538–555.

Rasch, G. (1960 [1980]). *Probabilistic models for some intelligence and attainment tests*. Copenhagen: Danmarks Paedagogiske Institute (Reprinted by University of Chicago, 1980).

Rastle, K., & Davis, M. H. (2008). Morphological decomposition based on the analysis of orthography. *Language and Cognitive Processes*, *23*(7–8), 942–971.

Rastle, K., Davis, M. H., Marslen-Wilson, W. D., & Tyler, L. K. (2000). Morphological and semantic effects in visual word recognition: A time-course study. *Language and Cognitive Processes*, *15*(4–5), 507–537.

Rastle, K., Davis, M. H., & New, B. (2004). The broth in my brother's brothel: Morpho-orthographic segmentation in visual word recognition. *Psychonomic Bulletin & Review*, *11*(6), 1090–1098.

Raveh, M., & Schiff, R. (2008). Morphology in word reading and spelling: Evidence from Hebrew. *Reading and Writing: An Interdisciplinary Journal*, *21*(8), 779–794.

Richlan, F., Kronbichler, M., & Wimmer, H. (2009). Functional abnormalities in the dyslexic brain: A quantitative meta-analysis of neuroimaging studies. *Human Brain Mapping*, *30*(10), 3299–3308. https://doi.org/10.1002/hbm.20752

Richlan, F., Kronbichler, M., & Wimmer, H. (2011). Meta-analyzing brain dysfunctions in dyslexic children and adults. *NeuroImage*, *56*(3), 1735–1742. https://doi.org/10.1016/j.neuroimage.2011.02.040

Ricketts, J., Nation, K., & Bishop, D. V. M. (2007). Vocabulary is important for some, but not all reading skills. *Scientific Studies of Reading*, *11*(3), 235–257.

Robertson, E. K., & Joanisse, M. F. (2010). Spoken sentence comprehension in children with dyslexia and language impairment: The roles of syntax and working memory. *Applied PsychoLinguistics*, *31*(1), 141–165.

Roman, A., Kirby, J., Parrila, R., Wade-Woolley, L., & Deacon, S. H. (2009). Towards a comprehensive view of the skills involved in word reading in grades 4, 6, and 8. *Journal of Experimental Child Psychology*, *102*, 96–113.

Rose, L. T., & Rouhani, P. (2012). Influence of verbal working memory depends on vocabulary: Oral reading fluency in adolescents with dyslexia. *Mind, Brain, and Education*, *6*(1), 1–9. http://doi.org/10.1111/j.1751-228X.2011.01135.x

Roth, F. P., Speece, D. L., & Cooper, D. H. (2002). A longitudinal analysis of the connection between oral language and early reading. *The Journal of Educational Research*, *95*(5), 259–272.

Rüsseler, J., Becker, P., Johannes, S., & Münte, T. F. (2007). Semantic, syntactic, and phonological processing of written words in adult developmental dyslexic readers: An event-related brain potential study. *BMC Neuroscience*, *8*, 52. https://doi.org/10.1186/1471-2202-8-52

Sachs, J. S. (1967). Recognition of semantic, syntactic, and lexical changes in sentences. *Psychonmic Bulletin*, *1*, 17–18.

Salmelin, R., Service, E., Kiesilä, P., Uutela, K., & Salonen, O. (1996). Impaired visual word processing in dyslexia revealed with magnetoencephalography. *Annals of Neurology*, *40*(2), 157–162.

Scarborough, H. S. (2005). Development of early literacy: Toward a unified model of reading. In S. B. Neuman & D. K. Dickinson (Eds.), *Handbook of early literacy research* (Vol. 1, pp. 97–110). New York, NY: Guilford Press.

Schiff, R., & Raveh, M. (2007). Deficient morphological processing in adults with developmental dyslexia: Another barrier to efficient word recognition? *Dyslexia*, *13*(2), 110–129.

Seidenberg, M. S. (2006). Connectionist models of reading. In G. Gaskell (Ed.), *The Oxford handbook of psycholinguistics* (pp. 235–250). Oxford: Oxford University Press.

Seidenberg, M. S., & McClelland, J. L. (1989). A distributed, developmental model of word recognition and naming. *Psychological Review*, *96*(4), 523.

Seigneuric, A., & Ehrlich, M.-F. (2005). Contribution of working memory capacity to children's reading comprehension: A longitudinal investigation. *Reading and Writing*, *18*(7–9), 617–656.

Semel, E., Wiig, E. H., & Secord, W. A. (2003). *Clinical evaluation of language fundamentals, fourth edition (CELF-4)*. Toronto, Canada: The Psychological Corporation/A Harcourt Assessment Company.

Sénéchal, M., Ouellette, G., & Rodney, D. (2006). The misunderstood giant: On the predictive role of early vocabulary to future reading. In S. B. Neuman & D. K. Dickinson (Eds.), *Handbook of early literacy research* (Vol. 2, pp. 173–182). New York, NY: Guilford Press.

Share, D. L. (1995). Phonological recoding and self-teaching: Sine qua non of reading acquisition. *Cognition*, *55*(2), 151–218.

Share, D. L., & Leikin, M. (2004). How reading begins: A study of preschoolers' print identification strategies. *Developmental Psychology*, *40*(6), 875–889.

Share, D. L., & Silva, P. A. (1987). Language deficits and specific reading retardation: Cause or effect? *British Journal of Disorders of Communication*, *22*, 219–226.

Shaywitz, B. A., Shaywitz, S. E., Pugh, K. R., Mencl, W. E., Fulbright, R. K., Skudlarski, P., Constable, R. T., Marchione, K. E., Fletcher, J. M., Lyon, G. R., & Gore, J. C. (1998). Functional disruption in the organization of the brain for reading in dyslexia. *Proceedings of the National Academy of Sciences of the United States of America*, *95*(5), 2636–2641. https://doi.org/10.1073/pnas.95.5.2636

Silva, M., & Cain, K. (2015). The relations between lower and higher level comprehension skills and their role in prediction of early reading comprehension. *Journal of Educational Psychology*, *107*(2), 321.

Singson, M., Mahony, D., & Mann, V. (2000). The relation between reading ability and morphological skills: Evidence from derivational morphology. *Reading and Writing: An Interdisciplinary Journal*, *12*(3), 219–252.

Snowling, M. J. (2000). *Dyslexia* (2nd ed.). Oxford, UK: Blackwell Publishers.

Snowling, M. J., & Melby-Lervåg, M. (2016). Oral language deficits in familial dyslexia: A meta-analysis and review. *Psychological Bulletin*, *142*(5), 498–545. http://doi.org/10.1037/bul0000037

Sparks, E., & Deacon, S. H. (2015). Morphological awareness and vocabulary acquisition: A longitudinal examination of their relationship in English-speaking children. *Applied PsychoLinguistics*, *36*(2), 299–321.

Stanovich, K. E. (1986). Matthew effects in reading: Some consequences of individual differences in the acquisition of literacy. *Reading Research Quarterly*, *21*(4), 360–407.

Swanson, H. L., & Hsieh, C. J. (2009). Reading disabilities in adults: A selective meta-analysis of the literature. *Review of Educational Research*, *79*(4), 1362–1390.

Tan, Y., Anton, J.-L., Chanoine, V., & Cavalli, E. (2022). Neural representations of morphological, orthographic, and semantic information during visual word recognition: An fMRI representational similarity analysis. *Frontiers in Human Neuroscience*, *16*, 108390.

Taylor, J. S. H., Duff, F. J., Woollams, A. M., Monaghan, P., & Ricketts, J. (2013). How word meaning influences word reading development: The role of semantic knowledge in the development of word reading skill. *Cognition*, *127*(1), 26–38.

Templeton, S., & Scarborough-Franks, L. (1985). The spelling's the thing: Knowledge of derivational morphology in orthography and phonology among older students. *Applied PsychoLinguistics*, *6*(4), 371–389.

Tong, X., Deacon, S. H., Kirby, J. R., Cain, K., & Parrila, R. (2011). Morphological awareness: A key to understanding poor reading comprehension in English. *Journal of Educational Psychology*, *103*(3), 523–534.

Tops, W., Callens, M., Bijn, E., & Brysbaert, M. (2012). Spelling in adolescents with dyslexia: Errors and modes of assessment. *Journal of Learning Disabilities*, *47*, 295–306.

Torppa, M., Lyytinen, P., Erskine, J., Eklund, K., & Lyytinen, H. (2010). Language development, literacy skills, and predictive connections to reading in Finnish children with and without familial risk for dyslexia. *Journal of Learning Disabilities*, *43*(4), 308–321.

Tsesmeli, S. N., & Seymour, P. H. (2006). Derivational morphology and spelling in dyslexia. *Reading and Writing*, *19*(6), 587–625.

Tunmer, W. E. (1989). The role of language-related factors in reading disability. In A. M. Galaburda (Ed.), *From reading to neurons* (pp. 91–131). MIT Press.

Tunmer, W. E., & Chapman, J. W. (2012a). Does set for variability mediate the influence of vocabulary knowledge on the development of word recognition skills? *Scientific Studies of Reading*, *16*(2), 122–140. https://doi.org/10.1080/10888438.2010.542527

Tunmer, W. E., & Chapman, J. W. (2012b). The simple view of Reading Redux. *Journal of Learning Disabilities*, *45*(5), 453–466. https://doi.org/10.1177/0022219411432685

Vandermosten, M., Boets, B., Poelmans, H., Sunaert, S., Wouters, J., & Ghesquiere, P. (2012). A tractography study in dyslexia: Neuroanatomic correlates of orthographic, phonological and speech processing. *Brain*, *135*, 935e948.

Vellutino, F. R., Scanlon, D. M., & Spearing, D. (1995). Semantic and phonological coding in poor and normal readers. *Journal of Experimental Child Psychology*, *59*(1), 76–123.

Verhoeven, L., & Perfetti, C. A. (2008). Morphological processing in reading acquisition: A cross-linguistic perspective. *Applied PsychoLinguistics*, *29*(3), 353–367.

Verhoeven, L., & van Leeuwe, J. (2012). The simple view of second language reading throughout the primary grades. *Reading and Writing*, *25*(8), 1805–1818.

Walley, A. C., Metsala, J. L., & Garlock, V. M. (2003). Spoken vocabulary growth: Its role in the development of phoneme awareness and early reading ability. *Reading and Writing: An Interdisciplinary Journal*, *16*(1–2), 5–20.

Welbourne, S. R., Woollams, A. M., Crisp, J., & Ralph, L. M. A. (2011). The role of plasticity-related functional reorganization in the explanation of central dyslexia. *Cognitive Neuropsychology*, *28*, 65–108.

Whiting, C., Shtyrov, Y., & Marslen-Wilson, W. D. (2015). Real-time functional architecture of visual word recognition. *Journal of Cognitive Neuroscience*, *27*(3), 475–491.

Wilson-Fowler, E. B., & Apel, K. (2015). Influence of morphological awareness on college students' literacy skills: A path analytic approach. *Journal of Literacy Research, 47*(3), 405–432.

Wiseheart, R., & Altmann, L. J. P. (2017). Spoken language production in college students with dyslexia: Effects of working memory and vocabulary. *International Journal of Language and Communication Disorders, 61*(6), 1521–1531.

Wiseheart, R., Altmann, L. J. P., Park, H., & Lombardino, L. J. (2009). Sentence comprehension in young adults with developmental dyslexia. *Annals of Dyslexia, 59*(2), 151. https://doi.org/10.1007/s11881-009-0028-7

Woollams, A. M., Ralph, M. A., Plaut, D. C., & Patterson, K. (2010). SD-squared revisited: Reply to Coltheart, Tree, and Saunders (2010). *Psychological Review, 117*, 273–281.

4
VISUO-ORTHOGRAPHIC PROCESSING IN DYSLEXIC ADULTS

Nadège Doignon-Camus and Anne Bonnefond

4.1 Introduction

Visuo-orthographic processing corresponds to the visual coding of orthographic information, from which written words are recognised. This coding can be defined as the ability to activate a mental representation of the sequence of letters corresponding to the visual stimulus. Skilled readers show a great facility for processing visuo-orthographic information and do this in a very short time: starting from an ocular fixation, their visual attention is distributed across all the letters in the written word, allowing them to identify simultaneously each of the letters making up the word and their order, leading to recognition of the written word. The visuo-orthographic processing abilities of readers, therefore, depend partly on the quality and span of attentional allocation, partly on the quality of the mental representations of letters and letter groups and finally, on access to these representations stored in long-term memory.

It is over the course of learning to read that a child develops orthographic knowledge and visuo-orthographic processing skills, the purpose of the learning process being the automatisation of these visuo-orthographic processing skills. Even before explicit instruction about the alphabetic principle (i.e. the relationship between written and spoken language), a child learns to identify individual letters. This orthographic knowledge about the fundamental units of written language is a prerequisite for learning to read; it involves recognition of the shape of a letter and its name (Treiman, Pennington, Shriberg, & Boada, 2008; Treiman, Tincoff, Rodriguez, Mouzaki, & Francis, 1998). Through this learning process, the child constructs abstract mental representations of letters, allowing them to recognise letters in both cases (upper and lower) and in different fonts. While the child initially processes words letter by letter, thereafter the child develops a mechanism for the parallel identification of letters, allowing them to process orthographic sequences (Grainger & Ziegler, 2011); their orthographic knowledge will then incorporate sensitivity to graphotactic regularities, in other words, regularities relating to the order of the letters. Their lexical orthographic knowledge will gradually increase to attain a level of expertise with simple words during the fourth year of acquisition (Adams, 1990; Stanovich, 1980). The skills which allow children's orthographic knowledge to develop are, on the one hand, phonological decoding skills (Share, 1995) and phonological awareness (Vellutino, Fletcher, Snowling, & Scanlon, 2004), and on the other, word spelling, partly due to exhaustive letter-by-letter processing and to the motor-kinaesthetic modality contributing to the representation of the word in memory (Bosse, 2015). Together, this orthographic knowledge will then enable the child to recognise written words rapidly, without necessarily applying the phonological decoding process and, as a result, freeing up attentional resources for understanding what is read.

From a neurofunctional perspective (Figure 4.1), the visual coding of orthographic information depends on the interaction of the dorsal and ventral pathways. The dorsal pathway is the extension of the visual magnocellular

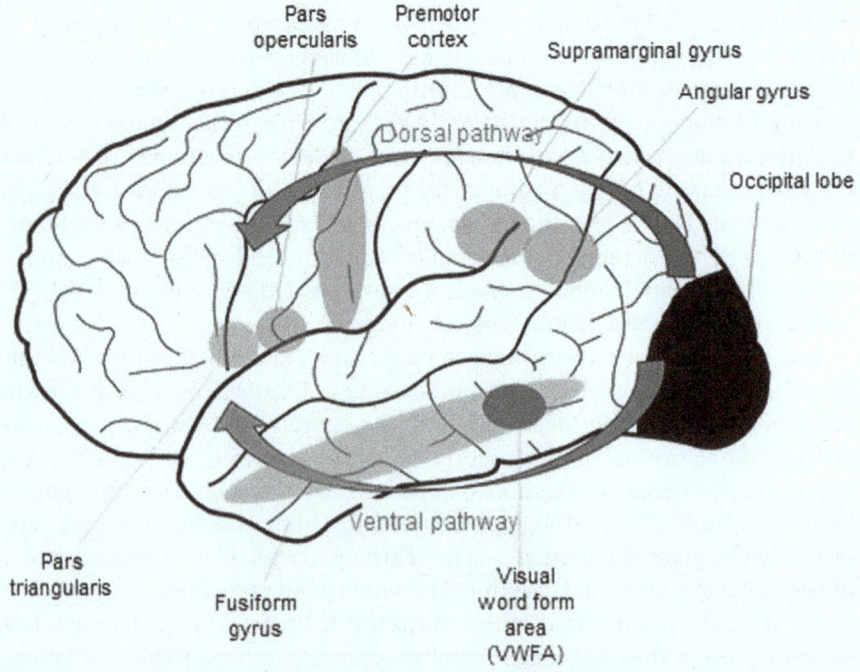

FIGURE 4.1 Mapping of the ventral and dorsal visual pathways used for the visual recognition of words. (Adapted from Curzietti, 2017.)

pathway, from the primary visual cortex to bilateral parietal regions, notably the supramarginal gyrus and the angular gyrus, and also including the premotor cortex and the pars opercularis of the left inferior frontal cortex. The pathway is involved in localising visual objects in space and underpins the process of allocating visual attention along a row of letters (Vidyasagar & Pammer, 2010), as well as phonological processing (Pugh et al., 2001). In the case of written word processing, the attention allocated to a row of letters, subtended by the dorsal pathway, makes it possible to segment this sequence into letter groups, to locate the letters or letter groups to be decoded and identified (Vidyasagar, 1999; Ziegler, Perry, & Zorzi, 2013).

Once the information has been processed in the parietal region, a message is sent back to the primary visual cortex and occipito-temporal structures, enabling individual letters to be identified and their order to be processed (Vidyasagar & Pammer, 2010). The identification of visual objects in space is, in fact, underpinned by regions of the ventral pathway, the extension of the visual parvocellular pathway that comprises the anterior, medial and left fusiform gyri, as well as the pars triangularis of the left inferior frontal gyrus. In the case of word processing, the visual word form area in the medial part of the left fusiform gyrus constitutes the region specialised for the identification of letters, letter groups and written words (Cohen et al., 2000).

In summary, visuo-orthographic processing depends both on the attentional processing allocated to orthographic information, underpinned by the dorsal pathway, and the accurate identification of the orthographic information, underpinned by the ventral pathway. Several studies have highlighted the conditions under which the dorsal pathway is most strongly implicated (e.g. serial reading, degraded visual presentation of letter sequences to skilled readers, reading acquisition phase), and those in which the role of the ventral pathway is privileged (normal presentation of letter sequences) (Cohen, Dehaene, Vinckier, Jobert, & Montavont, 2008; Rosazza, Cai, Minati, Paulignan, & Nazir, 2009). However, even though the description of these two pathways distinguishes the role of each, the complementarity and interaction of these two pathways remain fundamental to the successful coding of visual-orthographic information and written word recognition (Boros et al., 2016; Rosazza et al., 2009; Vidyasagar & Pammer, 2010).

Among readers who suffer from dyslexia, several studies have reported impairments in the visual coding of orthographic information and weaker orthographic knowledge, since acquisition of this knowledge partially depends on the phonological skills widely impaired among dyslexics (Bruck, 1990; Manis, Custodio, & Szeszulski, 1993; Vellutino et al., 2004). The aim of the two sections to follow is to present the visuo-orthographic processing difficulties linked to deficient attentional processing and impairment of the structures in the dorsal pathway, first of all, and then those associated with impaired letter identification underpinned by structures in the ventral pathway.

4.2 Visuo-orthographic Attentional Processing Underpinned by the Dorsal Parieto-occipital Pathway

According to Vidyasagar and Pammer (2010), dyslexics show a specific deficit in shifting the attentional spotlight along arrays of letters during ocular fixation, underpinned by the dorsal pathway. Such a deficit would be manifested as impaired orthographic coding with difficulties in segmenting letter sequences (Pammer & Vidyasagar, 2005; Vidyasagar, 2004). From a cognitive perspective, the perception of an array of letters requires the coding of the identity and position of each of the letters, with firstly the coding of letter location in relation to the point of ocular fixation and secondly the coding of the relative location of the letters in the word (Grainger, Dufau, & Ziegler, 2016). Even though letters are slightly better identified in the initial position, the processing of letter identity is performed in parallel (Grainger, 2017; Grainger & Ziegler, 2011; Stevens & Grainger, 2003). The precision of coding the identity and position of each of the letters is influenced by visual and attentional factors such as visual acuity, interference from adjacent letters and spatial attention (Leibnitz, Grainger, Muneaux, & Ducrot, 2016).

4.2.1 The Lateral Masking Effect

A widely studied phenomenon in the literature on typical adult readers and dyslexic adults is the lateral masking effect (or *crowding*), shown by slower and less accurate identification of a target letter when it is flanked by adjacent letters (which serve as distractors) than when it is presented in isolation. This lateral masking, which reduces the quality of visuo-orthographic information, is dependent on the distance between the ocular fixation point and the target letter to be identified, the distance between adjacent letters and the visual similarity of the letters (Callens, Whitney, Tops, & Brysbaert, 2013). Among adults with dyslexia, several studies have reported a larger effect of lateral masking than among typical readers (Cassim, Talcott, & Moores, 2014; Goolkasian & King, 1990; Klein, Berry, Briand, D'Entremont, & Farmer, 1990; Martelli, Filippo, Spinelli, & Zoccolotti, 2009; Moores, Cassim, & Talcott, 2011; Pernet, Valdois, Celsis, & Démonet, 2006; Shovman & Ahissar, 2006). It is important, however, to note that this lateral masking effect is sensitive to the conditions under which items are presented and the nature of the task (Castet, Descamps, Denis-Noël, & Colé, 2017; Doron, Manassi, Herzog, & Ahissar, 2015). Under certain experimental conditions, the difference between dyslexic and typical readers disappears, for example, when item duration is increased (Martelli et al., 2009; Moll & Jones, 2013), when the letters presented are unfamiliar (Shovman & Ahissar, 2006) or when the memory load imposed by the task is reduced (Hawelka & Wimmer, 2008).

Among dyslexic readers only, the impact of lateral masking on target letter identification is negatively correlated with their reading level: the more difficulty dyslexic readers have in recognising words and in decoding pseudowords, the more susceptible they are to lateral masking (Callens et al., 2013), suggesting a link between the interference of distractor letters on target letter identification and the reading level of dyslexic adults. Two studies have also confirmed the benefits of increasing the spaces between letters on the reading of words in text among dyslexic adults (Marinus et al., 2016; Sjoblom, Eaton, & Stagg, 2016): dyslexic readers read more rapidly and more accurately when the spacing between the letters was increased by 2.5 points than when the spacing between the letters corresponded to the usual conditions for presenting written words.

4.2.2 Interpretive Hypotheses for the Multi-Element Processing Deficit

As the effect of lateral masking is larger among adults with dyslexia than among typical readers, this demonstrates the difficulty that adults with dyslexia have in identifying a target element among a group of elements and highlights a deficit in the simultaneous processing of groups of elements. This multi-element processing deficit has given rise to several interpretive hypotheses, based on deficits in visual feature integration, spatial coding or processing speed. According to Pernet et al. (2006), the lateral masking effect among adults with dyslexia could be due to an impairment in visual feature integration, to the extent that it is more evident in target categorisation tasks, specifically requiring feature integration processes to form a perceptual representation and for comparison with the representation stored in memory, than in target discrimination tasks requiring only a visual analysis of features. According to other authors, difficulty in the simultaneous processing of a letter array might result more directly from a deficit in coding the spatial configuration of the letter array, that is, in the positional coding of letters (Collis, Kohnen, & Kinoshita, 2013; Hawelka, Huber, & Wimmer, 2006; Hawelka & Wimmer, 2005). Indeed, adults with dyslexia make more errors and/or require a longer processing time for an array than typical readers when they have to detect a target within an array of several elements. Finally, other authors believe that the difficulty for dyslexics in processing a letter array is due to a deficit in the speed of visual perceptual processing (Bogon, Finke, & Stenneken, 2014; Stenneken et al., 2011). Dyslexics need more time to extract the same amount of visual information as typical readers. This deficit would lead to slower processing of the orthographic units making up the word and non-automated access to lexical representations, producing a sequential reading strategy, based on sublexical units. This visual processing speed deficit has also been encountered among other patients affected by a disorder in processing multiple elements (Duncan et al., 2003).

A final hypothesis more widely studied in the literature views the deficit in the simultaneous processing of groups of elements among dyslexic readers as the result of a reduced visuo-attentional window. This hypothesis, according to which dyslexics process a limited amount of visual information due to a reduced visuo-attentional span, has been largely studied among the population of dyslexic children. The visuo-attentional span is defined as the number of distinct visual elements that can be processed simultaneously in a configuration of several elements (Bosse, Tainturier, & Valdois, 2007). For adults, the task measuring visuo-attentional span consists of presenting an array of six consonants for 200 ms centred on the screen fixation point and asking participants to report orally either all of the letters (global report) or a target letter (partial report). Results for dyslexic adults show a smaller visuo-attentional span than in typical readers (Castet, Descamps, Denis-Noël, & Colé, 2017; Lobier, Peyrin, Pichat, Le Bas, & Valdois, 2014; Reilhac, Peyrin, Démonet, & Valdois, 2013; Valdois, 2022, for a review in children and adults with dyslexia). From a neurofunctional perspective, the mechanisms involved in the parallel processing of several visual elements are supported bilaterally by the superior parietal lobule (Reilhac et al., 2013). Among adults with dyslexia showing a reduced visuo-attentional span, the bilateral activation of the superior parietal lobule is reduced in comparison to typical readers in target categorisation tasks (Lobier et al., 2014; Peyrin et al., 2012). From a cognitive perspective, a reduction in visuo-attentional span impedes the construction of memory traces for the written words encountered (Ans, Carbonnel, & Valdois, 1998), producing a lower quality of mental representation for letter sequences. According to the model of Ans et al. (1998), insofar as the visuo-attentional deficit limits the size of the attentional window, it prevents both the automatic and rapid recognition of written words and the sequential shifting of the visuo-attentional window necessary for the processing of rare or unfamiliar words. The visuo-attentional deficit hypothesis, therefore, offers an explanation of dyslexic difficulties in identifying letters and written words. Moreover, this hypothesis supports the idea that visuo-attentional deficits are independent of phonological deficits, since two case studies of adults with dyslexia have demonstrated a double dissociation between the two deficits (Peyrin et al., 2012): one of whom presented impaired phonological skills associated with lower activation of the left inferior frontal gyrus and supramarginal gyrus, and preserved visuo-attentional skills associated with normal bilateral activation of the parietal network; the other participant showed the opposite pattern, namely, preserved phonological skills associated with normal activation of the left phonological network, and impaired visuo-attentional skills associated with lower bilateral activation of the parietal lobe.

4.2.3 Link between the Visuo-orthographic Attentional Deficit and the Phonological Deficit?

Methodologically, all of these results reporting adult dyslexic difficulties in processing arrays of multiple elements are still under debate, since the elements to be processed in the tasks are very frequently orthographic in nature (e.g. letter sequences) and responses must be given orally. Several authors have questioned the possible impact of the phonological processing involved in these tasks (i.e. phonological coding of the letters or the numbers to be processed; involvement of phonological short-term memory in the oral response) (Collis et al., 2013; Hawelka & Wimmer, 2008; Shovman & Ahissar, 2006; Ziegler, Pech-Georgel, Dufau, & Grainger, 2010). Recently, a longitudinal study has shown that the ability of prereaders to process multiple non-verbal elements predicts later speed at reading long and rare words (Onochie-Quintanilla, Defior, & Simpson, 2017), testifying to a link between multi-element processing and the speed of phonological decoding. Among dyslexic adults, visual search performance correlates positively with phonological performance (i.e. nonword reading and rapid naming) (Jones, Branigan, & Kelly, 2008). More generally, Vidyasagar and Pammer (2010) make an explicit link between visuo-orthographic attentional problems and the phonological deficit, in suggesting that weak orthographic segmentation skills cause difficulties in converting orthographic units into phonological units. However, by limiting the involvement of phonological representations in experimental tasks or by virtue of the absence of correlation between multi-letter processing and phonological performances, several studies have suggested the presence of a visuo-attentional deficit independent of skill at accessing phonological representations (Cassim et al., 2014; Peyrin et al., 2012; Romani, Tsouknida, di Betta, & Olson, 2011).

In summary, the difficulties in processing letter sequences associated with visuo-attentional difficulties among adults with dyslexia, which were described previously, are assumed to reflect impairments to the bilateral parietal structures of the dorsal pathway (Lobier et al., 2014; Pernet et al., 2006; Peyrin et al., 2012; Vidyasagar, 1999; Vidyasagar & Pammer, 2010). These difficulties then have repercussions for the information passed on by the dorsal parietal structures towards the ventral occipito-temporal structures. The attentional processes underpinned by the dorsal pathway, in fact, directly influence the activity of the left fusiform gyrus within the ventral pathway (Vogel, Miezin, Petersen, & Schlaggar, 2012). A modified specialisation of the left ventral occipito-temporal area appears compromised for the processing of writing in the event of lower quality feedback from the dorsal to the ventral areas (Maurer & McCandliss, 2008; McCandliss & Noble, 2003).

4.3 Identification of Letters and Letter Sequences Supported by the Left Ventral Occipito-temporal Pathway

Assuming that the reading difficulties of dyslexic adults are attributable to impairments in visuo-attentional processing, further work has highlighted specific difficulties in the identification of letter sequences due to impairment of the left occipito-temporal region of the ventral pathway. Within this region, it is the activation of the visual word form area that seems to be particularly affected. According to the Neuronal Recycling hypothesis (Dehaene & Cohen, 2007), the visual word form area specialises during the acquisition of reading to support written language processing. This hypothesis suggests that cultural inventions like reading entail a modification to the initial functions of certain neural networks to convert to the new functions required for these inventions. The specialisation of the visual word form area would then involve modifying the initial neural coding of visual objects into a neural coding of letters and letter combinations (Dehaene, Cohen, Sigman, & Vinckier, 2005; Dehaene-Lambertz, Monzalvo, & Dehaene, 2018). An empirical argument in favour of this hypothesis is the presence of activation of the left ventral occipito-temporal region in illiterate participants when processing photos of faces and objects such as checkerboards or utensils, and the absence of activation of this region in the same participants when processing written language (Dehaene, Pegado, et al., 2010; Dehaene, Cohen, Morais, & Kolinsky, 2015; Feng, Monzalvo, Dehaene, & Dehaene-Lambertz, 2022; but see Hervais-Adelman, Kumar, et al., 2019).

One consequence of neural recycling and of the specialisation of this region is that it learns to differentiate letters that have a perfectly symmetrical shape (e.g. b and d). For all visual objects that we process, we are able to recognise them through a mirror-invariance mechanism. This mirror-invariance mechanism (or mirror generalisation) enables us to judge that objects remain exactly the same despite their change of position. In the case of reversed letters, such as "b" and "d", our ventral system must learn, as we learn to read, that the letters with a symmetrical shape are two different letters (Dehaene, Nakamura, et al., 2010; Pegado, Nakamura, Cohen, & Dehaene, 2011; Pegado, 2022). According to Dehaene, readers must unlearn invariance by symmetry when processing written language. Nevertheless, the skilled reader always remains sensitive to the existence of the mirror images and must inhibit the mirror generalisation process (Borst, Ahr, Roell, & Houdé, 2015). In the case of developmental dyslexia, several studies show that the children retain the mirror generalisation process for a longer time, the process of unlearning symmetry appearing to be slower to set up (Fernandes & Leite, 2017; Fernandes, Vale, Martins, Morais, & Kolinsky, 2014; Lachmann & van Leeuwen, 2007).

4.3.1 Study of the Neural Specialisation of the Visual Word Form Area by Means of the N170 Component: Delayed, Impaired or Preserved in Dyslexics?

The neural specialisation of the left ventral occipito-temporal region, testifying to the expertise of readers in processing written language, can be observed through the recording of visual evoked potentials and the study of the N170 component. The N170 component is a negative variation in voltage observed in the left occipito-temporal region approximately 170 ms after the presentation of a written word (Figure 4.2). Due to studies combining EEG and fMRI (Brem et al., 2006; Cohen et al., 2000; Dale et al., 2000), the N170 component has been linked to activity in the left fusiform gyrus within the ventral pathway (i.e. the visual word form area). Numerous studies in adult typical readers have reported modulation of the amplitude of the N170 component as a function of stimulus familiarity: the component has a larger negative amplitude when evoked by an array of letters than by an array of symbols or alphanumeric characters (Araújo, Faísca, Bramão, Reis, & Petersson, 2015; Bentin, Mouchetant-Rostaing, Giard, Echallier, & Pernier, 1999; Brem et al., 2006; Curzietti, Bonnefond, Staub, Vidailhet, & Doignon-Camus, 2017; Maurer, Brandeis, & McCandliss, 2005; Maurer, Brem, Bucher, & Brandeis, 2005). This result has been interpreted as an indication of readers' skill in processing written language and the neural specialisation of the left occipito-temporal region for this processing. Letters, symbols and alphanumeric characters alike are made up of the same visual features. It is the combination of these visual features that differentiates them: in the course of learning to read, letters become the basic units of the larger units that are words (Grainger, 2017). Visual skill in processing written language, shown by the difference in the amplitude of the N170 component following the presentation of letters and symbols, emerges in the

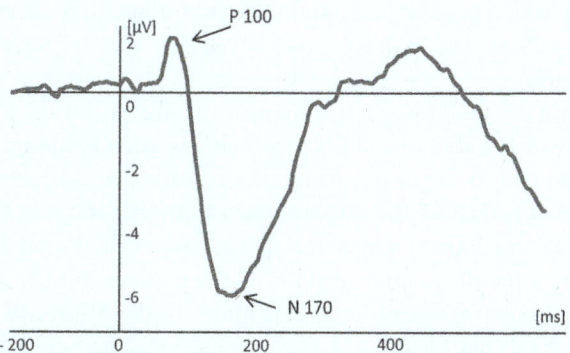

FIGURE 4.2 Early evoked potentials (P100 and N170) in processing a letter array.

course of learning to read, especially after the first two years (Maurer et al., 2006; Maurer, Brandeis, et al., 2005). In the population of dyslexic readers, however, results seem to show delayed or impaired skills. Among young Portuguese developmental dyslexics aged between 9 and 11 years (mean = 10.7 years), visual skill in processing written language was not observed in the N170 component (Araújo, Bramão, Faísca, Petersson, & Reis, 2012). Later in adulthood, similar results were observed despite many years of remediation (on average, 5.7 years, in the sample): dyslexic adults showed similar neural electrophysiological activity for the processing of letter arrays and symbol arrays in the initial stages of processing these stimuli (Mahé, Bonnefond, Gavens, Dufour, & Doignon-Camus, 2012). A second study tested whether the absence of this skill resulted from the low reading level of adults with dyslexia or from dyslexia itself, by comparing these adults with dyslexia with a group of adult poor readers closely matched on reading level (Mahé, Bonnefond, & Doignon-Camus, 2013). The poor readers did not show either a diagnosis of dyslexia or a reading disorder, but were lower in socio-economic status than the adults with dyslexia. In contrast to the adults with dyslexia, the modulation of the N170 component according to the alphabetic nature of the stimuli (letter vs. symbol arrays), lateralised to the left, was preserved among the adult poor readers, suggesting that the absence of neural specialisation in processing written language is a characteristic of dyslexia and not of a low reading level. However, this result has to be qualified, particularly depending on whether the adults with dyslexia are at university or not. By selecting a sample of 22 university students displaying developmental dyslexia, a study in progress reveals similar modulation of the N170 component as a function of stimulus type (letters vs. symbols) to that of students who are typical readers, suggesting preservation of the neural specialisation in the occipito-temporal region for processing written language (Cheviet, Bonnefond, Bertrand, Maumy-Bertrand, & Doignon-Camus, 2022). This finding suggests that the population of adults with dyslexia who succeed in pursuing higher education displays different characteristics from the average adult dyslexic, with preserved visual-orthographic skills.

In the literature, two alternative hypotheses are proposed to account for the emergence of the visual skill for processing written language during reading acquisition and for its impairment among adults with dyslexia. The dominant hypothesis is that of the Phonological Mapping theory (McCandliss & Noble, 2003), according to which the specialisation of the visual word form area depends on the phonological skills of the readers and the attention they focus on the associations between letters and sounds (Maurer & McCandliss, 2008). Thus, the difficulties that dyslexic readers show in constructing correspondences between letters and sounds would have a negative impact on the specialisation of the visual word form area. The alternative hypothesis to the McCandliss and Noble (2003) model is that of Lobier et al. (2014), according to which the specialisation of the visual word form area depends on attentional processes (sequential and attentional processing of letter sequences) underpinned by parietal structures. Atypical activation of the inferior parietal lobule bilaterally linked to the impaired attentional processes observed among adults with dyslexia (Richlan, 2012) would result in a lack of left occipito-temporal region specialisation for processing writing. While the neural specialisation of the visual word form area for the processing of written language appears impaired among a proportion of adults with dyslexia, this still remains to be explored more thoroughly to determine the reasons for a weaker specialisation and interindividual differences, especially in academic performance and in the range of compensatory strategies employed (Miller-Shaul, 2005). A first study recently provided evidence of a contribution of phonological but not visuo-attentional skills on the N170 component (Cheviet et al., 2022).

4.3.2 Impaired Activation of the Visual Word Form Area in Dyslexics and Access to the Lexicon

The left occipito-temporal region, recycled and specialised for the processing of writing during learning, is activated following the visual perception of a letter sequence. Numerous studies have shown that this region is less activated in the average dyslexic adult than in adults who are typical readers during written word processing tasks. For example, with the magnetoencephalography (MEG) technique, the usual activation of the left occipito-temporal region associated with the presentation of a letter array approximately 150 ms after its presentation was not observed among a group of dyslexic adults, in contrast to a group of young non-dyslexic adults (Helenius, Tarkiainen, Cornelissen, Hansen, & Salmelin, 1999). Using the same MEG technique, Cavalli et al. (2017) explored the activation of this left occipito-temporal region during the automatic activation of early orthographic representations by the orthographic priming paradigm (e.g. the target word OURS [bear] primed by the word OURSIN [sea urchin], which shares orthographic features with the target word or primed by the word GESIER [gizzard], which does not share any orthographic features with the target word). Unlike the data from typical readers, the data from dyslexic adults did not show an early orthographic priming effect (around 100ms) in the left occipito-temporal region. Based on nine fMRI studies, the meta-analysis by Richlan, Kronbichler, and Wimmer (2011) clearly shows left occipito-temporal dysfunction among dyslexic adults, with marked under-activation of this region when dyslexics perceive written words (see also Paz-Alonso, Oliver et al., 2018). This under-activation, especially of the medial and posterior portion of the left fusiform gyrus, is even more marked among dyslexic adults than dyslexic children. In conjunction with this left occipito-temporal under-activation reflecting impairment of the specific process of written word identification, Wimmer et al. (2010) observed an over-activation of the visual occipital regions among dyslexic adolescents and adults, reflecting prolonged processing of visuo-orthographic information (Richlan, 2012).

From a cognitive perspective, the left occipito-temporal region, specialised for the processing of written words, most notably supports the storage of lexical and sublexical orthographic mental representations, and access to these representations for the automatic recognition of written words. Dysfunction of this left occipito-temporal region in dyslexic adults, therefore, creates the difficulties in accessing the lexicon that are seen from the initial stages of processing written words. In adults who are typical readers, the traces of lexical access are reflected in the modulation of cerebral electrophysiological activity in the left occipito-temporal regions from 100 ms after the presentation of a written stimulus (P100 and N170 components; Figure 4.2) as a function of the lexicality of the stimulus (word vs. pseudoword) or its lexical frequency (frequent word vs. rare word) (Araújo et al., 2015; Hauk et al., 2006; Hauk, Coutout, Holden, & Chen, 2012; Kim & Straková, 2012; Sereno, Rayner, & Posner, 1998). In contrast, in adults with dyslexia, no modulation of the early components P100 and N170 is observed as a function of lexicality or word frequency (Mahé et al., 2012; Taroyan & Nicolson, 2009). Only a lexicality effect was found for the N170 component lateralised to the right (Mahé et al., 2012), in keeping with the over-activation of right hemisphere regions observed in dyslexic readers (Shaywitz et al., 1998). Similar results have been reported while manipulating orthographic neighbourhood as a variable. The orthographic neighbour of a target word is a word that shares all the letters of the target word in the same position except for a single letter (e.g. *dupe* [fool] is the orthographic neighbour of *jupe* [skirt]). The orthographic neighbourhood thus reflects the orthographic similarities between the target word and the other words stored in the lexicon and its manipulation makes it possible to investigate the activation processes for lexical candidates and lexical competition. In the typical reader, during the processing of letter sequences, cerebral electrophysiological responses are affected by orthographic neighbourhood from the first 100 ms (Hauk, Pulvermüller, Ford, Marslen-Wilson, & Davis, 2009), whereas in adults with dyslexia, no trace of the activation of orthographic neighbours is observed early on (Savill & Thierry, 2011). This result suggests that orthographic cues at the word form level are not processed either rapidly or efficiently by adults with dyslexia. In a similarity judgment task about two written words, typical readers respond more rapidly when the words are written vertically than when they are inverted (i.e. with a 180° rotation, the letters being upside down and the words reversed left to right). In adult dyslexic readers, this effect of degradation on response speed is less strong, indicating impaired automatisation in extracting cues from the visual form of words and a heavy reliance on a global reading strategy (Conway, Brady, & Misra, 2017).

4.3.3 Activation of the Visual Word Form Area and Pre-lexical Orthographic Processing

In addition to processing the visual form of the word at a lexical level, the perception of a written word generates orthographic coding at the sub-lexical level. This coding notably involves the ability to process the statistical properties of orthographic redundancy, that is, the frequency of occurrence of letters and letter groups in the written language. The distribution of letters in the language is not a random effect; certain combinations of letters are much more frequent than others: a widely used measure of orthographic redundancy is the frequency of bigrams (i.e. groups of two letters). The coding of orthographic redundancy is underpinned by the visual word form area, within which a posterior–anterior gradient has been demonstrated: it is the most anterior regions of the visual word form occipito-temporal system that are the most selective for letter sequences made up of frequent bigrams while the most posterior regions respond preferentially to letter sequences containing rare bigrams (Binder, Medler, Westbury, Liebenthal, & Buchanan, 2006; Vinckier et al., 2007). Two studies have been conducted, on dyslexic children only, and have reported an altered spatial organisation of the posterior-anterior gradient (Olulade, Flowers, Napoliello, & Eden, 2015; van der Mark et al., 2009).

Among adults with dyslexia as well, only a few studies have been conducted. In a behavioural approach, Pitchford, Ledgeway, & Masterson (2009) used a task of searching for a target letter within an array of letters while manipulating the positional frequency of the letters. In this task, typical readers detected the target letter more rapidly when located in its most frequent position than when located in its least frequent position. This result, providing evidence of the encoding of the positional frequency of letters in written language, was not observed among adults with dyslexia. The sensitivity of dyslexics to the positional frequency of letters seems to be limited to the initial position, since only one negative correlation was observed between letter detection time and the frequency of letters in the initial position; no correlation was observed for the other positions. More generally, by simply manipulating the legality of bigrams (an illegal bigram being a group of two letters that never occurs in the written language), Araújo et al. (2015) found an orthographic processing impairment among dyslexics. During the perception of a letter array, the authors observed an absence of modulation of the early components P100 and N170 according to whether an illegal bigram was present or not, contrary to what is observed among adult typical readers. This result shows that from the very first stages of processing letter arrays, sub-lexical orthographic analysis of the properties of letter arrays and the processing of this visuo-orthographic information is impaired among dyslexic adults. Sensitivity to the legality or the frequency of letter groups in written language emerges during reading acquisition through repeated exposure to written language and the implicit learning process. Since the two studies of Pitchford et al. (2009) and Araújo et al. (2015) were conducted with adults with dyslexia pursuing higher education, it seems unlikely that their performance is linked to an impoverished orthographic lexicon and less exposure to written language (Cavalli et al., 2016). The hypothesis advanced by Pitchford et al. (2009), however, assumes an impairment to the implicit learning process that enables orthographic statistical regularities to be extracted from repeated exposure to written material. A large number of empirical arguments have been reported in the literature in favour of this hypothesis. Using an implicit learning task with an artificial grammar and written material (Kahta & Schiff, 2016), or an implicit learning task with sequences of oral syllables (Gabay, Thiessen, & Holt, 2015) or even a statistical learning task with non-orthographic visual forms (Sigurdardottir et al., 2017), studies have reported weaker implicit learning performances in dyslexic adults compared to typical readers (Samara & Caravolas, 2017; but see Doignon-Camus, Seigneuric, Perrier, Sisti, & Zagar, 2013 with dyslexic children, and van Witteloostuijn, Boersma, Wijnen, & Rispens, 2017 with dyslexic adults). On the other hand, as soon as dyslexics are made aware of the presence of a rule for the generation of the sequences of stimuli and learning thereby becomes explicit, their performances no longer differ from those of typical readers (Kahta & Schiff, 2016).

4.3.4 *What If Orthographic Skills Were Preserved or Compensated?*

So far, we have reported visuo-attentional and visuo-orthographic deficits in dyslexic adults. However, there are other results in the literature that show evidence of preserved or compensated orthographic skills in this population of adults with dyslexia. The study by Miller-Shaul (2005) is particularly informative in that it compares the orthographic skills of dyslexics to those of typical readers, in two groups of participants, children in their fourth year of primary school and adult university students. In the task administered, participants had to judge whether the pair of words that they heard had the same orthographic features (the study was in Hebrew). Two major results were reported: firstly, dyslexic performance in terms of accuracy and speed of response was better in adults than in children, suggesting an improvement in orthographic skills during development; and secondly, no significant differences were observed between the dyslexics and typical readers in adulthood, suggesting the implementation of compensation procedures based on orthographic processing by dyslexics, enabling them to overcome the difficulties observed in childhood. Miller-Shaul (2005) also reported that while the difference between the orthographic skills of dyslexics and those of typical readers decreases with age, the difference between the two groups in terms of their phonological skills increases. As a result of their impaired phonological performance, dyslexic readers focus their attention more on the visuo-orthographic form than on the pronunciation of written words (Martin et al., 2010). It is important to note that, as in the study by Cheviet et al. (2022), in which preservation of visual skill for processing written language was reported, the sample of adult participants in the study by Miller-Shaul (2005) consisted only of university students.

These arguments in favour of compensation via orthographic skills can be supplemented by those from reading training studies, focused on orthographic processing. The first studies were conducted on dyslexic children (Breznitz, 1997a), and the training consisted of sentence reading under time pressure, that is, they had to read more rapidly than usual (through the progressive erasure of the items to be read, letter by letter). This forced accelerated reading procedure was combined with the auditory presentation of a distractor (i.e. auditory masking): during sentence reading, dyslexics heard a familiar song, saturating the phonological route, in other words, blocking the phonological recoding of written words. This experimental situation resulted in a decrease in reading errors among dyslexic children and an increase in comprehension scores. According to the author, the reduced recourse to the use of phonological decoding seems to enable a greater attentional focus on visuo-orthographic and semantic information, benefiting the dyslexic children (Breznitz, 1997b). Similar results have recently been observed among a population of dyslexic university students, for whom accelerated reading by means of the progressive erasure of letters improved comprehension and written word decoding performances, in the short and long (6 months later) term (Breznitz et al., 2013). A hypothesis proposed by several authors suggests that this accelerated reading programme leads to an improvement in cognitive skills such as working memory: by forcing rapid reading, the programme makes the reader process and store larger orthographic units in working memory, at a lexical level, thereby freeing up cognitive resources for understanding what is read (Breznitz et al., 2013; Horowitz-Kraus, Cicchino, Amiel, Holland, & Breznitz, 2014).

4.4 Conclusion

The study of the cognitive and neural mechanisms associated with written language processing in adults with developmental dyslexia has made it possible to identify two major characteristics of visuo-orthographic processing. Firstly, these readers show visuo-attentional deficits in processing letter sequences, connected to an impairment of bilateral parietal structures, causing difficulties in localising letters and in the segmentation of letter arrays. Secondly, adults with dyslexia show specific deficits in letter identification, the coding of orthographic statistical regularities and access to the lexicon, associated with a dysfunction of the visual word form area in the left occipito-temporal region. Two key non-independent areas could be investigated more closely in future studies: (a) the exploration of the interindividual differences within the population of dyslexic adults, by distinguishing those who succeed in pursuing university studies from those who do not; and (b) the exploration of the cognitive and neural adaptive or compensatory mechanisms that dyslexic adults have developed. The objective in these future studies would be to contribute to a more global definition of developmental dyslexia in adulthood, based on deficits but also on the adaptive alternative mechanisms implemented by these readers.

From a clinical perspective, the assessment of all the skills necessary for the process of visual word recognition seems essential, especially due to the heterogeneity of adults suffering from developmental dyslexia. Only a complete assessment of skills makes it possible to determine the precise deficit shown by the dyslexic reader and to envisage the most suitable method of remediation and/or possible adjustments. In particular, the assessment of visuo-orthographic skills seems especially important given that, as we saw in this chapter, developmental dyslexia in adults is associated with specific features in orthographic processing. Visuo-orthographic processing assessments should include assessment of both the visuo-attentional processes enlisted during the activity of reading (e.g., assessment of visuo-attentional span, which is known to predict reading performance, Franceschini, Gori, Ruffino, Pedrolli, & Facoetti, 2012) and the specific processes of letter and written word identification.

From the point of view of possible remediation techniques, the work of Breznitz (1997a) and Breznitz et al. (2013) suggests that accelerated reading is an effective tool for improving both reading and comprehension performance among dyslexic readers. From the results of other studies using phonological training, we can hypothesise that orthographic training may lead to a reorganisation of brain circuits. Indeed, a study conducted among adult dyslexic readers has shown that training in phonological skills leads to both improved reading performance and to neuroanatomical changes, with increased activation in the areas usually activated by typical readers and in new areas reflecting compensatory mechanisms (Eden et al., 2004). Other types of training than accelerated reading could be effective and may constitute avenues for remediation, but, in the absence of studies providing evidence of their effectiveness, it is impossible to give accurate recommendations about other methods for remediation of visuo-orthographic skills in adult dyslexic readers.

In addition to remediation methods for reading difficulties in dyslexic adults, it is important not to overlook possible adjustments to offer to dyslexic readers during the activity of reading. In the literature, two adjustments have been tested: increasing inter-letter spacing and using a different font. Several studies have demonstrated the benefits of increased spacing between letters for dyslexic readers, children and adults, especially in the accuracy and speed of reading (Hakvoort, van den Boer, Leenaars, Bos, & Tijms, 2017; Marinus et al., 2016; Sjoblom et al., 2016; Zorzi et al., 2012). Increasing the space between letters reduces the interference from adjacent letters in the letter array and allows better identification of each letter: letter identification being the first step in the visual recognition of words. In contrast, studies testing the effectiveness of specific fonts (Dyslexie or OpenDyslexic) on reading performance do not show any benefit (Kuster, van Weerdenburg, Gompel, & Bosman, 2017; Marinus et al., 2016; Wery & Diliberto, 2017). It is not the shape of the letters that makes the layout relevant for dyslexic readers, but the space between them.

In conclusion, while the majority of the studies conducted on dyslexic readers have focused on phonological skills, it appears that dyslexic problems cannot be reduced to a phonological deficit. The visuo-orthographic skills of adult dyslexic readers must be taken into account if the extent of their neurodevelopmental disorder is to be characterised accurately.

References

Adams, M. J. (1990). *Beginning to read: Thinking and learning about print*. Cambridge, MA: MIT Press.

Ans, B., Carbonnel, S., & Valdois, S. (1998). A connectionist multiple-trace memory model for polysyllabic word reading. *Psychological Review*, *105*(4), 678–723.

Araújo, S., Bramão, I., Faísca, L., Petersson, K. M., & Reis, A. (2012). Electrophysiological correlates of impaired reading in dyslexic pre-adolescent children. *Brain and Cognition*, *79*(2), 79–88. https://doi.org/10.1016/j.bandc.2012.02.010

Araújo, S., Faísca, L., Bramão, I., Reis, A., & Petersson, K. M. (2015). Lexical and sublexical orthographic processing: An ERP study with skilled and dyslexic adult readers. *Brain and Language*, *141*, 16–27. https://doi.org/10.1016/j.bandl.2014.11.007

Bentin, S., Mouchetant-Rostaing, Y., Giard, M. H., Echallier, J. F., & Pernier, J. (1999). ERP manifestations of processing printed words at different psycholinguistic levels: Time course and scalp distribution. *Journal of Cognitive Neuroscience*, *11*(3), 235–260.

Binder, J. R., Medler, D. A., Westbury, C. F., Liebenthal, E., & Buchanan, L. (2006). Tuning of the human left fusiform gyrus to sublexical orthographic structure. *NeuroImage*, *33*(2), 739–748. https://doi.org/10.1016/j.neuroimage.2006.06.053

Bogon, J., Finke, K., & Stenneken, P. (2014). TVA-based assessment of visual attentional functions in developmental dyslexia. *Frontiers in Psychology*, *5*. https://doi.org/10.3389/fpsyg.2014.01172

Boros, M., Anton, J.-L., Pech-Georgel, C., Grainger, J., Szwed, M., & Ziegler, J. C. (2016). Orthographic processing deficits in developmental dyslexia: Beyond the ventral visual stream. *NeuroImage*, *128*, 316–327.

Borst, G., Ahr, E., Roell, M., & Houdé, O. (2015). The cost of blocking the mirror generalization process in reading: Evidence for the role of inhibitory control in discriminating letters with lateral mirror-image counterparts. *Psychonomic Bulletin & Review*, *22*(1), 228–234. https://doi.org/10.3758/s13423-014-0663-9

Bosse, M.-L. (2015). Learning to read and spell: How children acquire word orthographic knowledge. *Child Development Perspectives*, *9*(4), 222–226.

Bosse, M.-L., Tainturier, M. J., & Valdois, S. (2007). Developmental dyslexia: The visual attention span deficit hypothesis. *Cognition*, *104*(2), 198–230. https://doi.org/10.1016/j.cognition.2006.05.009

Brem, S., Bucher, K., Halder, P., Summers, P., Dietrich, T., Martin, E., & Brandeis, D. (2006). Evidence for developmental changes in the visual word processing network beyond adolescence. *NeuroImage*, *29*(3), 822–837. https://doi.org/10.1016/j.neuroimage.2005.09.023

Breznitz, Z. (1997a). Effects of accelerated reading rate on memory for text among dyslexic readers. *Journal of Educational Psychology*, *89*(2), 289–297. https://doi.org/10.1037/0022-0663.89.2.289

Breznitz, Z. (1997b). Reading rate acceleration: Developmental aspects. *The Journal of Genetic Psychology*, *158*(4), 427–441. https://doi.org/10.1080/00221329709596680

Breznitz, Z., Shaul, S., Horowitz-Kraus, T., Sela, I., Nevat, M., & Karni, A. (2013). Enhanced reading by training with imposed time constraint in typical and dyslexic adults. *Nature Communications*, *4*, 1486. https://doi.org/10.1038/ncomms2488

Bruck, M. (1990). Word-recognition skills of adults with childhood diagnoses of dyslexia. *Developmental Psychology*, *26*(3), 439–454.

Callens, M., Whitney, C., Tops, W., & Brysbaert, M. (2013). No deficiency in left-to-right processing of words in dyslexia but evidence for enhanced visual crowding. *Quarterly Journal of Experimental Psychology*, *66*(9), 1803–1817.

Cassim, R., Talcott, J. B., & Moores, E. (2014). Adults with dyslexia demonstrate large effects of crowding and detrimental effects of distractors in a visual tilt discrimination task. *PLoS One*, *9*(9), e106191. https://doi.org/10.1371/journal.pone.0106191

Castet, E., Descamps, M., Denis-Noël, A., & Colé, P. (2017). Letter and symbol identification: No evidence for letter-specific crowding mechanisms. *Journal of Vision*, *17*(11), 2. https://doi.org/10.1167/17.11.2

Cavalli, E., Casalis, S., Ahmadi, A. E., Zira, M., Poracchia-George, F., & Colé, P. (2016). Vocabulary skills are well developed in university students with dyslexia: Evidence from multiple case studies. *Research in Developmental Disabilities*, *51*, 89–102. https://doi.org/10.1016/j.ridd.2016.01.006

Cavalli, E., Colé, P., Pattamadilok, C., Badier, J.-M., Zielinski, C., Chanoine, V., & Ziegler, J. C. (2017). Spatiotemporal reorganization of the reading network in adult dyslexia. *Cortex*, *92*(Supplement C), 204–221. https://doi.org/10.1016/j.cortex.2017.04.012

Cheviet, A., Bonnefond, A., Bertrand, F., Maumy-Bertrand, M., & Doignon-Camus, N. (2022). How visual attention span and phonological skills contribute to N170 print tuning: An EEG study in French dyslexic students. *Brain and Language*, *234*, 105176. https://doi.org/10.1016/j.bandl.2022.105176

Cohen, L., Dehaene, S., Naccache, L., Lehéricy, S., Dehaene-Lambertz, G., Hénaff, M.-A., & Michel, F. (2000). The visual word form area: Spatial and temporal characterization of an initial stage of reading in normal subjects and posterior split-brain patients. *Brain*, *123*(2), 291–307. https://doi.org/10.1093/brain/123.2.291

Cohen, L., Dehaene, S., Vinckier, F., Jobert, A., & Montavont, A. (2008). Reading normal and degraded words: Contribution of the dorsal and ventral visual pathways. *NeuroImage*, *40*(1), 353–366. https://doi.org/10.1016/j.neuroimage.2007.11.036

Collis, N. L., Kohnen, S., & Kinoshita, S. (2013). The role of visual spatial attention in adult developmental dyslexia. *Quarterly Journal of Experimental Psychology (2006)*, *66*(2), 245–260. https://doi.org/10.1080/17470218.2012.705305

Conway, A., Brady, N., & Misra, K. (2017). Holistic word processing in dyslexia. *PLoS One*, *12*(11), e0187326.

Curzietti, M. (2017, Octobre 3). *La reconnaissance visuelle des mots écrits chez les patients souffrant de schizophrénie*. de Strasbourg.

Curzietti, M., Bonnefond, A., Staub, B., Vidailhet, P., & Doignon-Camus, N. (2017). The effects of age on visual expertise for print. *Brain and Language*, *169*, 48–56. https://doi.org/10.1016/j.bandl.2017.03.001

Dale, A. M., Liu, A. K., Fischl, B. R., Buckner, R. L., Belliveau, J. W., Lewine, J. D., & Halgren, E. (2000). Dynamic statistical parametric mapping: Combining fMRI and MEG for high-resolution imaging of cortical activity. *Neuron*, *26*(1), 55–67.

Dehaene, S., & Cohen, L. (2007). Cultural recycling of cortical maps. *Neuron*, *56*(2), 384–398. https://doi.org/10.1016/j.neuron.2007.10.004

Dehaene, S., Cohen, L., Morais, J., & Kolinsky, R. (2015). Illiterate to literate: Behavioural and cerebral changes induced by reading acquisition. *Nature Reviews. Neuroscience*, *16*(4), 234–244. https://doi.org/10.1038/nrn3924

Dehaene, S., Cohen, L., Sigman, M., & Vinckier, F. (2005). The neural code for written words: A proposal. *Trends in Cognitive Sciences*, *9*(7), 335–341. https://doi.org/10.1016/j.tics.2005.05.004

Dehaene, S., Nakamura, K., Jobert, A., Kuroki, C., Ogawa, S., & Cohen, L. (2010). Why do children make mirror errors in reading? Neural correlates of mirror invariance in the visual word form area. *NeuroImage*, *49*(2), 1837–1848. https://doi.org/10.1016/j.neuroimage.2009.09.024

Dehaene, S., Pegado, F., Braga, L. W., Ventura, P., Nunes Filho, G., Jobert, A., ... Cohen, L. (2010). How learning to read changes the cortical networks for vision and language. *Science (New York, N.Y.)*, *330*(6009), 1359–1364. https://doi.org/10.1126/science.1194140

Dehaene-Lambertz, G., Monzalvo, K., & Dehaene, S. (2018). The emergence of the visual word form: Longitudinal evolution of category-specific ventral visual areas during reading acquisition. *PLoS Biology*, *16*(3), e2004103. https://doi.org/10.1371/journal.pbio.2004103

Doignon-Camus, N., Seigneuric, A., Perrier, E., Sisti, A., & Zagar, D. (2013). Evidence for a preserved sensitivity to orthographic redundancy and an impaired access to phonological syllables in French developmental dyslexics. *Annals of Dyslexia*, *63*(2), 117–132. https://doi.org/10.1007/s11881-012-0075-3

Doron, A., Manassi, M., Herzog, M. H., & Ahissar, M. (2015). Intact crowding and temporal masking in dyslexia. *Journal of Vision*, *15*(14), 13–13. https://doi.org/10.1167/15.14.13

Duncan, J., Bundesen, C., Olson, A., Humphreys, G., Ward, R., Kyllingsbæk, S., & Chavda, S. (2003). Attentional functions in dorsal and ventral simultanagnosia. *Cognitive Neuropsychology*, *20*(8), 675–701. https://doi.org/10.1080/02643290342000041

Eden, G. F., Jones, K. M., Cappell, K., Gareau, L., Wood, F. B., Zeffiro, T. A., & Flowers, D. L. (2004). Neural changes following remediation in adult developmental dyslexia. *Neuron*, *44*(3), 411–422. https://doi.org/10.1016/j.neuron.2004.10.019

Feng, X., Monzalvo, K., Dehaene, S., & Dehaene-Lambertz, G. (2022). Evolution of reading and face circuits during the first three years of reading acquisition. *NeuroImage*, *259*, 119394. https://doi.org/10.1016/j.neuroimage.2022.119394

Fernandes, T., & Leite, I. (2017). Mirrors are hard to break: A critical review and behavioral evidence on mirror-image processing in developmental dyslexia. *Journal of Experimental Child Psychology*, *159*(Supplement C), 66–82. https://doi.org/10.1016/j.jecp.2017.02.003

Fernandes, T., Vale, A. P., Martins, B., Morais, J., & Kolinsky, R. (2014). The deficit of letter processing in developmental dyslexia: Combining evidence from dyslexics, typical readers and illiterate adults. *Developmental Science*, *17*(1), 125–141. https://doi.org/10.1111/desc.12102

Franceschini, S., Gori, S., Ruffino, M., Pedrolli, K., & Facoetti, A. (2012). A causal link between visual spatial attention and reading acquisition. *Current Biology: CB*, *22*(9), 814–819. https://doi.org/10.1016/j.cub.2012.03.013

Gabay, Y., Thiessen, E. D., & Holt, L. L. (2015). Impaired statistical learning in developmental dyslexia. *Journal of Speech, Language, and Hearing Research: JSLHR*, *58*(3), 934–945. https://doi.org/10.1044/2015_JSLHR-L-14-0324

Goolkasian, P., & King, J. (1990). Letter identification and lateral masking in dyslexic and average readers. *The American Journal of Psychology*, *103*(4), 519–538.

Grainger, J. (2017). Orthographic processing: A "mid-level" vision of Reading. *The Quarterly Journal of Experimental Psychology*, 1–72. https://doi.org/10.1080/17470218.2017.1314515

Grainger, J., Dufau, S., & Ziegler, J. C. (2016). A vision of Reading. *Trends in Cognitive Sciences, 20*(3), 171–179. https://doi.org/10.1016/j.tics.2015.12.008

Grainger, J., & Ziegler, J. C. (2011). A dual-route approach to orthographic processing. *Frontiers in Psychology, 2*. https://doi.org/10.3389/fpsyg.2011.00054

Hakvoort, B., van den Boer, M., Leenaars, T., Bos, P., & Tijms, J. (2017). Improvements in reading accuracy as a result of increased interletter spacing are not specific to children with dyslexia. *Journal of Experimental Child Psychology, 164*, 101–116. https://doi.org/10.1016/j.jecp.2017.07.010

Hauk, O., Coutout, C., Holden, A., & Chen, Y. (2012). The time-course of single-word reading: Evidence from fast behavioral and brain responses. *NeuroImage, 60*(2), 1462–1477. https://doi.org/10.1016/j.neuroimage.2012.01.061

Hauk, O., Patterson, K., Woollams, A., Watling, L., Pulvermüller, F., & Rogers, T. T. (2006). [Q:] when would you prefer a SOSSAGE to a SAUSAGE? [a:] at about 100 msec. ERP correlates of orthographic typicality and lexicality in written word recognition. *Journal of Cognitive Neuroscience, 18*(5), 818–832. https://doi.org/10.1162/jocn.2006.18.5.818

Hauk, O., Pulvermüller, F., Ford, M., Marslen-Wilson, W. D., & Davis, M. H. (2009). Can I have a quick word? Early electrophysiological manifestations of psycholinguistic processes revealed by event-related regression analysis of the EEG. *Biological Psychology, 80*(1), 64–74. https://doi.org/10.1016/j.biopsycho.2008.04.015

Hawelka, S., Huber, C., & Wimmer, H. (2006). Impaired visual processing of letter and digit strings in adult dyslexic readers. *Vision Research, 46*(5), 718–723. https://doi.org/10.1016/j.visres.2005.09.017

Hawelka, S., & Wimmer, H. (2005). Impaired visual processing of multi-element arrays is associated with increased number of eye movements in dyslexic reading. *Vision Research, 45*(7), 855–863. https://doi.org/10.1016/j.visres.2004.10.007

Hawelka, S., & Wimmer, H. (2008). Visual target detection is not impaired in dyslexic readers. *Vision Research, 48*(6), 850–852. https://doi.org/10.1016/j.visres.2007.11.003

Helenius, P., Tarkiainen, A., Cornelissen, P., Hansen, P. C., & Salmelin, R. (1999). Dissociation of normal feature analysis and deficient processing of letter-strings in dyslexic adults. *Cerebral Cortex (New York, N.Y.: 1991), 9*(5), 476–483.

Hervais-Adelman, A., Kumar, U., Mishra, R. K., Tripathi, V. N., Guleria, A., Singh, J. P., Eisner, F., & Huettig, F. (2019). Learning to read recycles visual cortical networks without destruction. *Science Advances, 5*(9), eaax0262. https://doi.org/10.1126/sciadv.aax0262

Horowitz-Kraus, T., Cicchino, N., Amiel, M., Holland, S. K., & Breznitz, Z. (2014). Reading improvement in English- and Hebrew-speaking children with reading difficulties after reading acceleration training. *Annals of Dyslexia, 64*(3), 183–201. https://doi.org/10.1007/s11881-014-0093-4

Jones, M. W., Branigan, H. P., & Kelly, M. L. (2008). Visual deficits in developmental dyslexia: Relationships between non-linguistic visual tasks and their contribution to components of reading. *Dyslexia (Chichester, England), 14*(2), 95–115. https://doi.org/10.1002/dys.345

Kahta, S., & Schiff, R. (2016). Implicit learning deficits among adults with developmental dyslexia. *Annals of Dyslexia, 66*(2), 235–250. https://doi.org/10.1007/s11881-016-0121-7

Kim, A. E., & Straková, J. (2012). Concurrent effects of lexical status and letter-rotation during early stage visual word recognition: Evidence from ERPs. *Brain Research, 1468*, 52–62. https://doi.org/10.1016/j.brainres.2012.04.008

Klein, R., Berry, G., Briand, K., D'Entremont, B., & Farmer, M. (1990). Letter identification declines with increasing retinal eccentricity at the same rate for normal and dyslexic readers. *Perception & Psychophysics*, *47*(6), 601–606. https://doi.org/10.3758/BF03203112

Kuster, S. M., van Weerdenburg, M., Gompel, M., & Bosman, A. M. T. (2017). Dyslexie font does not benefit reading in children with or without dyslexia. *Annals of Dyslexia*. https://doi.org/10.1007/s11881-017-0154-6

Lachmann, T., & van Leeuwen, C. (2007). Paradoxical enhancement of letter recognition in developmental dyslexia. *Developmental Neuropsychology*, *31*(1), 61–77. https://doi.org/10.1207/s15326942dn3101_4

Leibnitz, L., Grainger, J., Muneaux, M., & Ducrot, S. (2016). Processus Visuo-attentionnels et lecture: Une synthèse. *L'Année Psychologique*, *116*(4), 597–622. https://doi.org/10.4074/S0003503316000403

Lobier, M. A., Peyrin, C., Pichat, C., Le Bas, J.-F., & Valdois, S. (2014). Visual processing of multiple elements in the dyslexic brain: Evidence for a superior parietal dysfunction. *Frontiers in Human Neuroscience*, *8*. https://doi.org/10.3389/fnhum.2014.00479

Mahé, G., Bonnefond, A., & Doignon-Camus, N. (2013). Is the impaired N170 print tuning specific to developmental dyslexia? A matched reading-level study with poor readers and dyslexics. *Brain and Language*, *127*(3), 539–544. https://doi.org/10.1016/j.bandl.2013.09.012

Mahé, G., Bonnefond, A., Gavens, N., Dufour, A., & Doignon-Camus, N. (2012). Impaired visual expertise for print in French adults with dyslexia as shown by N170 tuning. *Neuropsychologia*, *50*(14), 3200–3206. https://doi.org/10.1016/j.neuropsychologia.2012.10.013

Manis, F. R., Custodio, R., & Szeszulski, P. A. (1993). Development of phonological and orthographic skill: A 2-year longitudinal study of dyslexic children. *Journal of Experimental Child Psychology*, *56*(1), 64–86. https://doi.org/10.1006/jecp.1993.1026

Marinus, E., Mostard, M., Segers, E., Schubert, T. M., Madelaine, A., & Wheldall, K. (2016). A special font for people with dyslexia: Does it work and, if so, why? *Dyslexia (Chichester, England)*, *22*(3), 233–244. https://doi.org/10.1002/dys.1527

Martelli, M., Filippo, G. D., Spinelli, D., & Zoccolotti, P. (2009). Crowding, reading, and developmental dyslexia. *Journal of Vision*, *9*(4), 14–14. https://doi.org/10.1167/9.4.14

Martin, J., Colé, P., Leuwers, C., Casalis, S., Zorman, M., & Sprenger-Charolles, L. (2010). Reading in French-speaking adults with dyslexia. *Annals of Dyslexia*, *60*(2), 238–264. https://doi.org/10.1007/s11881-010-0043-8

Maurer, U., Brandeis, D., & McCandliss, B. D. (2005). Fast, visual specialization for reading in English revealed by the topography of the N170 ERP response. *Behavioral and Brain Functions: BBF*, *1*, 13. https://doi.org/10.1186/1744-9081-1-13

Maurer, U., Brem, S., Bucher, K., & Brandeis, D. (2005). Emerging neurophysiological specialization for letter strings. *Journal of Cognitive Neuroscience*, *17*(10), 1532–1552. https://doi.org/10.1162/089892905774597218

Maurer, U., Brem, S., Kranz, F., Bucher, K., Benz, R., Halder, P., & Brandeis, D. (2006). Coarse neural tuning for print peaks when children learn to read. *NeuroImage*, *33*(2), 749–758. https://doi.org/10.1016/j.neuroimage.2006.06.025

Maurer, U., & McCandliss, B. D. (2008). The development of visual expertise for words: The contribution of electrophysiology. In *Single word reading: Behavioral and biological perspectives* (Vol. 4, pp. 43–64). Mahwah, NJ: Lawrence Erlbaum Associates.

McCandliss, B. D., & Noble, K. G. (2003). The development of reading impairment: A cognitive neuroscience model. *Mental Retardation and Developmental Disabilities Research Reviews*, *9*(3), 196–204. https://doi.org/10.1002/mrdd.10080

Miller-Shaul, S. (2005). The characteristics of young and adult dyslexics readers on reading and reading related cognitive tasks as compared to normal readers. *Dyslexia (Chichester, England)*, *11*(2), 132–151. https://doi.org/10.1002/dys.290

Moll, K., & Jones, M. (2013). Naming fluency in dyslexic and nondyslexic readers: Differential effects of visual crowding in foveal, parafoveal, and peripheral vision. *The Quarterly Journal of Experimental Psychology, 66*(11), 2085–2091. https://doi.org/10.1080/17470218.2013.840852

Moores, E., Cassim, R., & Talcott, J. B. (2011). Adults with dyslexia exhibit large effects of crowding, increased dependence on cues, and detrimental effects of distractors in visual search tasks. *Neuropsychologia, 49*(14), 3881–3890. https://doi.org/10.1016/j.neuropsychologia.2011.10.005

Olulade, O. A., Flowers, D. L., Napoliello, E. M., & Eden, G. F. (2015). Dyslexic children lack word selectivity gradients in occipito-temporal and inferior frontal cortex. *NeuroImage. Clinical, 7*, 742–754. https://doi.org/10.1016/j.nicl.2015.02.013

Onochie-Quintanilla, E., Defior, S., & Simpson, I. C. (2017). Visual multi-element processing as a pre-reading predictor of decoding skill. *Journal of Memory and Language, 94*(Supplement C), 134–148. https://doi.org/10.1016/j.jml.2016.11.003

Pammer, K., & Vidyasagar, T. R. (2005). Integration of the visual and auditory networks in dyslexia: A theoretical perspective. *Journal of Research in Reading, 28*(3), 320–331.

Paz-Alonso, P. M., Oliver, M., Lerma-Usabiaga, G., Caballero-Gaudes, C., Quiñones, I., Suárez-Coalla, P., Duñabeitia, J. A., Cuetos, F., & Carreiras, M. (2018). Neural correlates of phonological, orthographic and semantic reading processing in dyslexia. *NeuroImage. Clinical, 20*, 433–447. https://doi.org/10.1016/j.nicl.2018.08.018

Pegado, F. (2022). Written language acquisition is both shaped by and has an impact on brain functioning and cognition. *Frontiers in Human Neuroscience, 16*, 819956. https://doi.org/10.3389/fnhum.2022.819956

Pegado, F., Nakamura, K., Cohen, L., & Dehaene, S. (2011). Breaking the symmetry: Mirror discrimination for single letters but not for pictures in the visual word form area. *NeuroImage, 55*(2), 742–749. https://doi.org/10.1016/j.neuroimage.2010.11.043

Pernet, C., Valdois, S., Celsis, P., & Démonet, J.-F. (2006). Lateral masking, levels of processing and stimulus category: A comparative study between normal and dyslexic readers. *Neuropsychologia, 44*(12), 2374–2385. https://doi.org/10.1016/j.neuropsychologia.2006.05.003

Peyrin, C., Lallier, M., Démonet, J. F., Pernet, C., Baciu, M., Le Bas, J. F., & Valdois, S. (2012). Neural dissociation of phonological and visual attention span disorders in developmental dyslexia: FMRI evidence from two case reports. *Brain and Language, 120*(3), 381–394. https://doi.org/10.1016/j.bandl.2011.12.015

Pitchford, N. J., Ledgeway, T., & Masterson, J. (2009). Reduced orthographic learning in dyslexic adult readers: Evidence from patterns of letter search. *Quarterly Journal of Experimental Psychology (2006), 62*(1), 99–113. https://doi.org/10.1080/17470210701823023

Pugh, K. R., Mencl, W. E., Jenner, A. R., Katz, L., Frost, S. J., Lee, J. R., & Shaywitz, B. A. (2001). Neurobiological studies of reading and reading disability. *Journal of Communication Disorders, 34*(6), 479–492.

Reilhac, C., Peyrin, C., Démonet, J.-F., & Valdois, S. (2013). Role of the superior parietal lobules in letter-identity processing within strings: FMRI evidence from skilled and dyslexicreaders. *Neuropsychologia, 51*(4), 601–612. https://doi.org/10.1016/j.neuropsychologia.2012.12.010

Richlan, F. (2012). Developmental dyslexia: Dysfunction of a left hemisphere reading network. *Frontiers in Human Neuroscience, 6*. https://doi.org/10.3389/fnhum.2012.00120

Richlan, F., Kronbichler, M., & Wimmer, H. (2011). Meta-analyzing brain dysfunctions in dyslexic children and adults. *NeuroImage, 56*(3), 1735–1742. https://doi.org/10.1016/j.neuroimage.2011.02.040

Romani, C., Tsouknida, E., di Betta, A. M., & Olson, A. (2011). Reduced attentional capacity, but normal processing speed and shifting of attention in developmental dyslexia: Evidence from a serial task. *Cortex; A Journal Devoted to the Study of the Nervous System and Behavior, 47*(6), 715–733. https://doi.org/10.1016/j.cortex.2010.05.008

Rosazza, C., Cai, Q., Minati, L., Paulignan, Y., & Nazir, T. A. (2009). Early involvement of dorsal and ventral pathways in visual word recognition: An ERP study. *Brain Research, 1272,* 32–44. https://doi.org/10.1016/j.brainres.2009.03.033

Samara, A., & Caravolas, M. (2017). Artificial grammar learning in dyslexic and non-dyslexic adults: Implications for orthographic learning. *Scientific Studies of Reading, 21*(1), 76–97. https://doi.org/10.1080/10888438.2016.1262865

Savill, N. J., & Thierry, G. (2011). Reading for sound with dyslexia: Evidence for early orthographic and late phonological integration deficits. *Brain Research, 1385,* 192–205. https://doi.org/10.1016/j.brainres.2011.02.012

Sereno, S. C., Rayner, K., & Posner, M. I. (1998). Cognitive neuroscience. *Neuroreport, 9,* 2195–2200.

Share, D. L. (1995). Phonological recoding and self-teaching: Sine qua non of reading acquisition. *Cognition, 55*(2), 151–218.

Shaywitz, S. E., Shaywitz, B. A., Pugh, K. R., Fulbright, R. K., Constable, R. T., Mencl, W. E., & Gore, J. C. (1998). Functional disruption in the organization of the brain for reading in dyslexia. *Proceedings of the National Academy of Sciences, 95*(5), 2636–2641.

Shovman, M. M., & Ahissar, M. (2006). Isolating the impact of visual perception on dyslexics' reading ability. *Vision Research, 46*(20), 3514–3525. https://doi.org/10.1016/j.visres.2006.05.011

Sigurdardottir, H. M., Danielsdottir, H. B., Gudmundsdottir, M., Hjartarson, K. H., Thorarinsdottir, E. A., & Kristjánsson, Á. (2017). Problems with visual statistical learning in developmental dyslexia. *Scientific Reports, 7*(1), 606. https://doi.org/10.1038/s41598-017-00554-5

Sjoblom, A. M., Eaton, E., & Stagg, S. D. (2016). The effects of letter spacing and coloured overlays on reading speed and accuracy in adult dyslexia. *The British Journal of Educational Psychology, 86*(4), 630–639. https://doi.org/10.1111/bjep.12127

Stanovich, K. E. (1980). Toward an interactive-compensatory model of individual differences in the development of Reading fluency. *Reading Research Quarterly, 16*(1), 32–71. https://doi.org/10.2307/747348

Stenneken, P., Egetemeir, J., Schulte-Körne, G., Müller, H. J., Schneider, W. X., & Finke, K. (2011). Slow perceptual processing at the core of developmental dyslexia: A parameter-based assessment of visual attention. *Neuropsychologia, 49*(12), 3454–3465. https://doi.org/10.1016/j.neuropsychologia.2011.08.021

Stevens, M., & Grainger, J. (2003). Letter visibility and the viewing position effect in visual word recognition. *Perception & Psychophysics, 65*(1), 133–151.

Taroyan, N. A., & Nicolson, R. I. (2009). Reading words and pseudowords in dyslexia: ERP and behavioural tests in English-speaking adolescents. *International Journal of Psychophysiology: Official Journal of the International Organization of Psychophysiology, 74*(3), 199–208. https://doi.org/10.1016/j.ijpsycho.2009.09.001

Treiman, R., Pennington, B. F., Shriberg, L. D., & Boada, R. (2008). Which children benefit from letter names in learning letter sounds? *Cognition, 106*(3), 1322–1338. https://doi.org/10.1016/j.cognition.2007.06.006

Treiman, R., Tincoff, R., Rodriguez, K., Mouzaki, A., & Francis, D. J. (1998). The foundations of literacy: Learning the sounds of letters. *Child Development, 69*(6), 1524–1540.

Valdois, S. (2022). The visual-attention span deficit in developmental dyslexia: Review of evidence for a visual-attention-based deficit. *Dyslexia, 28*(4), 397–415. https://doi.org/10.1002/dys.1724

van der Mark, S., Bucher, K., Maurer, U., Schulz, E., Brem, S., Buckelmüller, J., & Brandeis, D. (2009). Children with dyslexia lack multiple specializations along the visual word-form (VWF) system. *NeuroImage*, *47*(4), 1940–1949. https://doi.org/10.1016/j.neuroimage.2009.05.021

van Witteloostuijn, M., Boersma, P., Wijnen, F., & Rispens, J. (2017). Visual artificial grammar learning in dyslexia: A meta-analysis. *Research in Developmental Disabilities*, *70*, 126–137. https://doi.org/10.1016/j.ridd.2017.09.006

Vellutino, F. R., Fletcher, J. M., Snowling, M. J., & Scanlon, D. M. (2004). Specific reading disability (dyslexia): What have we learned in the past four decades? *Journal of Child Psychology and Psychiatry, and Allied Disciplines*, *45*(1), 2–40.

Vidyasagar, T. R. (1999). A neuronal model of attentional spotlight: Parietal guiding the temporal. *Brain Research Reviews*, *30*(1), 66–76.

Vidyasagar, T. R. (2004). Neural underpinnings of dyslexia as a disorder of visuo-spatial attention. *Clinical and Experimental Optometry*, *87*(1), 4–10.

Vidyasagar, T. R., & Pammer, K. (2010). Dyslexia: A deficit in visuo-spatial attention, not in phonological processing. *Trends in Cognitive Sciences*, *14*(2), 57–63. https://doi.org/10.1016/j.tics.2009.12.003

Vinckier, F., Dehaene, S., Jobert, A., Dubus, J. P., Sigman, M., & Cohen, L. (2007). Hierarchical coding of letter strings in the ventral stream: Dissecting the inner organization of the visual word-form system. *Neuron*, *55*(1), 143–156. https://doi.org/10.1016/j.neuron.2007.05.031

Vogel, A. C., Miezin, F. M., Petersen, S. E., & Schlaggar, B. L. (2012). The putative visual word form area is functionally connected to the dorsal attention network. *Cerebral Cortex (New York, N.Y.: 1991)*, *22*(3), 537–549. https://doi.org/10.1093/cercor/bhr100

Wery, J. J., & Diliberto, J. A. (2017). The effect of a specialized dyslexia font, OpenDyslexic, on reading rate and accuracy. *Annals of Dyslexia*, *67*(2), 114–127. https://doi.org/10.1007/s11881-016-0127-1

Wimmer, H., Schurz, M., Sturm, D., Richlan, F., Klackl, J., Kronbichler, M., & Ladurner, G. (2010). A dual-route perspective on poor reading in a regular orthography: An fMRI study. *Cortex*, *46*(10), 1284–1298. https://doi.org/10.1016/j.cortex.2010.06.004

Ziegler, J. C., Pech-Georgel, C., Dufau, S., & Grainger, J. (2010). Rapid processing of letters, digits and symbols: What purely visual-attentional deficit in developmental dyslexia? *Developmental Science*, *13*(4), F8–F14. https://doi.org/10.1111/j.1467-7687.2010.00983.x

Ziegler, J. C., Perry, C., & Zorzi, M. (2013). Modelling reading development through phonological decoding and self-teaching: Implications for dyslexia. *Philosophical Transactions of the Royal Society B: Biological Sciences*, *369*(1634), 20120397. https://doi.org/10.1098/rstb.2012.0397

Zorzi, M., Barbiero, C., Facoetti, A., Lonciari, I., Carrozzi, M., Montico, M., & Ziegler, J. C. (2012). Extra-large letter spacing improves reading in dyslexia. *Proceedings of the National Academy of Sciences of the United States of America*, *109*(28), 11455–11459. https://doi.org/10.1073/pnas.1205566109

5
EXECUTIVE FUNCTIONS IN ADULTS WITH DYSLEXIA

James H. Smith-Spark

5.1 Executive Functioning

The term executive functioning describes a range of complex cognitive abilities that allow an individual to plan, control, and monitor their goal-directed behaviour (e.g., Miyake et al., 2000), particularly in non-routine situations. The executive functions allow individuals to react in a flexible, strategic, and controlled manner to changes in either their internal needs or in their environmental surroundings. Miyake et al. (2000) have argued for both the unity and the diversity of executive functions in their theoretical framework (see also Miyake & Friedman, 2012), in which three specific executive functions, namely inhibition, updating, and set shifting, are identified. These executive functions are viewed as intercorrelated but separable. Inhibition describes the ability to prevent automatic, habitual, or dominant responses to stimuli and, instead, to produce more context-specific, task-appropriate behaviour that is more in keeping with an individual's current goals (e.g., Diamond, 2013). Updating relates to the ability to update the contents of working memory. Set shifting (or task switching; for a review, see Monsell, 2003) refers to the capacity to move effectively between different types of cognitive operation or between different representational sets, adapting flexibly to changes in task demands or environmental conditions (e.g., Miyake et al., 2000). From this core set of executive functions, higher-level executive functions (such as problem-solving, reasoning, and planning) can be constructed (Diamond, 2013). Fisk and Sharp (2004) have argued for the addition of a further core executive function, namely access, which relates to the ability to access information in long-term memory in a flexible, controlled manner.

DOI: 10.4324/9781003491125-6

Zelazo and Müller (2002) have proposed that there is a continuum along which executive functions run, from "cool" to "hot". "Cool" executive functions tend to be employed when faced with abstract tasks lacking in a real-world context, such as those experienced under laboratory conditions. In contrast, "hot" executive functions are called upon when tasks are significantly motivational to the individuals, involve rewards, and when emotions need to be controlled consciously. When working on real-world problems, these two types of executive function are typically brought together to achieve a solution (e.g., Zelazo, 2015).

Of particular relevance to dyslexia researchers and practitioners, executive functioning has been linked to language processing. For example, executive functioning has been found to have a predictive relationship with reading comprehension (for recent reviews, see Butterfuss & Kendeou, 2017; Follmer, 2017). Follmer's meta-analytic review indicates that stronger executive functions remain moderately associated with better reading comprehension skills into adulthood. Sesma, Mahone, Levine, Eason, and Cutting (2009) identify a number of ways in which executive function is argued to be involved in reading comprehension: allowing the reader to engage simultaneously in multiple processes (such as decoding unfamiliar words, accessing semantic information about familiar words, recalling the content of text presented earlier in a passage, and anticipating the direction of the text to come), strategy usage, planning, reasoning, and critical analysis. In a more recent study, Georgiou and Das (2018), using Miyake et al.'s (2000) tripartite theoretical framework of executive function, found that different executive function components had different relationships with reading outcomes in young adults. Only set shifting was found to have a direct predictive relationship with reading comprehension.

Executive functioning has also been linked to writing processes (e.g., Graham, Harris, & Olinghouse, 2007; Hayes & Flower, 1980), although most of the general literature in this area relates to children rather than adults. Drijbooms, Groen, and Verhoeven (2015) highlight the ways in which specific executive functions are likely to be involved in the writing of text. For example, they would be drawn upon when selecting appropriate grammatical and lexical representations, organizing ideas, and inhibiting the expression of irrelevant material, updating the mental representation of the text as it develops, and keeping track of where the writer is in the current sentence and in the text as a whole.

5.2 Dyslexia and Executive Functioning

The adverse effects of dyslexia on the executive functioning of children have been well studied (for meta-analytical reviews, see Booth, Boyle, & Kelly, 2010, and Lonergan et al., 2019), but executive functioning abilities continue to develop into early adulthood (e.g., Taylor, Barker, Heavey, & McHale, 2013).

Research literature on executive functioning in adults with dyslexia also exists, albeit smaller than that relating to children with the condition. This work on adults is considered in the present chapter. Firstly, evidence from laboratory studies is considered. Secondly, the impact of executive functioning deficits on day-to-day life is addressed. Possible approaches to improving executive functioning abilities are then discussed. The need for theoretical accounts of dyslexia to consider executive functioning deficits is considered briefly in the Conclusion.

5.3 Executive Functions under Laboratory Conditions

The executive functions covered in this section are those of inhibition, set shifting, fluency, planning, problem-solving, and dual-task performance. Each of these executive functions will be covered in its own subsection, with laboratory evidence obtained from adults with dyslexia being considered. As already stated, executive functioning in adult samples with dyslexia is not so well explored as it is in children with dyslexia. The amount of research exploring the effects of dyslexia on different executive functions, therefore, varies quite widely. This variation is reflected in the length of the subsections dedicated to each. A further executive function, updating (or working memory; e.g., Miyake et al., 2000), is not considered here given the coverage of memory in Chapter 6.

5.3.1 Inhibition

The Stroop task (Stroop, 1935) and the Go/No Go task (Luria, 1966) are two well-established measures of inhibition.

On the Stroop task, participants are presented with words one at a time. They are asked to name out loud the colour of the ink in which each word is printed. On congruent trials, the name of the colour matches the ink colour (e.g., the word "green" presented in a green font). On incongruent trials, there is a mismatch between the colour name and the colour of the font in which it is printed (e.g., the word "green" displayed in a blue font). Individuals are generally faster and more accurate to respond on congruent trials than to incongruent trials. The degree to which they are slowed or more error-prone on the incongruent trials indicates how well they can inhibit an automatic response arising from it being more a usual (or automatic) response to read words than to process other information about them, such as the colour in which they are printed. This slowing or reduced accuracy is known as the Stroop interference effect. Proulx and Elmasry (2015) have found evidence to indicate that problems with Stroop interference persist into adulthood in dyslexia. Abo-elhija, Farah, and Horowitz-Kraus (2022), meanwhile, have suggested that slower Stroop performance by adults with dyslexia might arise from a combination of executive function and reading difficulties.

On the Go/No Go task, participants need to make a motor response when presented with a particular stimulus (such as a line drawing of a house) while refraining from making a motor response when a different stimulus is presented (such as a picture of a car). After receiving these instructions, the participants are then presented with a significant number of stimuli in succession, all of which require a motor response (e.g., 40 drawings of a house in a row). This builds up a certain level of expectation as to what the response to the next stimulus to be presented is likely to be. This stimulus now represents the habituated or pre-potent response. Without a change being obvious to participants, a mixture of habituated and non-habituated stimuli is then presented, although with a much higher proportion of habituated stimuli being shown. Inhibition is measured by the success with which the participant is able to withhold responses to the non-habituated response (the picture of a car in the above example). Smith-Spark, Henry, Messer, Edvardsdottir, and Zięcik (2016) tested inhibition in adults with and without dyslexia. They administered a variant on the Go/No Go task, which required motor responses to both the habituated and non-habituated stimuli. When processing the habituated stimulus, there was no group difference in either reaction time or accuracy. However, the group with dyslexia showed a deficit in inhibition as they were less accurate when responding to the non-habituated stimulus.

Inhibition in adults with dyslexia has also been studied using other tasks. Poorer inhibition has been found in adults with dyslexia by Brosnan et al. (2002) using the Group-Embedded Figures Test. This task required participants to identify a simple shape (e.g., a triangle) that makes up a part of a larger complex figure (e.g., a kite), with further parallel and perpendicular lines being superimposed on this larger image. Inhibition is needed to avoid processing the surrounding distracting context. Brosnan et al.'s adults with dyslexia were less accurate in identifying the target simple shapes. Dyslexia-related deficits in auditory interference control and conflict resolution have also been reported in adults by Gabay, Gabay, Schiff, and Henik (2020), using the Simon task. In this task, the participants had to respond with an appropriate keypress to a series of high or low pitch tones presented through headphones, while ignoring the left/right ear spatial location of each tone, which might be congruent or incongruent with the side of the keyboard needed to indicate the tone's pitch.

Mahé, Doignon-Camus, Dufour, and Bonnefond (2014) used a flanker task in which participants had to indicate the direction of arrows while ignoring flanking stimuli. Event-related potentials were taken to measure levels of brain activation when carrying out the task. At a behavioural level, adults with and without dyslexia were both slowed when responding to targets that were flanked by incongruent stimuli. However, only the group with dyslexia performed less accurately on incongruent trials. Based on event-related potentials, Mahé et al. argued that adults with dyslexia had impaired conflict monitoring and attentional allocation. However, the authors concluded that inhibition itself was unimpaired in dyslexia and that any differences that are found are due to co-occurring attention deficit–hyperactivity disorder (ADHD) in samples with dyslexia.

Dyslexia-related deficits in inhibition have been found, therefore, across several different tasks. However, issues of co-occurrence with ADHD need to be acknowledged. The presence of ADHD in participants with dyslexia needs to be checked, and steps taken to account for its potential influence on the findings. For example, Smith-Spark et al. (2016) checked the educational psychologist reports for each of their participants with dyslexia. No issues with co-occurrence were identified in these reports. The absence of co-occurring ADHD was further supported by the authors' finding no evidence of group differences on a clinical measure designed to assess attentional difficulties.

5.3.2 Set Shifting

Set shifting can be measured by the Plus–Minus task (Jersild, 1927), in which participants are presented with three lists of two-digit numbers. In response to the first list, they are asked to add three to each of the numbers presented. On the second list, they have to subtract three from each of the numbers presented. The time to complete each of the two lists is recorded, and a mean completion time is calculated. The third list requires participants to alternate between adding and subtracting three from each two-digit number presented. Performance is again timed. The time taken to complete the alternating list is subtracted from the mean time to complete the first two lists. This provides a switch cost value, indicating the extent to which performance is slowed by having to switch between mathematical operations. Amongst their battery of executive functioning measures, Smith-Spark et al. (2016) administered the Plus–Minus task to short-form IQ-matched adults with and without dyslexia. Greater switch costs were produced by the adults with dyslexia. Indeed, the mean switch cost was around 2.5 times greater than that found in the adults without dyslexia.

On the other hand, no problems were found by Stoet, Markey, and Lopez (2007) in adults with dyslexia on a set shifting task, which involved switching between the requirement to distinguish stimuli based on their colour or their shape. Stoet et al. concluded that there were no problems with shifting attention in terms of central cognitive processing; rather, any dyslexia-related problems that were evident were related to difficulties at a perceptual level. However, Poljac et al. (2010) have raised methodological concerns about this study, arguing that stimulus congruence might have played a role in reducing switch cost. Moreover, the sample size was relatively small for both groups, thereby making differences more difficult to detect statistically. Furthermore, over 700 trials were presented, meaning that there was likely to have been reduced novelty to task demands by the end of testing. Extended testing may have washed out any group effects, given the importance of task novelty to executive functioning (e.g., Phillips, 1997; Rabbitt, 1997).

There is, therefore, only a very small amount of research on switching in adults with dyslexia. Moreover, the results of the little research that exists are rather equivocal. Dyslexia-related differences in set shifting may thus depend on the specific task, stimuli, and number of trials employed.

5.3.3 Fluency

Fluency is well-recognized as a measure of executive functioning (e.g., Pennington & Ozonoff, 1996). It reflects the ability to generate items in a set time while adhering to certain rules. As stated previously, Fisk and Sharp (2004) identified verbal fluency as a core executive function to add to the three incorporated within Miyake et al.'s (2000) framework. However, fluency can also be assessed using non-verbal tasks. Both verbal and non-verbal measures are considered in the current section.

Verbal fluency provides a measure of an individual's ability to gain controlled and flexible access to information in long-term memory and, thus, relates to Fisk and Sharp's (2004) core executive function of access. Verbal fluency tasks require an individual to name out loud as many items as they can that conform to specific rules within a given timeframe (usually 1 minute in duration). There are two main categories of verbal fluency tasks, namely phonemic fluency and semantic fluency. On phonemic fluency tasks, individuals are asked to name as many words as they can that begin with a certain letter, such as F, A, or S (e.g., Borkowski, Benton, & Spreen, 1967). They are required to generate items verbally and to do this without repetition, the production of proper nouns, or pluralizing words that have already been generated. Similar rules apply to semantic fluency, where individuals are asked to produce words belonging to a certain semantic category, such as types of fruit or species of animal (e.g., Newcombe, 1969).

Executive functioning abilities are needed to respond successfully to verbal fluency tasks. Demands are made, for example, upon cognitive flexibility, the production of non-habitual responses, the suppression of previously generated responses, error-monitoring, and strategic planning (e.g., Phillips, 1997; Rosen & Engle, 1997). Of the two types of verbal fluency tasks, phonemic fluency is argued to call more heavily upon executive functions than semantic fluency (e.g., Ardila, Ostrosky-Solís, & Bernal, 2006), as generating semantic associates is a more usual activity with existing schemata upon which to draw (e.g., Troyer, Moscovitch, & Winocur, 1997). Leggio, Silveri, Petrosini, and Molinari (2000) have also identified the novel and non-automatized searches required by phonemic fluency, which make it more cognitively complex than semantic fluency. Indeed, as stated previously, dealing with task novelty is a very important aspect of executive functions (Phillips, 1997; Shallice & Burgess, 1991). Further to this, Riva, Nichelli, and Devoti (2000) have highlighted the additional complexity of phonemic fluency, given the much greater number of category subsets that can be explored in performing the task.

Reduced phonemic fluency abilities are well established in adults with dyslexia. Relative to adults without dyslexia, adults with dyslexia have been found to produce a smaller number of words in the time allowed (e.g., Hatcher, Snowling, & Griffiths, 2002; Kinsbourne, Rufo, Gamzu, Palmer, & Berliner, 1991; Miller-Shaul, 2005; Moore, Brown, Markee, Theberge, & Zvi, 1995; Smith-Spark, Henry, Messer & Zięcik, 2017; Snowling, Nation, Moxham, Gallagher, & Frith, 1997; Wilson & Lesaux, 2001). This lowered output rate stands in contrast to their typically unimpaired semantic fluency performance (Frith, Landerl, & Frith, 1995; Reid, Szczerbinski, Iskierka-Kasperek, & Hansen, 2007; Smith-Spark, Henry et al., 2017; although see Snowling et al., 1997). Adults with dyslexia have also been found to be poorer at another fluency task, making heavier demands on phonological processing, called rhyme fluency, in which participants must generate items that rhyme with a target word (Hatcher et al., 2002). As would be expected from the additional phonological processing abilities needed by this task, adults with dyslexia showed even greater difficulties with this task than they did on Hatcher et al.'s phonemic fluency task. The dyslexia-related difference between phonological and semantic fluency abilities is reflective of a broader dissociation between phonological and semantic skills, which persists into adulthood in dyslexia (e.g., Cavalli, Duncan, Elbro, El Ahmadi, & Colé, 2017).

As well as measuring the total number of items generated correctly, verbal fluency performance can also be analysed at a finer-grained level. This allows a more nuanced understanding of performance. Troyer et al. (1997) have identified two components of verbal fluency performance, namely clustering and switching. Clustering describes the generation of words in succession that belong to the same phonemic or semantic subcategory. These words are usually produced in spurts or temporal clusters with short intervals between each cluster (e.g., Henry & Crawford, 2004). Once all items from a subcategory are exhausted, the individual must search for a new subcategory to continue generating items. Switching provides a measure of the number of times that an individual has moved from one subcategory to another during performance (e.g., on the "F" task, producing a cluster of words beginning "Fa", then moving to words beginning "Fi" and subsequently moving to words starting "Fe"). Switches between clusters are argued to demand executive functioning resources. For example, they require strategic search, conscious control, and cognitive flexibility to shift between representational sets (e.g., Troyer, 2000). The production of items within clusters relies upon verbal memory and word storage processes and is fairly automatic even when individuals have lower working memory spans (Rosen & Engle, 1997).

A different approach to assessing verbal fluency is suggested by Crowe (1998) and Hurks et al. (2006). They have argued in favour of exploring output rate over the individual 15s quartiles of a 1-minute task, proposing that greater executive resources are called upon in later quartiles once the most typical exemplars (and, thus, the most easily accessible) have been exhausted.

Measures of verbal fluency can, thus, allow an understanding of the processes involved in task performance at different levels of detail. However, there is considerably less evidence relating to performance on these finer-grained measures of verbal fluency in dyslexia compared with the corpus of data relating to overall output rate. Indeed, to the best of the author's knowledge, only Smith-Spark, Henry et al. (2017) have explored such detailed measures in adults. They used hierarchical regressions to see whether the presence of dyslexia predicted verbal fluency performance, controlling statistically for IQ. On their phonemic fluency task, Smith-Spark et al. found that, in addition to lowered overall correct output, dyslexia predicted fewer switches between clusters but had no relationship with cluster size. The presence of dyslexia also predicted lowered performance in the first two and last 15s quartiles of the task. Dyslexia did not predict performance on any of the measures taken of semantic fluency, although the participants with dyslexia scored slightly worse than the group without dyslexia on every measure taken.

An alternative, non-verbal approach to measuring fluency also exists. Design (or figural) fluency tasks require participants to draw straight lines to join constellations of printed dots with the aim of producing as many novel patterns as possible within a set time limit (e.g., Ruff, Light, & Evans, 1987). Despite this approach allowing dyslexia researchers to explore executive processing independently from phonological processing, design fluency has hardly been studied in dyslexia, with only Smith-Spark, Henry et al. (2017) having investigated it in adults. They found no evidence that the presence of dyslexia affected performance at the level of overall output, concluding that dyslexia-related fluency deficits were most likely the result of the phonological processing difficulties associated with the condition. However, Smith-Spark, Henry et al. were not able to explore performance at a finer-grained level to determine whether dyslexia influenced performance in more subtle ways. Further research is thus needed to explore this issue in greater depth.

In conclusion, dyslexia-related executive fluency problems seem to be evident in adults only when significant phonological processing demands are also present. That is, in the absence of an explicit need to produce responses based on phonological characteristics, dyslexia does not have an influence on executive fluency abilities. Smith-Spark, Henry et al.'s (2017) use of finer-grained measures has furthered the understanding of executive fluency in adults with dyslexia, identifying the components of phonemic fluency that are affected by the condition and those that are not, as well as indicating that semantic fluency is unaffected by dyslexia even when more detailed performance indices are used. Furthermore, the authors found no evidence that design fluency was influenced by dyslexia. However, it should be acknowledged that executive demands may still differ between phonemic fluency and design fluency, given that phonemic fluency requires individuals with dyslexia to draw upon phonological processing skills as well as executive functioning abilities (thus combining two areas in which dyslexia-related deficits are well established; e.g., Brosnan et al., 2002; Castles & Friedmann, 2014). As mentioned previously, phonemic fluency is also regarded as being more cognitively complex than semantic fluency, since task demands are more novel (as searching memory for words by initial phoneme is a much less automated activity than searching for words that are associated semantically; e.g., Leggio et al., 2000) and a greater number of category subsets need to be searched (e.g., Ardila et al., 2006; Riva et al., 2000; Troyer et al., 1997). Therefore, as Smith-Spark et al. have argued, future research is needed to compare fluency performance across different types of fluency tasks once demands on executive processes have been fully equated.

5.3.4 Planning and Problem-Solving

More complex tests of executive functioning draw upon several different executive functions for their successful completion (e.g., Diamond, 2013). Problem-solving and planning tasks are good examples of such tests.

The Wisconsin Card Sorting Test (WCST; Berg, 1948) is a problem-solving task that measures the ability of participants to formulate and execute strategies according to a specific rule. Berg originally conceptualized the test as a measure of set shifting, but, as well as testing cognitive flexibility, the WCST requires strategy monitoring to ensure that the approach taken complies with task demands and is efficient in reaching a solution. The participants are asked to match cards that differ from one another along several dimensions (pattern, colour, and number of elements). However, they are not told the rule to follow to match the cards. Instead, they must determine for themselves the correct dimension along which to sort the cards (e.g., by colour). For each card that is sorted, the experimenter gives feedback as to whether or not the participant is correct. Once a particular rule has been acquired (judged by 10 consecutive correct sorting responses), the card-sorting rule is changed without the participant being informed. Weyandt, Rice, Linterman, Mitzlaff, and Emert (1998) reported more WCST errors being produced by adults with dyslexia relative to a control group. However, IQ matching of groups was not reported by Weyandt et al., and the extent to which the difference reflected an impairment of executive processes is open to question. Indeed, there is evidence to suggest that WCST performance is more closely tied to the role of phonological working memory in keeping the current rule highly active rather than reflecting executive processes (Dunbar & Sussman, 1995). In contrast to Weyandt et al., Smith-Spark (2000) found no evidence of dyslexia-related impairments on the Revised WCST (Heaton, Chelune, Talley, Kay, & Curtiss, 1993). Indeed, the participants with dyslexia performed slightly better on most measures taken than a short-form IQ-matched group without dyslexia. Seidman (2005) has argued that the WCST, which was originally designed predominantly to assess adults who had suffered significant brain damage, may not be sensitive enough to detect differences in subtler developmental disorders. This may explain the differing results of Weyandt et al. (1998) and Smith-Spark (2000), particularly when IQ is controlled.

Planning involves sequencing, organizing, and anticipating actions in order to achieve a particular goal (e.g., Ward & Morris, 2005). The Tower of Hanoi task (e.g., Shallice, 1982) is a disc transfer problem. The materials consist of three pegs and a number of discs that vary in size. Problem difficulty gradually increases as more discs are included in the problem. A start state is presented to the participants, with the discs being stacked on one or more pegs. The participants are asked to reach an end state in which the discs are stacked in descending order of size on a particular peg or pegs. This end state should be reached in the minimum number of moves possible. To perform optimally, participants must analyse the problem and plan their moves before making them. There are three rules that must be followed in moving from the start to the end state: (1) only one disc may be moved at a time, (2) all discs that are not in the process of being moved must be placed on a peg, and (3) a larger disc must not be placed on a smaller disc. Weyandt et al. (1998) found no difference in overall score on the Tower of Hanoi task. Similarly, Brosnan et al. (2002) also found no difference on the Stockings of Cambridge, a variant of the Tower of Hanoi task.

However, dyslexia-related deficits with the use of strategies to solve problems have been reported elsewhere in the literature. On a measure of visuospatial working memory, Bacon, Parmentier, and Barr (2013) found that adults with dyslexia had difficulties with the self-identification and adoption of successful, less cognitively demanding strategies. The authors argued that it was the executive demands of the task that made it difficult for their participants to identify a different, more optimal approach to remembering spatial information. More generally, Meltzer (1991) has argued that people with dyslexia may not possess the cognitive flexibility to gain access to metacognitive information that would help them to recognize the potential utility of alternative strategies.

5.3.5 Dual-task Performance

The ability to perform two different tasks at the same time has been identified as an executive function (e.g., Logie, Cocchini, Della Sala, & Baddeley, 2004).

Miyake et al. (2000) have identified dual-task performance as a complex executive functioning task (like the Tower of Hanoi and the WCST), likely to draw upon several executive functions.

Dyslexia research on adults has approached dual-task performance from the perspective of skill learning rather than as a "pure" measure of executive functioning. Needle, Fawcett, and Nicolson (2006) used dual-task conditions to investigate balancing ability. Their heel-to-toe balancing task required participants to position one foot in front of the other, with the heel of the front foot touching the toe of the rear foot in a straight line, while holding their arms out to the sides, for one minute with as little movement (or "wobble") as possible. In addition to measuring balancing ability on its own, their participants were given dual tasks. These involved counting up or down from certain numbers and also a choice reaction task involving tones of differing frequencies. Poorer balance performance was found in the group with dyslexia under dual-task conditions. Reduced secondary task performance was also found under the more cognitively demanding counting conditions. Such dyslexia-related impairments were consistent with Nicolson, Fawcett, and Dean's (1995) cerebellar deficit hypothesis, which will be returned to briefly in the Conclusion when considering how dyslexia theory can explain executive functioning deficits. Gabay, Schiff, and Vakil (2012) found that the motor skill learning of adults with dyslexia was more greatly disrupted by dual-task conditions. Both initial skill acquisition and consolidation in the group with dyslexia were adversely affected. The authors consider how executive control might influence performance.

The small body of evidence on dual-task performance in adults with dyslexia suggests that there is an executive functioning deficit in this area. However, more research is needed to explore this ability from an executive functioning perspective.

5.3.6 Summary of the Laboratory-based Evidence

Dyslexia-related difficulties have thus been identified across a range of executive functions, with lowered performance being found on most of the executive function abilities reviewed in this chapter. Less clear-cut differences on the clinical tests used to assess planning and problem-solving may arise from the relative bluntness of these tasks as measures of cognitive performance in neurologically intact individuals. While the laboratory evidence indicates that adults with dyslexia experience executive functioning problems, individual executive functions have often been investigated in a rather piecemeal fashion, such that only one or two are addressed in the same paper. This makes it more difficult to gain a full picture of the executive functioning profile of adults with dyslexia. The most complete assessments are those reported by Brosnan et al. (2002) and Smith-Spark et al. (2016).

5.4 Executive Functions in Everyday Life

While controlled laboratory studies are vital to understanding executive functioning performance in dyslexia and informing dyslexia theory, the tasks used are often rather artificial and, thus, detached from day-to-day cognition. Moreover, they require participants to strive to perform optimally, rather than assessing typical or "average" levels of performance in individuals (see Stanovich, 2009). For the outcomes of research on executive functioning to be of maximum benefit to adults with dyslexia, the effects of the condition on day-to-day living must also be considered. Highlighting areas where problems with executive functioning have an impact upon work or education is vital in providing the evidence base to support arguments in favour of reasonable adjustments being made.

Diamond (2013) has identified slips in habitual action as one way in which executive function failure can express itself in day-to-day life. Such problems occur when people do not attend consciously to the goal that they have set when going about a customary day-to-day activity and, as a result, actions sometimes do not proceed as intended. The Cognitive Failures Questionnaire (CFQ; Broadbent, Cooper, FitzGerald, & Parkes, 1982) is a self-report measure that probes these kinds of problems in daily life. It asks individuals to assess how frequently they have made a range of errors in their everyday cognition over the past six months. Smith-Spark, Fawcett, Nicolson, and Fisk (2004) administered the CFQ to adults with and without dyslexia. The respondents with dyslexia reported more problems with distractibility, word finding, and over-focusing their attentional resources. Self-reported issues with attentional control and controlled access to verbal information resonate with some of the laboratory findings on executive functions described previously. Smith-Spark et al. also presented the CFQ for others, a proxy-rating questionnaire, to family members and close friends of the respondents. The proxy respondents also rated the adults with dyslexia as being more prone to cognitive failures; of most relevance to the current chapter, they were rated as being more distractible and more disorganized. Leather, Hogh, Seiss, and Everatt (2011) have also found increased levels of cognitive failures being reported by adults with dyslexia on the CFQ. They also found a moderate correlation between CFQ score and planning scores (a measure of goal setting and the extent to which individuals reflected on tasks before starting them and after completing them).

However, this self-report evidence is indirect, only touching upon areas cognate with executive functioning. A direct approach to investigating executive functioning in daily life was taken by Smith-Spark et al. (2016). In addition to measuring executive functioning under laboratory conditions, the authors also asked their participants to complete the Behavior Rating Inventory of Executive Function–Adult Version (BRIEF-A; Roth, Isquith, & Gioia, 2005), a self-report questionnaire designed specifically to measure executive functioning.

The BRIEF-A requires respondents to rate the frequency with which they experienced certain types of problems with executive functioning over the past month. The questions contribute to nine scales measuring different aspects of executive functioning in everyday life. These scales, in turn, are subsumed by two indices. The Metacognition Index reflects how well an individual feels he or she acts in an organized, planned, and systematic way, deploying working memory to help solve problems. The Behavioral Regulation Index assesses the control and regulation of emotional responses and behaviour. Smith-Spark et al. found that the group with dyslexia rated their executive functions as being generally more prone to problems than the group without dyslexia. More specifically, the adults with dyslexia rated themselves as having more frequent difficulties with the aspects of everyday executive functioning probed by the Metacognition Index, being more frequently prone to problems with working memory, managing current and future task demands, and keeping track of their progress when solving problems. No differences between the respondents with and without dyslexia were found on the Behavioral Regulation Index. Giancola, Godlaski, and Roth (2012) have argued that the Metacognition Index is associated with "cool" EFs, while the Behavioral Regulation Index is related to "hot" EFs. From this point of view, Smith-Spark et al.'s findings indicate that, under everyday conditions, dyslexia is perceived by those with the condition to impair "cool" executive functions while having no effect on "hot" executive functions. In day-to-day situations, therefore, adults with dyslexia feel that it is their analytical executive functions rather than emotional ones that are affected.

Some of the items of Roth et al.'s (2005) BRIEF-A contribute towards a Negativity scale. This scale allows individuals who have an unusually negative view of themselves to be identified. In Smith-Spark et al.'s (2016) study, no individual participants had to be excluded from the analyses due to unusually high Negativity scores, nor were any group differences found on this measure. Based on this pattern of results, heightened self-reports of executive function problems in everyday life are not likely to be the result of a negative self-image arising from the lowered self-esteem often found in adults with dyslexia (e.g., Riddick, Sterling, Farmer, & Morgan, 1999).

Every day, difficulties with executive functioning have also been raised by adults with dyslexia in interviews. Of the university students interviewed by Mortimore and Crozier (2006), two-thirds reported problems with general organization, and around half of the sample identified difficulties with timekeeping. Difficulties with organization, planning, time management, and adaptation to change have been identified as problematic for adults with dyslexia by McLoughlin and Leather (2013). Doyle and McDowall (2015) also highlight problems in several areas related to executive functioning, namely organizational skills, time management, goal setting and prioritization, self-regulation, and the ability to cope in the face of distraction.

Difficulties with executive functioning are likely to have an impact in adult educational settings. Indeed, problems with planning have been self-reported in interviews by 28% of a sample of over 100 university students with dyslexia (Stack-Cutler, Parrila, Jokisaari, & Nurmi, 2015). Just over 17% of Further and Higher Education students with dyslexia interviewed by Kirby, Sugden, Beveridge, Edwards, and Edwards (2008) reported problems with various aspects of executive functioning. As mentioned previously, executive functions have been argued to play a role in writing processes (e.g., Graham et al., 2007). Executive functioning deficits could, therefore, explain the difficulties associated with essay writing in adult university students. Gilroy and Miles (1996) identified the problems that adult students with dyslexia have with the planning and structuring of essays. This point is further supported by interviews conducted with university students with dyslexia by Mortimore and Crozier (2006), 76% of whom reported problems with organizing essays. Some empirical support for dyslexia-related difficulties with essay planning is provided by Galbraith, Baaijen, Smith-Spark, and Torrance (2012). They asked university students with and without dyslexia to produce an outline of their ideas on the pros and cons of legalizing euthanasia before writing the ideas down in the form of a newspaper article. The students with dyslexia had greater difficulties in building a stable outline of their ideas before writing the article, in using their outlines effectively during writing, and in coordinating their initial goals with the text that they produced.

Problems with everyday executive functions may also have broader consequences for outcomes in further and higher education. Rabin, Fogel, and Nutter-Upham (2011) have found that seven BRIEF-A scales (Roth et al., 2005) predicted academic procrastination in university students. Five of these scales came from the Metacognition Index, on which Smith-Spark et al. (2016) found adults with dyslexia reported experiencing more frequent problems. People with poorer executive functions may postpone or delay revising for exams, writing coursework assessments, and doing the necessary background reading for their studies to a point at which it is unlikely that they will be able to perform to the best of their abilities. There may, thus, be a greater propensity to academic procrastination in adults with dyslexia, and support tutors need to be aware of this when addressing study skills.

At least some of these difficulties are likely to transfer to employment. For instance, Doyle and McDowall (2015) have argued that problems relating to executive functioning feature heavily amongst the difficulties experienced by the adult with dyslexia in workplace settings. Leather et al. (2011) found that better self-reported planning abilities and fewer cognitive failures were found to be predictive of greater self-efficacy and job satisfaction in adults with dyslexia. Smith-Spark, Gordon, and Jansari (2023) investigated work-based cognition using a non-immersive virtual office environment (the JEF©; Jansari et al., 2014). University students with and without dyslexia and naïve to office work were asked to imagine that they were on their first day in an office job and had to set up a room for a meeting. Several of the JEF©'s measures assessed executive function, with the group with dyslexia scoring lower on the planning and selective-thinking measures (but showing no differences on the prioritization, creativity, and adaptiveness measures). Of the two measures on which significant group differences were found, planning was more greatly affected by dyslexia. Planning required the ordering of objects or events according to logic rather than their relative importance. Selective thinking measured the participants' ability to draw upon acquired knowledge to make choices between two or more alternatives.

5.5 Improving Executive Functioning Abilities

Having identified a range of executive functions across which difficulties are experienced, the question becomes one of how to minimize the impact of these problems on adults with dyslexia. Ideally, these problems would be addressed through training and interventions in childhood, to ensure that individuals with dyslexia would be compensated in this area when reaching adulthood (see Diamond, 2014, for a general review of approaches). For many people with dyslexia, however, the time to have their executive functions ameliorated in childhood has passed. To be of benefit to such individuals, supporting and improving executive functions in adulthood has to be addressed. Less evidence exists to indicate how executive functions can be improved in early adulthood through cognitive training, although the results seem broadly favourable (see Diamond, 2013, for a review). To the best of the author's knowledge, there has, to date, been no investigation into the effects of training on executive functions in adults with dyslexia. However, Franceschini et al. (2013) have demonstrated that action video games can improve focused and distributed attention in children with dyslexia, so there is some reason to be optimistic about their potential impact. However, in the general literature, questions remain (e.g., Diamond, 2013) as to the effectiveness of cognitive training in terms of its longer-term benefits and its transferability to tasks, both those that are closely related to the trained task (i.e., near-transfer effects) and those that are more distantly related to the trained task (i.e., far-transfer effects). The extent to which the benefits are, firstly, long-lasting and, secondly, generalizable to other tasks or skills is of paramount importance when considering the merits of cognitive training in terms of the time and resources invested in running such programmes.

Technology can play a role in addressing problems with organization. Reid, Strnadová, and Cumming (2013) have identified the types of support that mobile technology can provide for the adult with dyslexia. These include assistance with planning tasks and remembering to do things at the time that they are required (cf., the role of executive processes in memory for delayed intentions or prospective memory; Smith-Spark, 2017). However, it should be noted that Smith-Spark, Zięcik, and Sterling (2017) have provided self-report evidence suggesting that more frequent use of tools and technology by adults with dyslexia does not mitigate effectively against the effects of the condition on cognition. The authors argue that explicit instruction in their use is required. They link this to the work of Meltzer (1991) and Bacon et al. (2013), identifying problems with strategy use. Rather than simply giving adults with dyslexia technology and then leaving them to work out how to use it to best effect, the ways in which technology can facilitate performance may need to be demonstrated to adults with dyslexia to ensure that they can use it to its full potential.

The people with whom an individual is in contact may also provide a means of assisting with executive functioning. Stack-Cutler et al. (2015) have suggested that the resources available within the social networks of university students with dyslexia can be utilized to facilitate goal setting, planning, and problem-solving. The authors argue that students with dyslexia should be encouraged to build relationships with others and to identify means of support available within their university and beyond it.

Another approach, which involves external, personal support, is suggested by coaching, in which a personal coach helps a learner to improve in a specified area through guidance and training. Doyle and McDowall (2015) argue that coaching is a beneficial approach to improving executive functions in adults with dyslexia. Their data suggest that, through coaching, improvements can be made to working memory, time management, and organizational skills.

5.6 Conclusion

As with most areas of cognition, the impact of dyslexia on executive functioning in adulthood is much less explored than it is in children. Overall, however, the evidence indicates that dyslexia continues to have a negative impact on executive functioning in adulthood (for a neuro-behavioural review of executive function in dyslexia from childhood to adulthood, see Farah, Ionta, & Horowitz-Kraus, 2021). This impact is observable under laboratory conditions (e.g., Brosnan et al., 2002; Smith-Spark et al., 2016; Smith-Spark, Henry et al., 2017) and, more importantly for the individuals concerned, is also self-reported as being experienced in everyday life (Smith-Spark et al., 2016; Stack-Cutler et al., 2015). Smith-Spark et al.'s (2016) findings link the two settings together, demonstrating executive functioning problems under both laboratory and everyday conditions in the same sample of adults with dyslexia.

Executive functioning deficits have been reported in adults with both ADHD (e.g., Boonstra, Oosterlaan, Sergeant, & Buitelaar, 2005) and developmental coordination disorder (e.g., Tal Saban, Ornoy, & Parush, 2014). Given the rates of co-occurrence that dyslexia has with these disorders (e.g., Pennington & Bishop, 2009), researchers need to reduce the chances of co-occurrence influencing the results of executive functioning studies where dyslexia is the sole focus of research. As stated previously in this chapter, in one of the most complete studies of executive functioning in adulthood to date, Smith-Spark et al. (2016) found no evidence of group differences on a clinical measure of attention or in self-reported emotional regulation. Differences in these measures would be indicative of the problems with emotional control associated with ADHD (e.g., Shaw, Stringaris, Nigg, & Leibenluft, 2014). Given that they were not found, it seems reasonably certain that the executive functioning problems uncovered are the result of dyslexia and not due to co-occurring neurodevelopmental conditions. Future research on executive functioning in dyslexia needs to screen actively for the presence of ADHD amongst the sample with dyslexia, noting the prevalence of co-occurrence, and taking steps to address it.

As mentioned previously in this chapter, different tasks purportedly assessing the same underlying executive function have at times yielded very different patterns of results. This reflects a general concern when measuring executive functions and is known as the task impurity problem (e.g., Burgess, 1997). Executive functions have their effects by operating on other, more basic cognitive processes related to the task in question. Thus, a low score on one specific measure may be indicative of a problem with the specific cognitive processes required by that task rather than the executive processes acting upon them. Indeed, Burgess (1997) has argued that even quite small changes to a task can have a similar effect on performance. Based on this concern, there is a strong argument for using at least two different tasks to assess each executive function under investigation to gain a clearer picture of the pattern of deficits. Performance on several tests of the same executive function can then be combined and analysed to determine whether group differences exist (e.g., Thompson & Green, 2013).

The range of executive functioning problems identified in this chapter needs to be explained by the dyslexia theory. Given their range and the absence of significant phonological processing demands on some tasks, this seems a particular challenge for theoretical approaches that focus on core deficits in phonological processing (see Castles & Friedmann, 2014). However, explanations that take a broader view of dyslexia have also not considered executive functioning difficulties explicitly within their frameworks. That said, Nicolson and Fawcett's (1990) Dyslexia Automatization Deficit hypothesis does consider a heightened need for the conscious allocation of attention in dyslexia, with dual-task performance and task novelty being considered. The Cerebellar Deficit Hypothesis (Nicolson et al., 1995) may also be able to explain executive functioning deficits, given that the cerebellum has been linked to executive processes (e.g., Bellebaum & Daum, 2007). Dealing most explicitly with executive functioning deficits, Smith-Spark and Fisk (2007) have argued that adults with dyslexia may struggle with task novelty relative to controls.

Smith-Spark and Fisk's (2007) proposition was based on the results of a visuospatial working memory task. Students with dyslexia performed more poorly over the first half of this task but improved to an equivalent level of recall accuracy to a group of age- and IQ-matched controls over the second half. Smith-Spark and Fisk argued that this pattern of performance might indicate a problem with setting up cognitive schemata to deal effectively with novel task demands, thereby implicating a dysfunction in the Supervisory Attentional System (SAS) component of Norman and Shallice's (1986) model of the control of action. The SAS coordinates, integrates, and controls information. It is called upon when task novelty is high or poorly learnt action sequences are required (e.g., Shallice & Burgess, 1991) and when attentional resources are needed to modulate behaviour. Within his highly influential multicomponent model of working memory, Baddeley (1986) has identified the SAS as a potential candidate for the central executive, an attentional control system responsible for the direction of attention to relevant information, strategy selection, and the control of ongoing actions.

The way in which dyslexia-related problems manifested themselves on Smith-Spark and Fisk's task highlights the importance of task novelty to executive functioning (Rabbitt, 1997). Researchers need to be aware of task length, since the contribution of the executive functions to performance is likely to be at its greatest when the task is at its most novel. Thus, group differences are likely to be at their most noticeable in the earliest interactions with a task.

Smith-Spark and Fisk's argument for SAS dysfunction in dyslexia explained a pattern of performance shown on a working memory task. The question remains as to whether SAS dysfunction can explain dyslexia-related deficits on tasks that measure other executive functions, although support for SAS dysfunction in dyslexia has come from the study of children with dyslexia (Varvara, Varuzza, Sorrentino, Vicari, & Menghini, 2014) and Smith-Spark and Gordon's (2022) theoretical review presents a detailed consideration of the role of the SAS in executive function difficulties in dyslexia. It is also interesting to note Mahé et al.'s (2014) identification of conflict resolution problems in adults with dyslexia, given the role of the SAS in this area. Further, the difficulties they found with the allocation of attention would fit well with both Nicolson and Fawcett's (1990) DAD hypothesis and SAS dysfunction.

As a final caveat, the studies reviewed in this chapter have tended to have been conducted on university students with dyslexia and are, thus, indicative of executive functioning in relatively high-achieving (and typically young) adults. It remains to be seen whether similar profiles are shown across the general working-age population with dyslexia. As the number of older individuals with officially diagnosed dyslexia increases over the next 20–30 years, this may provide an important and fertile ground for future research.

A range of executive functions are affected by dyslexia and, beyond the laboratory, have been found to have an impact on everyday life. Executive functioning problems need to be accounted for when supporting adults with dyslexia and considered when making reasonable adjustments in education and employment.

References

Abo-elhija, D., Farah, R., & Horowitz-Kraus, T. (2022). Stroop performance is related to reading profiles in Hebrew-speaking individuals with dyslexia and typical readers. *Dyslexia, 28*(2), 212–227.

Ardila, A., Ostrosky-Solís, F., & Bernal, B. (2006). Cognitive testing toward the future: The example of semantic verbal fluency (ANIMALS). *International Journal of Psychology, 41*, 324–332.

Bacon, A. M., Parmentier, F. B. R., & Barr, P. (2013). Visuospatial memory in dyslexia: Evidence for strategic deficits. *Memory, 21*, 189–209.

Baddeley, A. D. (1986). *Working memory*. Oxford: Clarendon Press.

Bellebaum, C., & Daum, I. (2007). Cerebellar involvement in executive control. *The Cerebellum, 6*, 184–192.

Berg, E. A. (1948). A simple objective test for measuring flexibility in thinking. *Journal of General Psychology, 39*, 15–22.

Boonstra, A. M., Oosterlaan, J., Sergeant, J. A., & Buitelaar, J. K. (2005). Executive functioning in adult ADHD: A meta-analytic review. *Psychological Medicine, 35*, 1097–1108.

Booth, J. N., Boyle, J. M. E., & Kelly, S. W. (2010). Do tasks make a difference? Accounting for heterogeneity of performance of children with reading difficulties on tasks of executive function: Findings from a meta-analysis. *British Journal of Developmental Psychology, 28*, 133–176.

Borkowski, J. G., Benton, A. L., & Spreen, O. (1967). Word fluency and brain damage. *Neuropsychologia, 5*, 135–140.

Broadbent, D. E., Cooper, P. F., FitzGerald, P., & Parkes, K. R. (1982). The cognitive failure questionnaire (CFQ) and its correlates. *British Journal of Clinical Psychology, 21*, 1–16.

Brosnan, M., Demetre, J., Hamill, S., Robson, K., Shepherd, H., & Cody, G. (2002). Executive functioning in adults and children with developmental dyslexia. *Neuropsychologia, 40*, 2144–2155.

Burgess, P. W. (1997). Theory and methodology in executive function research. In P. Rabbitt (Ed.), *Methodology of frontal and executive function* (pp. 81–116). Hove, East Sussex: Psychology Press.

Butterfuss, R., & Kendeou, P. (2017). The role of executive functions in reading comprehension. *Educational Psychology Review*. https://doi.org/10.1007/s10648-017-9422-6

Castles, A., & Friedmann, N. (2014). Developmental dyslexia and the phonological deficit hypothesis. *Mind and Language, 29*, 270–285.

Cavalli, E., Duncan, L. G., Elbro, C., El Ahmadi, A., & Colé, P. (2017). Phonemic—Morphemic dissociation in university students with dyslexia: An index of reading compensation? *Annals of Dyslexia, 67*, 63–84.

Crowe, S. F. (1998). Decrease in performance on the verbal fluency test as a function of time: Evaluation in a young healthy sample. *Journal of Clinical and Experimental Neuropsychology, 20*, 391–401.

Diamond, A. (2013). Executive functions. *Annual Review of Psychology, 64*, 135–168.

Diamond, A. (2014). Executive functions: Insights into ways to help more children thrive. *Zero to Three, 35*, 9–17.

Doyle, N., & McDowall, N. (2015). Is coaching an effective adjustment for dyslexic adults? *Coaching: An International Journal of Theory Research and Practice, 8*, 154–168.

Drijbooms, E., Groen, M. A., & Verhoeven, L. (2015). The contribution of executive functions to narrative writing in fourth grade children. *Reading and Writing, 28*, 989–1011.

Dunbar, K., & Sussman, D. (1995). Toward a cognitive account of the frontal lobe function: Simulating frontal lobe deficits in normal subjects. *Annals of the New York Academy of Sciences, 769*, 289–304.

Farah, R., Ionta, S., & Horowitz-Kraus, T. (2021). Neuro-behavioral correlates of executive dysfunctions in dyslexia over development from childhood to adulthood. *Frontiers in Psychology, 12*, 708863.

Fisk, J. E., & Sharp, C. A. (2004). Age-related impairment in executive functioning: Updating, inhibition, shifting, and access. *Journal of Clinical and Experimental Neuropsychology, 26*, 874–890.

Follmer, D. J. (2017). Executive function and reading comprehension: A meta-analytic review. *Educational Psychologist*. https://doi.org/10.1080/00461520.2017.1309295

Franceschini, S., Gori, S., Ruffino, M., Viola, S., Molteni, M., & Facoetti, A. (2013). Action video games make dyslexic children read better. *Current Biology, 23*, 462–466.

Frith, U., Landerl, K., & Frith, C. (1995). Dyslexia and verbal fluency: More evidence for a phonological deficit. *Dyslexia, 1*, 2–11.

Gabay, Y., Gabay, S., Schiff, R., & Henik, A. (2020). Visual and auditory interference control of attention in developmental dyslexia. *Journal of the International Neuropsychological Society, 26*(4), 407–417.

Gabay, Y., Schiff, R., & Vakil, E. (2012). Attentional requirements during acquisition and consolidation of a skill in normal readers and developmental dyslexics. *Neuropsychology, 26*, 744–757.

Galbraith, D., Baaijen, V., Smith-Spark, J., & Torrance, M. (2012). The effects of dyslexia on the writing processes of students in higher education. In M. Torrance, D. Alamargot, M. Castelló, F. Ganier, O. Kruse, A. Mangen, L. Tolchinsky, & L. van Waes (Eds.), *Learning to write effectively: Current trends in European research* (pp. 195–198). Brill Books Online. https://doi.org/10.1163/9781780529295_044

Georgiou, G. K., & Das, J. P. (2018). Direct and indirect effects of executive function on reading comprehension in young adults. *Journal of Research in Reading, 41*(2), 243–258.

Giancola, P. R., Godlaski, A. J., & Roth, R. M. (2012). Identifying component-processes of executive functioning that serve as risk factors for the alcohol-aggression relation. *Psychology of Addictive Behaviors, 26*, 201–211.

Gilroy, D. E., & Miles, T. R. (1996). *Dyslexia at college* (2nd ed.). London and New York: Routledge.

Graham, S., Harris, K. R., & Olinghouse, N. (2007). Addressing executive function problems in writing: An example from the self-regulated strategy development model. In L. Meltzer (Ed.), *Executive function in education* (pp. 216–236). New York: Guilford.

Hatcher, J., Snowling, M. J., & Griffiths, Y. M. (2002). Cognitive assessment of dyslexic students in higher education. *British Journal of Educational Psychology, 72*, 119–133.

Hayes, J. R., & Flower, L. S. (1980). Identifying the organization of writing processes. In L. W. Gregg & E. R. Steinberg (Eds.), *Cognitive processes in writing* (pp. 3–30). Mahwah, NJ: Erlbaum.

Heaton, R. K., Chelune, G. J., Talley, J. L., Kay, G. G., & Curtiss, G. (1993). *Wisconsin card sorting test manual: Revised and expanded*. Odessa, FL: Psychological Assessment Resources.

Henry, J. D., & Crawford, J. R. (2004). A meta-analytic review of verbal fluency performance following focal cortical lesions. *Neuropsychology, 18*, 284–295.

Hurks, P. P. M., Vles, J. S. H., Hendriksen, J. G. M., Kalff, A. C., Feron, F. J. M., Kroes, M., et al. (2006). Semantic category fluency versus initial letter fluency over 60 seconds as a measure of automatic and controlled processing in healthy school-aged children. *Journal of Clinical & Experimental Neuropsychology, 28*, 684–695.

Jansari, A. S., Devlin, A., Agnew, R., Akesson, K., Murphy, L., & Leadbetter, T. (2014). Ecological assessment of executive functions: A new virtual reality paradigm. *Brain Impairment, 15*(2), 71–87.

Jersild, A. T. (1927). Mental set and shift. *Archives of Psychology*, Whole No. 89.

Kinsbourne, M., Rufo, D. T., Gamzu, E., Palmer, R. L., & Berliner, A. K. (1991). Neuropsychological deficits in adults with dyslexia. *Developmental Medicine and Child Neurology, 33*, 763–775.

Kirby, A., Sugden, D., Beveridge, S., Edwards, L., & Edwards, R. (2008). Dyslexia and developmental co-ordination disorder in further and higher education-similarities and differences. Does the 'label' influence the support given? *Dyslexia, 14*, 197–213.

Leather, C., Hogh, H., Seiss, E., & Everatt, J. (2011). Cognitive functioning and work success in adults with dyslexia. *Dyslexia, 17*, 327–338.

Leggio, M. G., Silveri, M. C., Petrosini, L., & Molinari, M. (2000). Phonological grouping is specifically affected in cerebellar patients: A verbal fluency study. *Journal of Neurology, Neurosurgery & Psychiatry, 69*, 102–106.

Logie, R. H., Cocchini, G., Della Sala, S., & Baddeley, A. D. (2004). Is there a specific executive capacity for dual task coordination? Evidence from Alzheimer's disease. *Neuropsychology, 18*, 504–513.

Lonergan, A., Doyle, C., Cassidy, C., MacSweeney Mahon, S., Roche, R. A. P., Boran, L., & Bramham, J. (2019). A meta-analysis of executive functioning in dyslexia with consideration of the impact of comorbid ADHD. *Journal of Cognitive Psychology, 31*(7), 725–749.

Luria, A. R. (1966). *Higher cortical functions*. New York: Basic Books.

Mahé, G., Doignon-Camus, N., Dufour, A., & Bonnefond, A. (2014). Conflict control processing in adults with developmental dyslexia: An event related potentials study. *Clinical Neurophysiology, 125*, 69–76.

McLoughlin, D., & Leather, C. (2013). *The dyslexic adult*. Chichester, West Sussex: John Wiley.

Meltzer, L. (1991). Problem-solving strategies and academic performance in learning disabled students: Do subtypes exist? In L. V. Feagans, E. J. Short, & L. J. Meltzer (Eds.), *Subtypes of learning disabilities: Theoretical perspectives and research* (pp. 163–188). Hillsdale, NJ: Lawrence Erlbaum Associates.

Miller-Shaul, S. (2005). The characteristics of young and adult dyslexic readers on reading and reading related cognitive tasks as compared to normal readers. *Dyslexia, 11*, 132–151.

Miyake, A., & Friedman, N. P. (2012). The nature and organization of individual differences in executive functions: Four general conclusions. *Current Directions in Psychological Science, 21*, 8–14.

Miyake, A., Friedman, N. P., Emerson, M. J., Witzki, A. H., Howerter, A., & Wager, T. D. (2000). The unity and diversity of executive functions, and their contributions to complex "frontal lobe" tasks: A latent variable analysis. *Cognitive Psychology, 41*, 49–100.

Monsell, S. (2003). Task switching. *Trends in Cognitive Sciences, 7*, 134–140.

Moore, L. H., Brown, W. S., Markee, T. E., Theberge, D. C., & Zvi, J. C. (1995). Bimanual coordination in dyslexic adults. *Neuropsychologia, 33*, 781–793.

Mortimore, T., & Crozier, W. R. (2006). Dyslexia and difficulties with study skills in higher education. *Studies in Higher Education, 31*, 235–251.

Needle, J. L., Fawcett, A. J., & Nicolson, R. I. (2006). Balance and dyslexia: An investigation of adults' abilities. *European Journal of Cognitive Psychology, 18*, 909–936.

Newcombe, F. (1969). *Missile wounds of the brain*. London: Oxford University Press.
Nicolson, R. I., & Fawcett, A. J. (1990). Automaticity: A new framework for dyslexia research. *Cognition*, *35*, 159–182.
Nicolson, R. I., Fawcett, A. J., & Dean, P. (1995). Time estimation deficits in developmental dyslexia: Evidence of cerebellar involvement. *Proceedings of the Royal Society of London, Series B: Biological Sciences*, *259*(1354), 43–47.
Norman, D. A., & Shallice, T. (1986). Attention to action: Willed and automatic control of behaviour. In R. J. Davidson, G. E. Schwartz, & D. Shapiro (Eds.), *Consciousness and self-regulation: Advances in research and theory* (Vol. 4, pp. 1–18). New York: Plenum Press.
Pennington, B. F., & Bishop, D. V. M. (2009). Relations among speech, language and reading disorders. *Annual Review of Psychology*, *60*, 283–306.
Pennington, B. F., & Ozonoff, S. (1996). Executive functions and developmental psychopathology. *Journal of Child Psychology and Psychiatry*, *37*, 51–87.
Phillips, L. H. (1997). Do "frontal tests" measure executive function? Issues of assessment and evidence from fluency tests. In P. M. A. Rabbitt (Ed.), *Methodology of frontal and executive function* (pp. 191–213). Hove, East Sussex: Psychology Press.
Poljac, E., Simon, S., Ringlever, L., Kalcik, D., Groen, W. B., Buitelaar, J. K., & Bekkering, H. (2010). Impaired task switching performance in children with dyslexia but not in children with autism. *Quarterly Journal of Experimental Psychology*, *63*, 401–416.
Proulx, M. J., & Elmasry, H. -M. (2015). Stroop interference in adults with dyslexia. *Neurocase*, *21*, 413–417.
Rabbitt, P. (1997). Introduction: Methodologies and models in the study of executive function. In P. Rabbitt (Ed.), *Methodology of frontal and executive function* (pp. 1–38). Hove, UK: Psychology Press.
Rabin, L. A., Fogel, J., & Nutter-Upham, K. E. (2011). Academic procrastination in college students: The role of self-reported executive function. *Journal of Clinical and Experimental Neuropsychology*, *33*, 344–357.
Reid, A. A., Szczerbinski, M., Iskierka-Kasperek, E., & Hansen, P. (2007). Cognitive profiles of adult developmental dyslexics: Theoretical implications. *Dyslexia*, *13*, 1–24.
Reid, G., Strnadová, I., & Cumming, T. (2013). Expanding horizons for students with dyslexia in the 21st century: Universal design and mobile technology. *Journal of Research in Special Educational Needs*, *13*, 175–181.
Riddick, B., Sterling, C., Farmer, M., & Morgan, S. (1999). Self-esteem and anxiety in the educational histories of adult dyslexic students. *Dyslexia*, *5*, 227–248.
Riva, D., Nichelli, F., & Devoti, M. (2000). Developmental aspects of verbal fluency and confrontation naming in children. *Brain and Language*, *71*, 267–284.
Rosen, V. M., & Engle, R. W. (1997). The role of working memory capacity in retrieval. *Journal of Experimental Psychology: General*, *126*, 211–227.
Roth, R. M., Isquith, P. K., & Gioia, G. A. (2005). *BRIEF-A: Behavior rating inventory of executive function - adult version*. Lutz, FL: Psychological Assessment Resources.
Ruff, R. M., Light, R. H., & Evans, R. W. (1987). The Ruff figural fluency test: A normative study with adults. *Developmental Neuropsychology*, *3*, 37–51.
Seidman, L. J. (2005). Neuropsychological functioning in people with ADHD across the lifespan. *Clinical Psychology Review*, *26*, 466–485.
Sesma, H. W., Mahone, E. M., Levine, T., Eason, S. H., & Cutting, L. E. (2009). The contribution of executive skills to reading comprehension. *Child Neuropsychology*, *15*, 232–246.
Shallice, T. (1982). Specific impairments of planning. *Philosophical Transactions of the Royal Society of London*, *298*, 199–209.

Shallice, T., & Burgess, P. W. (1991). Deficits in strategy application following frontal lobe damage in man. *Brain*, *114*, 727–741.

Shaw, P., Stringaris, A., Nigg, J., & Leibenluft, E. (2014). Emotional dysregulation and attention-deficit/hyperactivity disorder. *American Journal of Psychiatry*, *171*, 276–293.

Smith-Spark, J. H. (2000). *Memory in adult dyslexics: An exploration of the working memory system*. Unpublished PhD thesis, University of Sheffield, UK.

Smith-Spark, J. H. (2017). A review of prospective memory impairments in developmental dyslexia: Evidence, explanations, and future directions. *The Clinical Neuropsychologist*. https://doi.org/10.1080/13854046.2017.1369571

Smith-Spark, J. H., Fawcett, A. J., Nicolson, R. I., & Fisk, J. E. (2004). Dyslexic students have more everyday cognitive lapses. *Memory*, *12*, 174–182.

Smith-Spark, J. H., & Fisk, J. E. (2007). Working memory functioning in developmental dyslexia. *Memory*, *15*, 34–56.

Smith-Spark, J. H., & Gordon, R. (2022). Automaticity and executive abilities in developmental dyslexia: A theoretical review. *Brain Sciences*, *12*, 446.

Smith-Spark, J. H., Gordon, R., & Jansari, A. S. (2023). The impact of developmental dyslexia on workplace cognition: Evidence from a virtual reality environment. *Behaviour & Information Technology*, *42*(3), 269–277.

Smith-Spark, J. H., Henry, L. A., Messer, D. J., Edvardsdottir, E., & Zięcik, A. P. (2016). Executive functions in adults with developmental dyslexia. *Research in Developmental Disabilities*, *53–54*, 323–341.

Smith-Spark, J. H., Henry, L. A., Messer, D. J., & Zięcik, A. P. (2017). Verbal and non-verbal fluency in adults with developmental dyslexia: Phonological processing or executive control problems? *Dyslexia*, *23*, 234–250.

Smith-Spark, J. H., Zięcik, A. P., & Sterling, C. (2017). Adults with developmental dyslexia show selective impairments in time-based and self-initiated prospective memory: Self-report and clinical evidence. *Research in Developmental Disabilities*, *62*, 247–258.

Snowling, M. J., Nation, K., Moxham, P., Gallagher, A., & Frith, U. (1997). Phonological processing skills of dyslexic students in higher education: A preliminary report. *Journal of Research in Reading*, *20*, 31–41.

Stack-Cutler, H. L., Parrila, R. K., Jokisaari, M., & Nurmi, J.-E. (2015). How university students with reading difficulties are supported in achieving their goals. *Journal of Learning Disabilities*, *48*, 323–334.

Stanovich, K. E. (2009). Distinguishing the reflective, algorithmic, and autonomous minds: Is it time for a tri-process theory? In J. S. B. T. Evans & K. Frankish (Eds.), *In two minds: Dual processes and beyond* (pp. 55–88). Oxford University Press.

Stoet, G., Markey, H., & Lopez, B. (2007). Dyslexia and attentional shifting. *Neuroscience Letters*, *427*, 61–65.

Stroop, J. R. (1935). Studies of interference in serial verbal reactions. *Journal of Experimental Psychology*, *18*, 643–662.

Tal Saban, M., Ornoy, A., & Parush, S. (2014). Executive function and attention in young adults with and without developmental coordination disorder – A comparative study. *Research in Developmental Disabilities*, *35*, 2644–2650.

Taylor, S. J., Barker, L. A., Heavey, L., & McHale, S. (2013). The typical developmental trajectory of social and executive functions in late adolescence and early adulthood. *Developmental Psychology*, *49*, 1253–1265.

Thompson, M. S., & Green, S. B. (2013). Evaluating between-group differences in latent variable means. In G. R. Hancock & R. O. Mueller (Eds.), *Quantitative methods in education and the behavioral sciences: Issues, research, and teaching. Structural equation modeling: A second course* (pp. 163–218). Charlotte, NC: IAP Information Age Publishing.

Troyer, A. K. (2000). Normative data for clustering and switching on verbal fluency tasks. *Journal of Clinical and Experimental Neuropsychology, 22*, 370–378.

Troyer, A. K., Moscovitch, M., & Winocur, G. (1997). Clustering and switching as two components of verbal fluency: Evidence from younger and older healthy adults. *Neuropsychology, 11*, 138–146.

Varvara, P., Varuzza, C., Sorrentino, A. C. P., Vicari, S., & Menghini, D. (2014). Executive functions in developmental dyslexia. *Frontiers in Human Neuroscience, 8*(120).

Ward, G., & Morris, R. (2005). Introduction to the psychology of planning. In R. Morris & G. Ward (Eds.), *The cognitive psychology of planning* (pp. 1–34). Hove, East Sussex: Psychology Press.

Weyandt, L. L., Rice, J. A., Linterman, I., Mitzlaff, L., & Emert, E. (1998). Neuropsychological performance of a sample of adults with ADHD, developmental reading disorder, and controls. *Developmental Neuropsychology, 14*, 643–656.

Wilson, A. M., & Lesaux, N. K. (2001). Persistence of phonological processing deficits in college students with dyslexia who have age-appropriate reading skills. *Journal of Learning Disabilities, 34*, 394–400.

Zelazo, P., & Müller, U. (2002). Executive function in typical and atypical development. In U. Goswami (Ed.), *Handbook of childhood cognitive development* (pp. 445–469). Oxford: Blackwell.

Zelazo, P. D. (2015). Executive function: Reflection, iterative reprocessing, complexity, and the developing brain. *Developmental Review, 38*, 55–68.

6
MEMORY IN ADULTS WITH DYSLEXIA

James H. Smith-Spark and Rebecca Gordon

6.1 Memory

Memory is a vital set of processes required for everyday living. It allows us to collect and store information either for immediate use or to be retrieved and applied in future situations. We need memory for behaviours that are performed routinely without our really thinking about them, for tasks that require the effortful recall of specific information and to recollect precious moments from our past. It pervades all aspects of our lives. Indeed, without the ability to encode, store and recall information, we would not be able to imagine or plan for a future (e.g. Schacter, Addis, & Buckner, 2007).

Memory is not a unitary construct but consists of several systems that provide varied and fundamental abilities. First, we can think of memory as transient but necessary for an immediate task. Such information is stored for a period of up to approximately 30 seconds (or longer if actively maintained through repetition) and then discarded if no longer required. This constitutes short-term memory and may be used when we wish to remember a phone number or a shopping list, but once we have dialled the number or written down the list, we no longer need to keep that information in mind. Equally, we may temporarily maintain visuospatial information to navigate ourselves around our immediate environment or to remember where objects have been placed. This kind of information is necessary for the task at hand and is usually discarded once it is no longer needed.

It is when information is required for future use that we create long-term memories. When we recall any experienced event, be it the moment we first met our spouse, how we celebrated our birthday last year, or what we ate for breakfast today, these are long-term episodic memories; a type of mental time travel

DOI: 10.4324/9781003491125-7

that allows us to relive moments from our own past. Recalling other, more subjective information, such as the capital city of France, or the date of our friend's birthday, is semantic long-term memory; a record of knowledge about the world, not the personal or "autobiographical" content of episodic memory. Nevertheless, both these types of memory are considered declarative as they are explicitly recalled; we are aware that we are retrieving the information.

There is, however, another type of long-term memory, which is non-declarative in nature. This consists of information that we have encoded and stored but that we recall implicitly; that is, we are not aware that we are retrieving it. It includes skills such as riding a bicycle, playing a musical instrument and other behaviours that do not require the active recall of knowledge. This is long-term procedural memory and is entirely separate from declarative memory; damage to, or complete removal of, a specific region of the brain can impair declarative memory severely, yet new procedural memories can still be formed, such as the learning of a new motor skill.

The multi-faceted structure of memory is not complete unless working memory and prospective memory are also considered. Although the placement of these two constructs within the memory model (see Figure 6.1) is much debated, the importance of their contribution to daily living is not. Using the example of a shopping list, imagine that you were unable to write down the items required but, instead, had to maintain that information in mind while walking around a supermarket. You would mentally 'tick off' items as you located them in the store and placed them in your shopping basket. At the same time, you would be navigating the aisles and focusing your attention on where certain items might be located. This simultaneous act of processing (locating the items), storage (remembering the list) and updating (ticking off items as they are placed in the shopping basket) is a good example of everyday working memory. These cognitive tasks are reliant on short-term memory to keep active the relevant verbal (shopping items) and visuospatial (location)

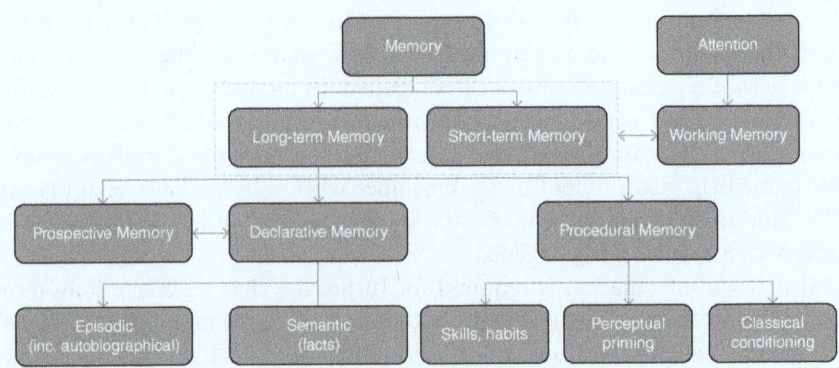

FIGURE 6.1   Schematic overview of memory systems.

information, and also reliant on attention to switch between these two activities and updating of the mental list (see Figure 6.1). Now, let us imagine that you are at work and realize that you need to do some shopping on the way home. The formation of this intention and the ability to remember to act upon it in the future call upon the prospective memory system.

In this chapter, the effects of dyslexia on each of these memory systems in adulthood will be considered. Short-term memory, working memory, long-term memory and prospective memory will be addressed in turn. In each case, general definitions will be provided prior to a discussion of their functioning in adults with dyslexia. As highlighted in Chapter 5, it is important not just to gauge optimal memory performance on one-off tests carried out under laboratory conditions. The typical, everyday levels of performance experienced over weeks, months or years also provide a very useful source of information about the ways in which dyslexia can affect memory. Indeed, it is very important to understand how memory problems are most likely to manifest themselves in educational and employment settings. This understanding can then be used to inform support plans and reasonable adjustments for adults with dyslexia in order to ensure that they are able to achieve their full potential. Therefore, where it exists, evidence arising from the everyday study of memory will also be considered. Finally, for each memory system that is addressed, methods to improve memory functioning or to minimize the effects of dyslexia on it will be considered.

6.2 Short-term Memory

Short-term memory describes the capacity for storing verbal and visuospatial information for short periods of time; however, information stored in this memory system can be quickly lost after approximately 30 seconds if not actively maintained (Atkinson & Shiffrin, 1971). Therefore, maintenance strategies play a key role in short-term memory capacity. Verbal information (such as a sequence of digits or a list of words) can be kept active by repeating the information vocally or sub-vocally. This is known as verbal rehearsal (Baddeley, Thomson, & Buchanan, 1975). Information held in visuospatial short-term memory (e.g. visually presented objects) suffers similar rapid decay, but sometimes it is possible to verbally recode the information (i.e. name the object) and then employ verbal rehearsal to maintain it for longer periods (Conrad & Hull, 1964). However, there is some debate as to whether this extends to spatial short-term memory, which may be more reliant on selective spatial attention (Awh, Jonides, & Reuter-Lorenz, 1998).

With regard to verbal short-term memory in adults with dyslexia, there are a large number of studies indicating that adults with dyslexia are able to remember a smaller number of letters, digits and words than adults without dyslexia (e.g. Brunswick, McCrory, Price, Frith, & Frith, 1999; Laasonen et al.,

2012; Pennington, Van Orden, Smith, Green, & Haith, 1990; Smith-Spark, Fisk, Fawcett, & Nicolson, 2003; Wilson & Lesaux, 2001). While a much smaller literature exists on visuospatial short-term memory in adults with dyslexia, the evidence suggests that it is not affected by dyslexia (e.g. Smith-Spark et al., 2003). More work to explore this dissociation between verbal and visuospatial short-term memory in dyslexia might give broader theoretical insights into how information is stored in temporary memory.

Riddick, Farmer, and Sterling (1997) have highlighted the extent to which the impact of short-term memory problems on the everyday life of adults with dyslexia is underexplored. This remains the case, with the vast majority of research being laboratory-based. Riddick et al. interviewed students with dyslexia about their experiences with cognition. The interviewees identified remembering telephone numbers, formulae, lists and names of people as being particular concerns.

6.3 Working Memory

Working memory is the cognitive system responsible for the concurrent storage, processing and updating of information in pursuit of short-term goals (e.g. Baddeley & Hitch, 1974; Cowan, 1999; Miyake & Shah, 1999). Also referred to as a component of executive function, this limited capacity system is vital to performance in thinking and reasoning tasks (e.g. Baddeley, 2007). There is much literature on the structure and underlying systems involved in working memory. The most enduring and influential approach has been provided by the multicomponent model of working memory (e.g. Baddeley & Hitch, 1974; see also Baddeley, 1986). There is considerable empirical evidence indicating that this system consists of two short-term stores (verbal and visuospatial) responsible for the storage and maintenance of information, together with a control mechanism known as the central executive that enables flexible switching between processing, storage and updating, while filtering out irrelevant information. In this model, a degree of attentional control is required to integrate information that may otherwise be susceptible to decay if it existed only in short-term memory (Allen, Baddeley, & Hitch, 2014). Greater importance is placed on the role of attention in the time-based resource-sharing (TBRS) account of working memory (Barrouillet, Bernardin, & Camos, 2004; Barrouillett, Portrat, & Camos, 2011). In this model, it is argued that processing places an attentional demand on cognitive resources. Since attention is a limited resource, this processing demand results in the reduced availability of attentional resources for the maintenance of stored information and, thus, the decay of the information that needs to be remembered. So, where Baddeley and Hitch (1974) posit a multi-component model with domain-specific maintenance, the TBRS account proposes a central attentional resource responsible for domain-general maintenance.

Impairments in working memory have been identified by McLoughlin, Fitzgibbon, and Young (1994) as a defining characteristic of dyslexia in adulthood. Consistent with this view, working memory is the most studied memory system in adults with dyslexia. Research on verbal and visuospatial working memory will now be considered in turn.

Verbal working memory deficits are well-documented in adults with dyslexia across a range of tasks (for example, see Beidas, Khateb, & Breznitz, 2013; Fostick & Revah, 2018; Łockiewicz, Bogdanowicz, Bogdanowicz, Karasiewicz, & Pąchalska, 2012; Tamboer, Vorst, & de Jong, 2017; Sela, Izzetoglu, Izzetoglu, & Onaral, 2012; Vasic, Lohr, Steinbrink, Martin, & Wolf, 2008; although Alloway, Wootan, & Deane, 2014, found no evidence for working memory span deficits).

Verbal working memory span tasks require the simultaneous storage and processing of numbers, words and letters. Smith-Spark and Fisk (2007) reported poorer performance on two verbal working memory span tasks. Their computation span task required participants to solve a series of arithmetic problems (selecting the correct answer from a choice of three) while also remembering the last digit of each problem for later recall. On Smith-Spark and Fisk's reading span task, the participants were asked to read sentences and answer a question about each one (again choosing the correct answer from a choice of three), while retaining the final word of the sentence for later serial recall. On both tasks, Smith-Spark and Fisk found that adults with dyslexia had lower verbal working memory spans than adults without dyslexia, being able to recall fewer words or digits successfully in the correct serial order. Smith-Spark, Henry, Messer, Edvardsdottir, and Zięcik (2016) used the Operation Span task (Conway et al., 2005) to compare the verbal working memory spans of adults with and without dyslexia. Like Smith-Spark and Fisk's computation span task, participants were required to solve a series of arithmetic problems while also remembering items for later serial recall. In the Operation Span task, they had to remember a letter presented after each problem rather than the last digit of each problem as required by Smith-Spark and Fisk's Computation Span task. Smith-Spark et al. found that adults with dyslexia performed worse than adults without dyslexia on the Operation Span task, with them showing significantly lower span lengths and recalling significantly fewer letters correctly.

In memory updating tasks, letters are presented one at a time to participants in varying (unknown) sequence lengths. On each trial, participants are required to remember the last six letters in the order in which they were presented. Smith-Spark et al. (2003) found that adults with dyslexia recalled fewer letters correctly than adults without dyslexia across a range of list lengths.

While some researchers have argued that dyslexia-related working memory difficulties are yoked to the phonological loop (e.g. Brosnan et al., 2002), dyslexia-related problems would seem to extend beyond the phonological domain in adulthood. Evidence for spatial working memory deficits has been reported on a range of different tasks (Bacon, Parmentier, & Barr, 2013; Smith-Spark, Henry, et al., 2016), especially when task demands are at their most taxing (Smith-Spark et al., 2003) or novel (Smith-Spark & Fisk, 2007).

On the spatial memory updating task used by Smith-Spark et al. (2003), participants were asked to remember the final four cells highlighted sequentially in a 5 × 5 matrix. On some trials, the number of cells to be highlighted was known to the participants, while on others, it was not. In contrast with their spatial short-term memory scores, the adults with dyslexia were significantly worse than the controls on the spatial updating task.

The spatial working memory span task used by Smith-Spark and Fisk (2007) required participants to indicate whether more cells were highlighted above or below a central dividing line on the monitor screen. In addition to this processing component, they were also asked to remember the position of a highlighted cell for subsequent serial recall. As discussed in Chapter 5, the group with dyslexia took longer to adapt to the task demands, showing lowered spatial working memory performance in the first half of the task but performing at a similar level to the control group in the second half.

The Symmetry Span task (e.g. Conway et al., 2005) requires participants to make judgments about whether black and white shapes were symmetrical. After each such shape, participants are shown a 5 × 5 matrix in which one cell is highlighted. The position of this cell needed to be remembered for later serial recall. Using this very well-established task, Smith-Spark, Henry, et al. (2016) found that adults with dyslexia recalled significantly fewer cells correctly.

The findings from visuospatial working memory tasks argue in favour of a modality-general executive processing deficit in dyslexia rather than working memory deficits being tied to the phonological processing system. However, the literature is quite small, and research has focused almost exclusively on spatial working memory to date. However, Beidas et al. (2013) found lowered visual working memory performance in Hebrew-speaking adults with dyslexia relative to neurotypical adults after controlling for differences in phonological skills. Further to this, Provazza, Adams, Giofrè, and Roberts (2019) have reported both visual and spatial working memory deficits in university students with dyslexia. Nevertheless, more research is needed to determine whether there is a dichotomy in performance between spatial and visual working memory tasks in adults with dyslexia. Firstly, it would help to pin down exactly which components of visuospatial working memory are affected by dyslexia and which task demands lead to dyslexia-related visuospatial working memory impairments. Secondly, and more generally, such work would be instructive in relation to the modality-general executive processing deficit argument considered in Chapter 5. This is especially the case given that working memory tasks are likely to draw upon a range of cognitive processes affected by dyslexia (such as information processing speed, shifting, interference control and attentional resource allocation). Considering these component processes, it would be interesting to see what light the TBRS approach of Barrouillet et al. (2004) would shed on the performance of adults with dyslexia.

Outside the laboratory setting, self-reports have indicated that adults with dyslexia experience a higher frequency of working memory problems in everyday life than adults without dyslexia (Smith-Spark, Henry, et al., 2016). In response to the Behavior Rating Inventory of Executive Function – Adult Version (BRIEF-A; Roth, Isquith, & Gioia, 2005), adults with dyslexia indicated that they had significantly more frequent problems with working memory in everyday situations compared with adults without dyslexia. Items contributing to this scale included questions probing difficulties in dealing with tasks that have more than one step, forgetting what is being done in the middle of carrying out tasks, staying on one topic when talking, forgetting instructions easily and doing more than one thing at a time.

In the context of adult educational settings, working memory deficits can have a considerable detrimental impact on the achievement of adults with dyslexia, affecting their ability to carry out study-related activities, such as understanding what they are reading, either at the level of sentences (e.g. Wiseheart, Altmann, Park, & Lombardino, 2009) or text passages (e.g. Simmons & Singleton, 2000), or doing mental arithmetic calculations (Simmons & Singleton, 2006).

6.3.1 Improving the Short-term and Working Memory Performance of Adults with Dyslexia

Impairments in short-term and working memory can have a negative impact on everyday life. Adults with dyslexia may achieve poorer grades in education (Connelly, Campbell, MacLean, & Barnes, 2006; Hatcher, Snowling, & Griffiths, 2002) and be less likely to advance in their careers (De Beer, Engels, Heerkens, & van der Klink, 2014). Therefore, it is necessary to address the causes of these disadvantages by minimizing the impact of cognitive impairments related to, and improving abilities dependent upon, working memory. The use of some strategies, known as mnemonics, has been shown to improve short-term and working memory performance. For example, Cowan (2010) found that people can hold approximately four items of information in short-term memory; however, grouping items into meaningful "chunks" so that each chunk then represents a single item can increase the number of items that can be maintained. Cowan gives the example of remembering a list of shopping items. In order to remember bread, pepper and milk, you might imagine a loaf of bread floating in some peppery milk. This would represent one chunk. You could then create more chunks, thereby increasing the total number of items that can be maintained in short-term and working memory.

It may also be possible to alleviate the load on working memory. This can be achieved by reducing the amount of information that needs to be temporarily maintained (e.g. by providing external resources such as tablet computers) and by reducing the length of time that information needs to be remembered (e.g. providing instructions in smaller units, using shorter sentences).

Improving working memory ability is a more controversial topic. There is research to suggest that working memory training in adults without dyslexia can lead to improved cognitive function (e.g. Richmond, Morrison, Chein, & Olson, 2011). Conversely, there is also considerable evidence to suggest that the opposite is true and that training on working memory tasks does not transfer to other abilities (such as reading) that rely on this cognitive resource (Owen et al., 2010). However, there is little direct work on working memory training in adults with dyslexia. Shiran and Breznitz (2011) report a successful working memory training in Hebrew-speaking university students with dyslexia. This six-week training improved their verbal and visuospatial working memory abilities and also their reading performance (in terms of decoding, reading rate and comprehension). Similar improvements were also found in their working memory-trained students without dyslexia.

6.4 Long-term Memory

Long-term memory is the memory system responsible for the encoding, consolidation and storage of information for future recall. For some types of information, this recall is neither effortful nor is it a process of which we are consciously aware. For example, when performing a learnt motor skill, such as riding a bike, we do not explicitly recall how to balance while pushing down on the pedals and turning the handlebars. Instead, the recall of this information is implicit and the information it relates to is non-declarative; that is, it cannot be expressed as a fact or event. This stands in contrast to declarative memory, which is concerned with information that is explicitly recalled. For example, when asked "What is the capital of France" or "What did you do at the weekend?", we will actively retrieve the relevant facts and events from long-term memory and will be able to state (or declare) them. However, as mentioned in the introduction to this chapter, declarative long-term memory can be further broken down into semantic and episodic memory. Knowing that Paris is the capital of France is a semantic memory, which transcends space and time (Tulving, 1972); for example, we are extremely likely to know that Paris is the capital city of France, while we are highly unlikely to know when we learnt this fact. Conversely, episodic memory represents personally experienced events with discrete spatial and temporal locations in one's past (e.g. Tulving, 2002), such as remembering our first visit to Paris. Episodic memory is thus aptly also referred to as "What-Where-When" memory (e.g. Clayton & Dickinson, 1998) or "mental time travel" (e.g. Eichenbaum & Cohen, 2001). The information stored by this system is autobiographical in nature.

6.4.1 Semantic Memory

There is a small literature on semantic memory in adults with dyslexia, with some difficulties or differences being reported across laboratory and real-world settings. These findings will now be considered.

Callens, Tops, and Brysbaert (2012) found lowered memory performance in university students with dyslexia who were questioned about a passage that they had had read out to them earlier in a testing session.

For verbal information, Obidziński and Nieznański (2022) have found deficits in item and context memory in adults with dyslexia. They highlight the potential difficulties arising from this in both education and the workplace, where adults with dyslexia may have difficulties with both retrieving important information (which may be highly technical and/or formalized) and also remembering the context in which it was first learned.

Problems with access to information in long-term memory have also been found in everyday life. Smith-Spark, Fawcett, Nicolson, and Fisk (2004) asked university students with and without dyslexia to respond to Broadbent, Cooper, FitzGerald, and Parkes' (1982) Cognitive Failures Questionnaire. Amongst other self-reported everyday difficulties with cognition, the students with dyslexia felt they experienced more frequent problems with not being able to remember something, but, instead, it being on "the tip of their tongue".

In educational settings, too, difficulties with accessing information stored in long-term memory have been reported. Interviews conducted by Riddick et al. (1997) indicated that university students with dyslexia reported experiencing problems with the recall of information under examination conditions, with them highlighting a lack of adequate prompts to facilitate the recollection of relevant information. The students also reported forgetting information under exam conditions that they otherwise knew. Similar concerns have been raised by female university students with dyslexia interviewed by Smith-Spark and Lewis (2023).

Dyslexia-related problems with semantic memory also have a negative impact on arithmetic abilities. For example, Simmons and Singleton (2006) found that students with dyslexia recalled a smaller number of multiplication and subtraction facts correctly. Furthermore, when they recalled addition and subtraction facts successfully, they did so more slowly than students without dyslexia. De Smedt and Boets (2010) also found that adults with dyslexia recalled fewer arithmetic facts and did so more slowly than adults without dyslexia matched for non-verbal IQ.

Smith-Spark and Moore (2009) found differences in the way that information about famous people was represented by university students with dyslexia.

Typically, people show a processing advantage for words, objects or people that they have learned about earlier in life compared with information learned later, being faster and more accurate to process and respond to it. This processing advantage is known as the age of acquisition effect. Smith-Spark and Moore found that, while students without dyslexia showed an age-of-acquisition effect in the speed with which famous faces could be named, students with dyslexia did not show any such processing advantage for famous people who had first been learned about earlier in life. This result suggests a difference in the way that information is represented in memory by adults with dyslexia. It may also relate to dyslexia-related problems with the consolidation of learning, as argued by Nicolson, Fawcett, Brookes, and Needle (2010) and discussed later in this chapter when procedural memory is considered.

6.4.2 Episodic Memory

Episodic memory is also very much underexplored in dyslexia, particularly in adults. One self-report study, however, has identified dyslexia-related difficulties with this memory system. Smith-Spark, Zięcik, and Sterling (2016a) administered the self-report Prospective and Retrospective Memory Questionnaire (PRMQ; Smith, Della Sala, Logie, & Maylor, 2000) to adults with and without dyslexia. Four of the eight PRMQ scales related to retrospective memory, which, in this context, referred to memory for personally experienced events in the past. The scales were further subdivided between self-cued and environmentally cued memory and also memory over the short-term (e.g. keeping track of characters between scenes of a television programme) and the long-term (over several days; e.g. telling the same story to the same individual on more than one occasion). The questions about self-cued retrospective memory asked respondents to rate how frequently they had forgotten things that they had been told or had done. Environmentally cued retrospective memory questions probed how environmental features might trigger memories (e.g. reading a prose passage but failing to realize that one had only recently read the very same text). The group with dyslexia reported experiencing significantly more frequent problems on three of the four retrospective memory scales, with more difficulties being experienced with short-term self-cued and environmentally cued memories and long-term self-cued memories. Smith-Spark, Zięcik et al. also administered the proxy-rating PRMQ (Crawford, Henry, Ward, & Blake, 2006) to close associates (such as family members or housemates), asking them also to rate the frequency of memory failures made by the PRMQ respondents. Their responses were broadly consistent with those of the PRMQ respondents themselves, indicating higher frequencies of retrospective memory problems on three of the four subscales (with long-term environmentally cued retrospective memory being the exception). Further to this, a positive predictive relationship between self-reports of dyslexia symptoms and the frequency of everyday memory difficulties (both retrospective and prospective) has been found in a community sample of adults (Protopapa & Smith-Spark, 2022). Finally, Smith-Spark and Lewis (2023) reported interviews with female university students with officially diagnosed dyslexia in which the interviewees felt that their memory for personally experienced events was less detailed than that of family or friends who experienced the same event and who did not have dyslexia.

6.4.3 Procedural Memory

As stated previously, the procedural memory system is responsible for the learning and execution of motor and cognitive skills and storing implicit knowledge about them (e.g. Lum, Ullman, & Conti-Ramsden, 2013). Nicolson and Fawcett (1990) proposed the Dyslexia Automatization Deficit hypothesis, which proposed that the phonological problems experienced by the individual with dyslexia are just one facet of a more general difficulty with any learning task, cognitive or motor. According to this hypothesis, the difficulty arises for the person with dyslexia in the final stage of skill acquisition, that of automatization of performance. This stage is reached when the skill has been fully proceduralized and can be performed so fluently and efficiently that it requires no consciously directed attentional resources. Nicolson and Fawcett postulated that individuals with dyslexia employ a strategy of "conscious compensation" to hide their automatization deficit by the allocation of extra attentional capacity to the task in which they are engaged. According to Fawcett and Nicolson (1994), four general types of skill are prone to disruption in dyslexia. These are (i) complex skills that require fluency in component subskills, (ii) time-dependent skills which call upon fast processing speed, (iii) multi-modality skills that involve the monitoring of different sources or modalities of information and (iv) vigilance tasks that demand concentration over time. The task demands made by each type of skill prevent the use of conscious compensation to support performance. While the hypothesis was based originally on data obtained from children, Needle, Fawcett, and Nicolson (2006) found problems with balance in adults with dyslexia, further supporting the automatization deficit hypothesis and indicating that dyslexia-related problems with basic skills persist into adulthood. The Dyslexia Automatization Deficit hypothesis was later developed into the Cerebellar Deficit theory (Nicolson, Fawcett, & Dean, 1995), which argues that the cerebellum, a structure in the hindbrain, is unable to support the complete acquisition of skill in dyslexia.

Ullman (2004) has also argued for procedural memory deficits in dyslexia. These dyslexia-related difficulties with procedural memory have led to the procedural deficit hypothesis (Ullman & Pierpont, 2005; Nicolson & Fawcett, 2011; although see West, Vadillo, Shanks, & Hulme, 2017, for a critique). Specifically in relation to dyslexia, Nicolson and Fawcett have argued that a deficit in parts of the procedural memory system which are related to the processing of language, especially that relating to phonology, can at least partly explain reading difficulties in dyslexia. The declarative memory system has been argued to compensate in part for at least some dyslexia-related procedural memory deficits (e.g. Nicolson & Fawcett, 1990, 2007). A meta-analysis of procedural learning in dyslexia by Lum et al. (2013), in which adult studies were included, indicates that procedural memory deficits are evident in dyslexia, although the effect size reduces with age. Lum et al. argue that this age-related reduction may reflect the use of the declarative memory system to compensate for procedural memory problems.

Nicolson et al. (2010) provide evidence from three studies, two involving university students and one involving adolescents, indicating dyslexia-related problems with procedural learning and indicating that these difficulties extended beyond the literacy domain. The studies involving adults showed problems with single-word reading under speeded conditions and the consolidation of the learning of a motor sequence over a 24-hour period. Nicolson et al. argued that the pattern of the data on the latter task indicated problems with consolidating new skills, while adults with dyslexia showed a "normal ability" (p. 204) to learn through extensive practice. Ozernov-Palchik, Qi, Beach, and Gabrieli (2023) have recently found that adults with dyslexia show no procedural memory deficits across multiple tasks, but reported a specific impairment in auditory statistical learning related to difficulties with reading.

6.4.4 Improving the Long-term Memory Abilities of Adults with Dyslexia

The benefits conferred on recall by using strategies to encode and consolidate information into long-term memory are well documented and robust. One such strategy is elaboration, the process of reconstructing and reframing information, which has been shown to greatly improve recall (McDaniel & Donnelly, 1996; Wong, 1985). There are many effective strategies using elaboration, such as describing a concept in detail either to yourself or someone else (Willoughby, Wood, & Khan, 1994). You could try this yourself by explaining to someone the structure of the memory system provided at the beginning of this chapter. Alternatively, you may create a story that contains information you need to remember. For example, if you were revising for a history exam and needed to remember that Mozart moved from Munich to Paris, you are more likely to remember this if you elaborate by adding details such as that Mozart wanted to leave Munich to avoid a romantic entanglement or that Mozart was intrigued by musical developments coming out of Paris (see Bradshaw & Anderson, 1982). The reason such strategies aid long-term memory is that the new information is integrated into existing concepts and experiences. This creates several routes into the new information, making it easier to reactivate and recall later

(Hunt & Worthen, 2006; Roediger & Butler, 2011). Other strategies are beneficial to long-term memory for similar reasons, such as dual-coding (Paivio, 1971). This describes the process of learning material through forming verbal associations with visual images. If you can create visual representations of information, you are more likely to be able to recall that information later (Mayer & Anderson, 1992). To use the earlier example of memory structure, you will probably find it easier to recall this information because we have provided a diagram (Figure 6.1). This is because, when you attempt to recall this information, you are able to picture the diagram, along with the descriptions associated with it (Paivio & Csapo, 1973). This method works particularly well for information related to structure and event sequences. For example, to aid in retaining information regarding the route to a new location, you could draw a rudimentary map rather than trying to remember the sequence of directions verbally. When you need to recall that information later, you are able to "picture" the map, as well as recall instructions such as "Turn left at the green building".

An alternative to these internal memory strategies is the use of cognitive offloading, which is the use of external mechanisms to reduce cognitive demand (for a review, see Risko & Gilbert, 2016). This is something that many people do automatically, and it relies on our awareness of our own memory capacity. That is, people are more likely to use external reminders when they need to remember larger amounts of information (e.g. longer shopping lists) or the information they need to retain is complex (Gilbert, 2015). A good example of cognitive offloading is the use of smartphones, which has been shown to be particularly effective for prospective memory, which is covered in the following section (Risko & Gilbert, 2016).

As noted by Morgan and Klein (2000), for example, the use of recording devices by students with dyslexia can help support memory when taking notes at work or in lectures. Moody (2006), in the context of employment, recommended the use of a small personal notebook to be carried around and used to note anything that needed to be remembered. She also suggested that adults with dyslexia who struggled to remember where they had put items (such as keys or diaries) in their working environment should always train themselves to put them in the same place. While some adults with dyslexia report excellent long-term memory (in contrast to their poor short-term memory), information is more likely to be remembered if it is personally meaningful rather than being factual information or concerning dates (Morgan & Klein, 2000). This would suggest an advantage for episodic over semantic memory in adults with dyslexia and also highlights the usefulness of using strategies that make information more meaningful. In the time that has elapsed since these publications, the capability of assistive technologies has increased substantially in terms of functionality and interactivity. Moreover, the relationships that people have with them have changed. Interview work exploring the way in which university students with dyslexia use technology to support their memory across different settings has been conducted (Smith-Spark & Lewis, 2023). Among other themes, the interviewees identified a reliance on technology to support their studies and experiencing anxiety if they forgot to take key equipment with them to classes, and also a preference for using traditional tools to support memory rather than using technological solutions.

From teaching Shakespeare to acting students, Whitfield (2015, 2017) has identified the benefits to memory gained from transmuting information that would otherwise have to be stored mentally into external representations (such as through bodily expression or as pictures). As well as reducing cognitive load, this approach has been argued to help release creativity.

6.5 Prospective Memory

The prospective memory system is responsible for memory for delayed intentions (Winograd, 1988). Prospective memory is called upon whenever there is a delay, no matter how small, between forming an intention to do something and having the opportunity to act upon that intention. It is, thus, concerned with "remembering to remember" (Mäntylä, 1994) to perform a task after a delay. Examples of such delayed intentions would be running out of milk at breakfast and forming the intention to buy a bottle of milk on the way home from work that evening, or forming the intention to pay an electricity bill by the end of the following week when it is due. A well-functioning prospective memory is very important for everyday life (e.g. McDaniel & Einstein, 2007), being called upon frequently for tasks that can be either mundane, habitual or potentially life-saving (such as carrying out safety checks or taking medication at the prescribed intervals).

For prospective memory to be successful, two components must function effectively (e.g. Einstein & McDaniel, 1996; Ellis, 1996). Firstly, there is a prospective (or planning) component. The function of this component is to remind the individual, at the appropriate moment, that there is an intention that needs to be acted upon. Secondly, there is a retrospective component which involves remembering what the intention itself was.

There are two main types of prospective memory, defined by the type of cue that should prompt memory of the delayed intention at the appropriate point in the future. In event-based prospective memory, intentions are cued by people or objects in their surrounding environment. For example, seeing a colleague should prompt the intention to pass on a message to him or her, or passing the postbox should cue the intention to post the letter carried in one's bag. Time-based prospective memory, on the other hand, is argued to be more reliant on internally generated cues to remember to carry out an intention at a particular time in the future (e.g. Einstein, McDaniel, Richardson, Guynn, & Cunfer, 1995), such as to return a call to a friend in 30 minutes' time.

In contrast to most areas of dyslexia research, prospective memory has, to date, been investigated more extensively in adults (Smith-Spark, Zięcik, & Sterling, 2016a, 2016b, 2017a, 2017b; see Smith-Spark, 2018, for a review) than in children. This work on adults will now be described, beginning with laboratory-based evidence and moving on to consider the impact of dyslexia on prospective memory in day-to-day settings.

Smith-Spark, Zięcik, and Sterling (2016b) found significantly less accurate prospective memory in adults with dyslexia on a computerized time-based task. To simulate the everyday need to break out from an ongoing activity in order to carry out an intention, the participants were asked to make ongoing judgements about arrays of famous faces. A prospective memory response was required every three minutes, requiring the participant to press a key on a computer that was out of his or her direct view. The participants were allowed to check a clock, also placed out of direct sight, as many times as they liked over the course of the task. Clock-checking behaviour was logged by a computer. The adults with dyslexia were less accurate overall in the accuracy of their prospective memory responses than the adults without dyslexia. They also made fewer clock checks, although the pattern of these checks (with their frequency increasing as the time of the prospective memory response approached) did not differ from that of the group without dyslexia. The authors also used secondary tasks to manipulate concurrent working memory load (both phonological and visuospatial), but did not find any interaction between participant group and working memory load. From these findings, it would seem that problems with time-based prospective memory are not related to dyslexia-related working memory deficits.

Smith-Spark et al. (2017a), using a well-established clinical measure of prospective memory, the Memory for Intentions Test (MIST; Raskin, Buckheit, & Sherrod, 2010), found that adults with dyslexia had less accurate prospective memory than adults without dyslexia overall. At a finer-grained level, their performance was also lower when responding to time-based cues but at an equivalent level to the adults without dyslexia when responses were required to event-based cues. After completing the MIST, adults with and without dyslexia did not differ in the accuracy with which they correctly recognized instructions for the eight prospective memory tasks. Based on this finding, Smith-Spark (2018) has suggested that it is the efficient access to the instructions at the time that they are required that may result in dyslexia-related problems. On the other hand, the instructions themselves seemed to have been successfully encoded and retained over the delay interval. This suggestion would also be in line with the argument made in this chapter about access to information in long-term memory under exam conditions, and also links to the executive processes covered in Chapter 5.

The studies summarized here indicate that dyslexia-related prospective memory problems are evident under laboratory conditions. Given the importance of understanding the real-world impact of memory problems in dyslexia, the prospective memory of adults with dyslexia has also been studied with more naturalistic task demands and under naturalistic conditions.

Still within the laboratory context, Smith-Spark, Zięcik, and Sterling (2016b) instructed their adult participants to remind the experimenter in 40 minutes' time to save a computer file, telling them that if they failed to do so, then the data would be lost. The group with dyslexia was significantly less likely to remember to remind the experimenter than the group without dyslexia.

Similar results were obtained when the opportunity to remember the intention was in the participants' everyday context and outside the controlled laboratory setting. Smith-Spark et al. (2017a) used the 24-hour delayed prospective memory task from Raskin et al.'s (2010) Memory for Intentions Test. This task required the participants to leave an answerphone message for the experimenter 24 hours after attending a laboratory session. Smith-Spark et al. found that the adults with dyslexia were significantly more likely to fail to leave the message than remember it successfully, while the adults without dyslexia were more likely to carry the task out successfully than fail to perform it.

A similar pattern of results was reported by Smith-Spark et al. (2017b) over the more extended delay period of one week. In this case, the authors used an event-based prospective memory task, which involved the participants being asked to respond to a blank SMS message that was sent to them one week after they had attended a laboratory session. Their response required the placement of a call to a mobile telephone number provided by the experimenter. Smith-Spark et al. found that the adults with dyslexia were less likely to respond to the prospective memory task correctly and more likely not to respond to it, while the reverse pattern was found in the adults without dyslexia. When questioned subsequently, no differences were found between the adults with and without dyslexia in self-reported motivation to carry out the task or in the number of times that they had thought about the task in the intervening interval. However, fewer adults with dyslexia reported remembering the task instructions, suggesting a reduced ability to remember the content of delayed intentions over extended periods of time.

These results are very useful in providing evidence of observable differences in prospective memory in adults with dyslexia under naturalistic conditions. Nonetheless, they required responses to one-off events, and the task requirements were still somewhat artificial and contrived. This section will now turn to consider typical levels of prospective memory accuracy over weeks or months, with self-report questionnaires mainly providing the evidence base.

As discussed previously in relation to declarative memory, Smith-Spark, Zięcik, and Sterling (2016a) administered the PRMQ (Smith et al., 2000) to adults with and without dyslexia. As well as their problems on the Retrospective

Memory scale, the adults with dyslexia reported more problems on the Prospective Memory scale overall and on each of the four prospective memory subscales, indicating pervasive problems with this type of memory over short and long delays and over self-cued and environmentally cued remembering. As with the retrospective memory findings, proxy ratings provided by close associates of the PRMQ respondents corroborated these findings, also indicating more frequent problems with prospective memory in the adults with dyslexia.

As well as the MIST (Raskin et al., 2010) already described in this section, Smith-Spark et al. (2017a) asked their participants also to complete the Prospective Memory Questionnaire (PMQ; Hannon, Adams, Harrington, Fries-Dias, & Gibson, 1995). On the PMQ's Techniques Used to Assist Recall subscale, the adults with dyslexia reported more frequent use of tools and techniques to support memory. Despite this increased level of support, they still reported significantly more frequent prospective memory problems on two of the three subscales relating to prospective memory, namely the Long-term Episodic and Internally cued subscales. The Long-term Episodic subscale assessed memory for intentions for infrequently occurring events, which needed to be retained over days or hours (e.g. missing scheduled appointments). The Self-Initiated subscale measured prospective memory in situations where there was no external cue to serve as a reminder to carry out the intention. No group difference was self-reported on the Short-term Habitual subscale, which related to memory for tasks that had to be performed regularly over short intervals (e.g. remembering to lock the door when leaving the house). Smith-Spark, Zięcik et al.'s study, therefore, found dyslexia-related prospective memory problems under both laboratory conditions and in self-reports of everyday functioning in the same sample of participants.

Morgan and Klein (2000) identify the challenges to prospective memory experienced by a working parent with dyslexia and the "toll" (p. 68) taken on her by having to remember the sequence of things that she needs to do after finishing work, even with the assistance of lists and a diary. This mother with dyslexia also talked about the household management problems that she experienced. She reported attempting to use lists to avoid forgetting items that needed to be bought during the weekly shop. However, she frequently forgot where she had put the list and had to start a new one, missing items that were on the original. In this case, we see problems with both retrospective and prospective memory having an impact on daily life.

In a review of prospective memory in dyslexia, Smith-Spark (2018) characterized prospective memory problems as being more likely when cues were time-based rather than event-based, when delays between forming an intention and being able to act upon it are longer rather than shorter, when the task to be performed is episodic (or one-off) rather than being performed habitually and when cues to remember the intention have to be self-initiated rather than environmentally supported.

6.5.1 Improving the Prospective Memory of Adults with Dyslexia

Smith-Spark (2018) identified several means by which the prospective memory performance of adults with dyslexia might be improved. Firstly, prolonged delays between the formulation of a delayed intention and the opportunity to act upon it should be avoided wherever possible. Secondly, prospective memory task instructions should be accurately recorded for later playback. Thirdly, the association between a prospective memory cue and an action should be strengthened as much as possible. Fourthly, time-based cues should be converted to event-based cues (or, in the light of Smith-Spark, Gordon, & Jansari's, 2023, results, action-based cues). These will now be considered in turn.

Given the evidence that dyslexia-related prospective memory problems are more likely over prolonged delay intervals, it would be beneficial, wherever possible, to reduce the delay between forming an intention and being in a position to act upon it. Where longer delays are unavoidable, frequent reminders of the still-to-be-performed task would be advisable. Related to this point, it would be beneficial for adults with dyslexia to aim to carry out the least salient (or most novel) part of a task first, thereby reducing the demands made on prospective memory and executive functioning resources. Given that adults with dyslexia do not feel that they have problems with habitual prospective memory (Smith-Spark et al., 2017a), this strategy would seem likely to play to their strengths.

With regard to making a note of prospective memory tasks and the instructions associated with them, Reid, Strnadová, and Cumming (2013) have identified the range of technological support available to the adult with dyslexia to help with organization, such as smartphones and tablets. However, it should be noted that Smith-Spark et al. (2017a) found that adults with dyslexia still reported significantly more frequent prospective memory problems despite an increased use of tools and strategies. Therefore, it may not be enough simply to provide individuals with dyslexia with technology to assist them, for example, at university. Instead, they may well need training in how to use this technology most effectively (Draffan, Evans, & Blenkhorn, 2007; Smith-Spark, 2018).

There are several ways in which the association between prospective memory cues and actions can be strengthened. Firstly, implementation intention (e.g. Gollwitzer, 1999) involves forming if-then plans to specify how, when and where an intention will be acted upon. Activating a mental representation of the future situation is argued to make both the prospective memory cue and the intended action more accessible and, thus, to make performance dependent on automatic processes rather than more cognitively demanding consciously controlled processes (e.g. Zimmermann & Meier, 2010). However, it should be noted that, in older adults, Burkard, Rochat, Van der Linden, Gold, and Van der Linden (2014) found that implementation intentions were only effective in improving prospective memory in people with higher working memory spans. Given the working memory problems highlighted earlier in this chapter, this approach may be of limited benefit to adults with dyslexia (although transforming cognitive demands from consciously controlled to automatic is an appealing prospect in the light of the executive functioning problems associated with dyslexia; see Chapter 5). Secondly, episodic future thinking involves the ability to project oneself mentally into a personally experienced future in which one imagines oneself performing the intended action. Altgassen, Kretschmer, and Schnitzspahn (2016) argue that benefits from this strategy could arise from deepening the encoding of the intention (and thus strengthening the memory trace for later access and retrieval) and more automatic retrieval of the intention as a result of a stronger association between the prospective memory cue and the context in which it should be acted upon. Thirdly, repeated-encoding techniques can be used to strengthen the memory traces associated with delayed intentions through repetition of the task instructions. In a comparison of episodic future thinking and repeated encoding, Altgassen et al. (2016) found that repeated encoding (in the form of the participants repeatedly reading the instructions) worked best for neurotypical young adults. The successful application of this approach to adults with dyslexia would be dependent on the format in which instructions could be repeated. Given their obvious difficulties with reading-related tasks, an audio recording of the instructions for repeated playback would seem a more appropriate medium.

Further to these approaches, the relative strength of adults with dyslexia in dealing successfully with event-based prospective memory demands (Smith-Spark, 2018) could be harnessed to compensate for weaknesses with time-based and self-initiated prospective memory. Wherever possible, therefore, it would seem advisable for adults with dyslexia to convert time-based prospective memory tasks into event-based tasks instead. This can be done by simple means and does not necessarily require the deployment of sophisticated technology to provide reminders. For example, if an individual needs to remember to take a letter with him or her when leaving the house (a time-based cue; i.e. upon leaving), putting the letter by the front door will change the nature of this prospective memory task from time-based to event-based. The placing of a physical object (such as the letter) in a very salient or unusual location thus creates an "event" in the individual's surrounding environment. This can then act as a prompt to remember a delayed intention. Such cues can be set up easily while one is engaged in other activities that need to be done before leaving the house. Furthermore, the act of walking by the object in the meantime is likely to strengthen the memory trace associated with the delayed intention (due to the additional cognitive processing involved in asking oneself what the object is doing in that unusual, salient location).

6.6 Conclusion

The information presented in this chapter has shown that adults with dyslexia present with deficits across different memory systems and processes. This chapter has explored the direct effects of dyslexia on different memory systems. It should be noted, of course, that problems with memory are likely to affect other areas of cognition in which memory processes are implicated and to have consequences for the cognitive profile of the adult with dyslexia as a whole. For example, issues with short-term and long-term memory (both explicit and implicit), working memory and prospective memory can lead to many daily challenges. Laboratory-based research has found that adults with dyslexia have problems maintaining small amounts of information for short periods of time, particularly whilst performing a concurrent task. Such deficits can mean difficulty in processing information in education settings and in the workplace; the knock-on effect of which is day-to-day failure in tasks that the neurotypical population takes for granted. Despite variability in findings, there is some promising research suggesting the benefits of cognitive training to improve working memory. Moreover, the ever-advancing technological resources can provide external memory aids to support short-term and working memory.

We have also seen how adults with dyslexia may have greater difficulty remembering events from their past, whether it be personal experiences or less subjective, but equally important, information. This can lead to daily problems remembering instructions or important, relevant details, such as those that might be obtained from discussions and meetings. Memory strategies can greatly improve recall of information, and technological devices (such as smartphones) can facilitate cognitive offloading to reduce the strain on internal memory systems. However, there are fewer solutions to impairments in procedural memory. The aforementioned research suggests that dyslexia involves a deficit in phonological learning and the ability to automate certain cognitive processes, thus leading to a greater reliance on the more effortful declarative memory.

Arguably, prospective memory presents the greatest challenge to adults with dyslexia in everyday contexts; however, recent research in this area is hopefully leading to a greater understanding of the needs of this population in education and the workplace. Studies looking at prospective memory outside the laboratory setting and in everyday contexts are especially important in informing programmes for reasonable adjustments and alternative approaches to the provision of instructions, training and day-to-day tasks to adults with dyslexia.

References

Allen, R. J., Baddeley, A. D., & Hitch, G. J. (2014). Evidence for two attentional components in visual working memory. *Journal of Experimental Psychology: Learning, Memory, and Cognition, 40*, 1499–1509.

Alloway, T. P., Wootan, S., & Deane, P. (2014). Investigating working memory and sustained attention in dyslexic adults. *International Journal of Educational Research, 67*, 11–17.

Altgassen, M., Kretschmer, A., & Schnitzspahn, K. M. (2016). Future thinking instructions improve prospective memory performance in adolescents. *Child Neuropsychology, 28*, 1–18.

Atkinson, R. C., & Shiffrin, R. M. (1971). The control of short-term memory. *Scientific American, 225*, 82–90.

Awh, E., Jonides, J., & Reuter-Lorenz, P. A. (1998). Rehearsal in spatial working memory. *Journal of Experimental Psychology: Human Perception and Performance, 24*, 780–790.

Bacon, A. M., Parmentier, F. B. R., & Barr, P. (2013). Visuospatial memory in dyslexia: Evidence for strategic deficits. *Memory, 21*, 189–209.

Baddeley, A. D. (1986). *Working memory*. Oxford: Clarendon Press.

Baddeley, A. D. (2007). *Working memory, thought, and action*. New York: Oxford University Press.

Baddeley, A. D., & Hitch, G. J. (1974). Working memory. In G. Bower (Ed.), *Recent advances in learning and motivation* (Vol. VIII, pp. 47–90). New York: Academic Press.

Baddeley, A. D., Thomson, N., & Buchanan, M. (1975). Word length and the structure of short term memory. *Journal of Verbal Learning and Verbal Behaviour, 14*, 575–589.

Barrouillet, P., Bernardin, S., & Camos, V. (2004). Time constraints and resource sharing in adults' working memory spans. *Journal of Experimental Psychology: General, 133*, 83–100.

Barrouillett, P., Portrat, S., & Camos, V. (2011). On the law relating processing speed to storage in working memory. *Psychological Review, 118*, 175–192.

Beidas, H., Khateb, A., & Breznitz, Z. (2013). The cognitive profile of adult dyslexics and its relation to their reading abilities. *Reading and Writing, 26*, 1487–1515.

Bradshaw, G. L., & Anderson, J. R. (1982). Elaborative encoding as an explanation of levels of processing. *Journal of Verbal Learning and Verbal Behavior, 21*, 165–174.

Broadbent, D. E., Cooper, P. F., FitzGerald, P., & Parkes, K. R. (1982). The cognitive failure questionnaire (CFQ) and its correlates. *British Journal of Clinical Psychology, 21*, 1–16.

Brosnan, M., Demetre, J., Hamill, S., Robson, K., Shepherd, H., & Cody, G. (2002). Executive functioning in adults and children with developmental dyslexia. *Neuropsychologia, 40*, 2144–2155.

Brunswick, N., McCrory, E., Price, C. J., Frith, C. D., & Frith, U. (1999). Explicit and implicit processing of words and pseudowords by adult developmental dyslexics. A search for Wernicke's Wortschatz? *Brain, 122*, 1901–1917.

Burkard, C., Rochat, L. J., Van der Linden, A.-C., Gold, G., & Van der Linden, M. (2014). Is working memory necessary for implementation intentions to enhance prospective memory in older adults with cognitive problems? *Journal of Applied Research in Memory and Cognition, 3*, 37–43.

Callens, M., Tops, W., & Brysbaert, M. (2012). Cognitive profile of students who enter higher education with an indication of dyslexia. *PLoS One, 7*(6), e38081.

Clayton, N. S., & Dickinson, A. (1998). Episodic-like memory during cache recovery by scrub jays. *Nature, 395*, 272–274.

Connelly, V., Campbell, S., MacLean, M., & Barnes, J. (2006). Contribution of lower order skills to the written composition of college students with and without dyslexia. *Developmental Neuropsychology, 29*, 175–196.

Conrad, R., & Hull, A. J. (1964). Information, acoustic confusion and memory span. *British Journal of Psychology, 55*, 429–432.

Conway, A. R. A., Kane, M. J., Bunting, M. F., Hambrick, D. Z., Wilhelm, O., & Engle, R. W. (2005). Working memory span tasks: A methodological review and user's guide. *Psychonomic Bulletin and Review*, *12*, 769–786.

Cowan, N. (1999). An embedded-processes model of working memory. In A. Miyake & P. Shah (Eds.), *Models of working memory: Mechanisms of active maintenance and executive control* (pp. 62–101). Cambridge: Cambridge University Press.

Cowan, N. (2010). The magical mystery four: How is working memory capacity limited, and why? *Current Directions in Psychological Science*, *19*, 51–57.

Crawford, J. R., Henry, J. D., Ward, L. A., & Blake, J. (2006). The prospective and retrospective memory questionnaire (PRMQ): Latent structure, normative data and discrepancy analysis for proxy-ratings. *British Journal of Clinical Psychology*, *45*, 83–104.

De Beer, J., Engels, J., Heerkens, Y., & van der Klink, J. (2014). Factors influencing work participation of adults with developmental dyslexia: A systematic review. *BMC Public Health*, *14*, 77.

De Smedt, B., & Boets, B. (2010). Phonological processing and arithmetic fact retrieval: Evidence from developmental dyslexia. *Neuropsychologia*, *48*, 3973–3981.

Draffan, E. A., Evans, D. G., & Blenkhorn, P. (2007). Use of assistive technology by students with dyslexia in post-secondary education. *Disability and Rehabilitation: Assistive Technology*, *2*, 105–116.

Eichenbaum, H., & Cohen, N. J. (2001). *Oxford psychology series; no. 35. From conditioning to conscious recollection: Memory systems of the brain*. New York: Oxford University Press.

Einstein, G. O., & McDaniel, M. A. (1996). Retrieval processes in prospective memory: Theoretical approaches and some new empirical findings. In M. Brandimonte, G. O. Einstein, & M. A. McDaniel (Eds.), *Prospective memory: Theory and application* (pp. 115–141). Mahwah, NJ: Erlbaum.

Einstein, G. O., McDaniel, M. A., Richardson, S. L., Guynn, M. J., & Cunfer, A. R. (1995). Aging and prospective memory: Examining the influences of self-initiated retrieval processes. *Journal of Experimental Psychology: Learning, Memory, and Cognition*, *21*, 996–1007.

Ellis, J. (1996). Prospective memory or realization of delayed intentions: A conceptual framework for research. In M. Brandimonte, G. O. Einstein, & M. A. McDaniel (Eds.), *Prospective memory: Theory and applications* (pp. 1–23). Mahwah, NJ: Lawrence Erlbaum Associates.

Fawcett, A. J., & Nicolson, R. I. (1994). Speed of processing, motor skill, automaticity and dyslexia. In A. J. Fawcett & R. I. Nicolson (Eds.), *Dyslexia in children: Multidisciplinary perspectives* (pp. 157–190). London: Harvester Wheatsheaf.

Fostick, L., & Revah, H. (2018). Dyslexia as a multi-deficit disorder: Working memory and auditory temporal processing. *Acta Psychologica*, *183*, 19–28.

Gilbert, S. J. (2015). Strategic offloading of delayed intentions into the external environment. *Quarterly Journal of Experimental Psychology*, *68*, 971–992.

Gollwitzer, P. M. (1999). Implementation intentions: Strong effects of simple plans. *American Psychologist*, *54*, 493–503.

Hannon, R., Adams, P., Harrington, S., Fries-Dias, C., & Gibson, M. (1995). Effects of brain injury and age on prospective memory self-rating and performance. *Rehabilitation Psychology*, *40*, 289–298.

Hatcher, J., Snowling, M. J., & Griffiths, Y. M. (2002). Cognitive assessment of dyslexic students in higher education. *British Journal of Educational Psychology*, *72*, 119–133.

Hunt, R. R., & Worthen, J. B. (Eds.) (2006). In *Distinctiveness and memory*. New York: Oxford University Press.

Laasonen, M., Virsu, V., Oinonen, S., Sandbacka, M., Salakari, A., & Service, E. (2012). Phonological and sensory short-term memory are correlates and both affected in developmental dyslexia. *Reading and Writing, 25*, 2247–2273.

Łockiewicz, M., Bogdanowicz, K. M., Bogdanowicz, M., Karasiewicz, K., & Pąchalska, M. (2012). Memory impairments in adults with dyslexia. *Acta Neuropsychologica, 10*, 215–229.

Lum, J. A., Ullman, M. T., & Conti-Ramsden, G. (2013). Procedural learning is impaired in dyslexia: Evidence from a meta-analysis of serial reaction time studies. *Research in Developmental Disabilities, 34*, 3460–3476.

Mäntylä, T. (1994). Remembering to remember: Adult age differences in prospective memory. *Journal of Gerontology, 49*, 276–282.

Mayer, R. E., & Anderson, R. B. (1992). The instructive animation: Helping students build connections between words and pictures in multimedia learning. *Journal of Educational Psychology, 84*, 444–452.

McDaniel, M. A., & Donnelly, C. M. (1996). Learning with analogy and elaborative interrogation. *Journal of Educational Psychology, 88*, 508.

McDaniel, M. A., & Einstein, G. O. (2007). *Prospective memory: An overview and synthesis of an emerging field*. London: Sage.

McLoughlin, D., Fitzgibbon, G., & Young, V. (1994). *Adult dyslexia: Assessment, counselling and training*. London: Whurr.

Miyake, A., & Shah, P. (1999). Toward unified theories of working memory: Emerging general consensus, unresolved theoretical issues, and future research directions. In A. Miyake & P. Shah (Eds.), *Models of working memory: Mechanisms of active maintenance and executive control* (pp. 442–481). New York: Cambridge University Press.

Moody, S. (2006). *Dyslexia: How to survive and succeed at work*. London: Vermilion.

Morgan, E., & Klein, C. (2000). *The dyslexic adult in a non-dyslexic world*. London: Whurr.

Needle, J. L., Fawcett, A. J., & Nicolson, R. I. (2006). Balance and dyslexia: An investigation of adults' abilities. *European Journal of Cognitive Psychology, 18*, 909–936.

Nicolson, R. I., & Fawcett, A. J. (1990). Automaticity: A new framework for dyslexia research. *Cognition, 35*, 159–182.

Nicolson, R. I., & Fawcett, A. J. (2007). Procedural learning difficulties: Reuniting the developmental disorders? *Trends in Neurosciences, 30*, 135–141.

Nicolson, R. I., & Fawcett, A. J. (2011). Dyslexia, dysgraphia, procedural learning and the cerebellum. *Cortex, 47*, 117–127.

Nicolson, R. I., Fawcett, A. J., Brookes, R. L., & Needle, J. (2010). Procedural learning and dyslexia. *Dyslexia, 16*, 194–212.

Nicolson, R. I., Fawcett, A. J., & Dean, P. (1995). Time estimation deficits in developmental dyslexia: Evidence of cerebellar involvement. *Proceedings of the Royal Society of London, Series B: Biological Sciences, 259*(1354), 43–47.

Obidziński, M., & Nieznański, M. (2022). Context and target recollection for words and pictures in young adults with developmental dyslexia. *Frontiers in Psychology, 13*, 993384.

Owen, A. M., Hampshire, A., Grahn, J. A., Stenton, R., Dajani, S., Burns, A. S., Howard, R. J., & Ballard, C. G. (2010). Putting brain training to the test. *Nature, 465*(7299), 775–778.

Ozernov-Palchik, O., Qi, Z., Beach, S. D., & Gabrieli, J. D. E. (2023). Intact procedural memory and impaired auditory statistical learning in adults with dyslexia. *Neuropsychologia, 188*, 108638.

Paivio, A. (1971). *Imagery and verbal processes*. New York: Holt, Rinehart and Winston.

Paivio, A., & Csapo, K. (1973). Picture superiority in free recall: Imagery or dual coding? *Cognitive Psychology, 5*, 176–206.

Pennington, B. F., Van Orden, G. C., Smith, S. D., Green, P. A., & Haith, M. M. (1990). Phonological processing skills and deficits in adult dyslexics. *Child Development, 61*, 1753–1778.

Protopapa, C., & Smith-Spark, J. H. (2022). Self-reported symptoms of developmental dyslexia predict impairments in everyday cognition in adults. *Research in Developmental Disabilities, 128*, 104288.

Provazza, S., Adams, A.-M., Giofrè, D., & Roberts, D. J. (2019). Double trouble – Visual and phonological impairments in English dyslexic readers. *Frontiers in Psychology, 10*, Article 2725.

Raskin, S., Buckheit, C., & Sherrod, C. (2010). *Memory for intentions test*. Lutz, FL: PAR.

Reid, G., Strnadová, I., & Cumming, T. (2013). Expanding horizons for students with dyslexia in the 21st century: Universal design and mobile technology. *Journal of Research in Special Educational Needs, 13*, 175–181.

Richmond, L. L., Morrison, A. B., Chein, J. M., & Olson, I. R. (2011). Working memory training and transfer in older adults. *Psychology and Aging, 26*, 813–822.

Riddick, B., Farmer, M., & Sterling, C. (1997). *Students and dyslexia: Growing up with a specific learning difficulty*. London: Whurr.

Risko, E. F., & Gilbert, S. J. (2016). Cognitive offloading. *Trends in Cognitive Sciences, 20*, 676–688.

Roediger, H. L., & Butler, A. C. (2011). The critical role of retrieval practice in long-term retention. *Trends in Cognitive Sciences, 15*, 20–27.

Roth, R. M., Isquith, P. K., & Gioia, G. A. (2005). *BRIEF-A: Behavior rating inventory of executive function - adult version*. Lutz, FL: Psychological Assessment Resources.

Schacter, D. L., Addis, D. R., & Buckner, R. L. (2007). Remembering the past to imagine the future: The prospective brain. *Nature Reviews. Neuroscience, 8*(9), 657–661.

Sela, I., Izzetoglu, M., Izzetoglu, K., & Onaral, B. (2012). A working memory deficit among dyslexic readers with no phonological impairment as measured using the N-back task: An fNIR study. *PLoS One, 7*, e46527.

Shiran, A., & Breznitz, Z. (2011). The effect of cognitive training on recall range and speed of information processing in the working memory of dyslexic and skilled readers. *Journal of Neurolinguistics, 24*, 524–537.

Simmons, F., & Singleton, C. (2000). The reading comprehension abilities of dyslexic students in higher education. *Dyslexia, 6*, 178–192.

Simmons, F. R., & Singleton, C. (2006). The mental and written arithmetic abilities of adults with dyslexia. *Dyslexia, 12*, 96–114.

Smith, G., Della Sala, S., Logie, R. H., & Maylor, E. A. (2000). Prospective and retrospective memory in normal ageing and dementia: A questionnaire study. *Memory, 8*, 311–321.

Smith-Spark, J. H. (2018). A review of prospective memory impairments in developmental dyslexia: Evidence, explanations, and future directions. *The Clinical Neuropsychologist, 32*, 816–835.

Smith-Spark, J. H., Fawcett, A. J., Nicolson, R. I., & Fisk, J. E. (2004). Dyslexic students have more everyday cognitive lapses. *Memory, 12*, 174–182.

Smith-Spark, J. H., & Fisk, J. E. (2007). Working memory functioning in developmental dyslexia. *Memory, 15*, 34–56.

Smith-Spark, J. H., Fisk, J. E., Fawcett, A. J., & Nicolson, R. I. (2003). Investigating the central executive in adult dyslexics: Evidence from phonological and visuospatial working memory performance. *European Journal of Cognitive Psychology, 15*, 567–587.

Smith-Spark, J. H., Gordon, R., & Jansari, A. S. (2023). The impact of developmental dyslexia on workplace cognition: Evidence from a virtual reality environment. *Behaviour & Information Technology, 42*(3), 269–277.

Smith-Spark, J. H., Henry, L. A., Messer, D. J., Edvardsdottir, E., & Zięcik, A. P. (2016). Executive functions in adults with developmental dyslexia. *Research in Developmental Disabilities*, *53–54*, 323–341.

Smith-Spark, J. H., & Lewis, E. G. (2023). Lived experiences of everyday memory in adults with dyslexia: A thematic analysis. *Behavioral Sciences*, *13*(10), 840.

Smith-Spark, J. H., & Moore, V. (2009). The representation and processing of familiar faces in dyslexia: Differences in age of acquisition effects. *Dyslexia*, *15*, 129–146.

Smith-Spark, J. H., Zięcik, A. P., & Sterling, C. (2016a). Self-reports of increased prospective and retrospective memory problems in adults with developmental dyslexia. *Dyslexia*, *22*, 245–262.

Smith-Spark, J. H., Zięcik, A. P., & Sterling, C. (2016b). Time-based prospective memory in adults with developmental dyslexia. *Research in Developmental Disabilities*, *49–50*, 34–46.

Smith-Spark, J. H., Zięcik, A. P., & Sterling, C. (2017a). Adults with developmental dyslexia show selective impairments in time-based and self-initiated prospective memory: Self-report and clinical evidence. *Research in Developmental Disabilities*, *62*, 247–258.

Smith-Spark, J. H., Zięcik, A. P., & Sterling, C. (2017b). The event-based prospective memory of adults with developmental dyslexia under naturalistic conditions. *Asia Pacific Journal of Developmental Differences*, *4*, 17–33.

Tambocr, P., Vorst, H. C. M., & de Jong, P. F. (2017). Six factors of adult dyslexia assessed by cognitive tests and self-report questions: Very high predictive validity. *Research in Developmental Disabilities*, *71*, 143–168.

Tulving, E. (1972). Episodic and semantic memory. *Organization of Memory*, *1*, 381–403.

Tulving, E. (2002). Episodic memory: From mind to brain. *Annual Review of Psychology*, *53*, 1–25.

Ullman, M. T. (2004). Contribution of memory circuits to language: The declarative/procedural model. *Cognition*, *92*, 231–270.

Ullman, M. T., & Pierpont, E. I. (2005). Specific language impairment is not specific to language: The procedural deficit hypothesis. *Cortex*, *41*, 399–433.

Vasic, N., Lohr, C., Steinbrink, C., Martin, C., & Wolf, R. C. (2008). Neural correlates of working memory performance in adolescents and young adults with dyslexia. *Neuropsychologia*, *46*, 640–648.

West, G., Vadillo, M. A., Shanks, D. R., & Hulme, C. (2017). The procedural learning deficit hypothesis of language learning disorders: We see some problems. *Developmental Science*, *21*, e12552.

Whitfield, P. (2015). Towards an emancipatory praxis of pedagogy: Supporting acting students with dyslexia when working on Shakespeare. *Voice and Speech Review*, *9*, 113–128.

Whitfield, P. (2017). The micro grasp and macro Gestus strategy as a facilitation of dyslexia in actor-training: Reconstructing the written text when performing. *Shakespeare, Theatre, Dance and Performance Training*, *8*(3), 329–347.

Willoughby, T., Wood, E., & Khan, M. (1994). Isolating variables that impact on or detract from the effectiveness of elaboration strategies. *Journal of Educational Psychology*, *86*, 279.

Wilson, A. M., & Lesaux, N. K. (2001). Persistence of phonological processing deficits in college students with dyslexia who have age-appropriate reading skills. *Journal of Learning Disabilities*, *34*, 394–400.

Winograd, E. (1988). Some observations on prospective remembering. In M. M. Gruneberg, P. E. Morris, & R. N. Sykes (Eds.), *Practical aspects of memory: Current research and issues* (Vol. 1, pp. 348–353). Chichester, UK: Wiley.

Wiseheart, R., Altmann, L. J. P., Park, H., & Lombardino, L. J. (2009). Sentence comprehension in young adults with developmental dyslexia. *Annals of Dyslexia, 59*, 151–167.

Wong, B. Y. (1985). Self-questioning instructional research: A review. *Review of Educational Research, 55*, 227–268.

Zimmermann, T. D., & Meier, B. (2010). The effect of implementation intentions on prospective memory performance across the lifespan. *Applied Cognitive Psychology, 24*, 645–658.

7
NEUROLOGICAL FUNCTION IN ADULT DYSLEXIA

Fabio Richlan

7.1 History of the Study of Neurological Function in Dyslexia

The study of neurological function and dysfunction in dyslexia has a relatively long history. Beginning in the 19th century, seminal neurological examinations on the neural basis of acquired reading problems – "word blindness" or pure alexia – were conducted by the famous French neurologist Joseph Jules Dejerine (1891, 1892). With respect to developmental reading problems, significant progress was made in the seventies and eighties of the last century with the histological post-mortem brain examinations by Albert Galaburda and colleagues. Specifically, Galaburda and Kemper (1979) found reduced left–right asymmetry of the planum temporale – localized on the dorsal bank of the superior temporal gyrus, posterior to Heschl's gyrus – in a post-mortem examination of the brain of a developmental dyslexia case. In addition, Galaburda, Sherman, Rosen, Aboitiz, and Geschwind (1985) and Humphreys, Kaufmann, and Galaburda (1990) reported findings of neuronal ectopias and architectural dysplasias in left perisylvian regions of a few additional dyslexia cases. These cerebral cortical anomalies were assumed to result from a disturbance during fetal brain development, specifically during prenatal neuronal migration. At least some of the eight cases examined by the Galaburda group, however, may have suffered from comorbid problems, which may have been reflected in the brain abnormalities identified ex vivo. Furthermore, it was suggested that the brains of the dyslexia cases had been stored for a longer period of time than those of the control group and, therefore, were more prone to suffering from cell shrinkage and other post-mortem structural alterations not directly related to reading problems (Heim & Keil, 2004).

7.2 Modern-day Neuroimaging and the Use of Voxel-Based Morphometry (VBM) to Study Gray Matter Abnormalities in Dyslexia

With the advent of modern-day neuroimaging technology such as computed tomography (CT) and magnetic resonance imaging (MRI), it became possible to study the structure of a larger number of brains in vivo. At the beginning of this development, analysis of these novel brain images was difficult and required manual tracing and measuring of specific regions of interest based on expert neuroanatomical knowledge. Statistical comparisons were mainly limited to these more or less subjectively and a priori defined regions (e.g., the planum temporale) and to rather coarse neuroanatomical measures such as global cerebral volume. This unsatisfactory state of affairs was overcome by statistical methods capable of analyzing differences between brain images in an unbiased and objective way, such as Statistical Parametric Mapping (Friston et al., 1990). A major advance in the analysis of structural T1-weighted MRI scans was the introduction of Voxel-Based Morphometry (VBM) by Ashburner and Friston (2000), and the subsequent optimization of this method in the following years (Mechelli, Price, Friston, & Ashburner, 2005).

VBM is an objective and powerful tool to study local tissue properties of the brain on the voxel-level (spatial resolution typically about $1 \times 1 \times 1$ mm), together with automatic segmentation of gray matter, white matter, and cerebrospinal fluid. The basic idea behind VBM is to identify a particular tissue type – usually gray matter – in the brain scan of each participant (segmentation) and to warp these tissue maps to a common three-dimensional space (normalization). The normalized tissue maps are then spatially blurred (smoothing), and a voxel-by-voxel statistical analysis of this preprocessed data is performed. VBM provides a general measure of local gray matter volume or density of a voxel, which is the product of several aspects of cortical architecture such as surface area, folding complexity, and cortical thickness (Hutton, Draganski, Ashburner, & Weiskopf, 2009). VBM is well-established in the field and has been used to investigate pre-reading children with and without a familial risk for dyslexia (e.g., Black et al., 2012; Raschle et al., 2017; Raschle, Chang, & Gaab, 2011), typically reading and dyslexic children (e.g., Eckert et al., 2005; Hoeft et al., 2007; Jednoróg et al., 2015; Krafnick, Flowers, Luetje, Napoliello, & Eden, 2014; Kronbichler et al., 2008), and typically reading and dyslexic adults (e.g., Brambati et al., 2004; Brown et al., 2001; Menghini et al., 2008; Pernet, Andersson, Paulesu, & Demonet, 2009a; Pernet, Poline, Demonet, & Rousselet, 2009b; Silani et al., 2005; Steinbrink et al., 2008; Vinckenbosch, Robichon, & Eliez, 2005).

7.3 Meta-analyses of VBM Studies on Dyslexia

Due to the substantial number of existing VBM studies on dyslexia, objective meta-analyses were used in order to identify and specify stable effects across studies. A quantitative coordinate-based meta-analysis of nine original VBM studies on gray matter abnormalities in developmental dyslexia identified consistent gray matter reduction in the right superior temporal gyrus (STG) and in the left superior temporal sulcus (STS) (Richlan, Kronbichler, & Wimmer, 2013). The right STG was also a focal point in a remarkable study by Carreiras et al. (2009), who compared ex-illiterates who did or did not learn to read as adults. The main finding was that learning to read was accompanied by increased gray matter volume in bilateral temporo-parietal (TP) and dorsal occipital regions. This finding points to the possibility that the right STG gray matter reduction found in the meta-analysis by Richlan et al. (2013) reflects the reduced reading experience of dyslexic readers and is thus a consequence rather than a cause of reading problems in developmental dyslexia.

Two VBM studies with pre-reading children at risk for dyslexia, however, support a different interpretation of the right STG gray matter reduction. Specifically, Raschle et al. (2011) found that children with a family risk for developmental dyslexia exhibited reduced gray matter in both left and right TP cortex even before formal reading instruction. In a similar study, Black et al. (2012) found maternal history of reading disability to be associated with reduced bilateral TP gray matter volume in a sample of 5- to 6-year-old beginning readers. For these young children, the reduction in gray matter volume can hardly be attributed to a reduced amount of reading experience. It will be interesting to see in follow-up studies how these early brain alterations shape later reading skills and whether or not they build the neurological basis for adult dyslexic brain abnormalities.

While the gray matter reduction in the right STG was a more or less unexpected finding of the meta-analysis, the gray matter reduction in the left STS was not. The left STS gray matter reduction is in line with a large body of evidence for left perisylvian cortical anomalies in dyslexia, as identified in the already mentioned post-mortem brain examinations (e.g., Galaburda et al., 1985; Humphreys et al., 1990), as well as in early neuroimaging studies (Eliez et al., 2000). Recently, the left STS was shown to be one of the most reliable regions identified with reduced gray matter volume in developmental dyslexia in a combined meta-analysis and multi-center study across different laboratories (Eckert, Berninger, Vaden Jr, Gebregziabher, & Tsu, 2016). Classically, neurological damage to the left STS was associated with a disruption in auditory speech comprehension (Wernicke's aphasia). In newer conceptions (e.g., Hickok & Poeppel, 2007), the left STS – as opposed to the bilateral STG, which is associated with auditory spectrotemporal analysis – is thought to be an important region for the representation and processing of phonological information. Thus, it is activated during both the perception and production of speech, as well as during active maintenance of phonemic information. These cognitive functions are particularly crucial for a successful start at the beginning of learning to read.

In functional neuroimaging studies of developmental dyslexia, the left STS is frequently identified with underactivation during reading or reading-related tasks (e.g., Blau et al., 2010; Meyler et al., 2007; Paulesu et al., 2001). In the dominant version of the phonological deficit explanation, a language-phonological deficit localized in the left STG/STS region is assumed to disturb the emergence of phoneme awareness at the beginning of learning to read, which constitutes the proximal cause for developmental dyslexia (e.g., Shaywitz & Shaywitz, 2005; Snowling, 2000; Vellutino & Fletcher, 2005). Other studies, however, suggest that the left STS plays a central role in the integration of auditory and visual information (e.g., Holloway, van Atteveldt, Blomert, & Ansari, 2015; Van Atteveldt, Formisano, Goebel, & Blomert, 2004). Therefore, during skilled reading and especially during reading acquisition, its main function may be more directly related to serial grapheme-to-phoneme conversion, and therefore to self-reliant sublexical reading. Dyslexic underactivation of this region in response to the demands of letter-speech sound integration was interpreted as resulting from a failure to develop neural systems specialized for efficient interactive processing of auditory and visual linguistic inputs (Blau et al., 2010). Taken together, left STS and right STG gray matter reductions are reliable neuroanatomical signatures of adult dyslexia, which might already exist even before the onset of formal reading instruction.

7.4 Limitations of VBM Studies on Dyslexia

One additional interesting but quite disappointing finding became evident in the meta-analysis of VBM studies on developmental dyslexia. That is, convergence across studies was generally limited, with only about half of the studies contributing to the most reliable meta-analytic clusters. This finding was recently investigated in more detail in the review article by Ramus, Altarelli, Jednoróg, Zhao, and Scotto di Covella (2017). They comprehensively analyzed and summarized existing research on the neuroanatomical basis of developmental dyslexia and came to rather sobering conclusions. They argue that most VBM studies on developmental dyslexia are based on too few and too heterogeneous participants, leading to a high number of false positive results in the primary literature and, therefore, little or no replicability of results across independent studies. This makes progress in the field extremely tedious and undermines the identification of reliable neuroanatomical markers of dyslexia. Sources of heterogeneity include dyslexia subtypes, cultures, languages, and sex. Future studies should pay attention to these sources of heterogeneity, including larger samples of typical and dyslexic readers, possibly from different research centers (see Eckert et al., 2016), and should rely on more careful, manual methods of data analysis rather than the more or less automated data processing used in VBM.

Although VBM has been extensively used in order to study structural brain abnormalities in various diseases, several potential limitations exist when comparing patients with a brain-based disorder to control participants. Specifically, the spatial normalization step during the VBM procedure was the subject of considerable debate (Ashburner & Friston, 2001; Bookstein, 2001; Mechelli et al., 2005). It was argued that abnormalities in the brain scans of patients may lead to systematic group-specific misregistration when attempting to match these images to an average brain template of healthy controls. As a result, the VBM method would produce results sensitive to this registration bias rather than to structural abnormalities per se. On the contrary, it was put forward that the normalization step relies on a relatively simple warping and scaling method, which attempts to find a global match between brain images (i.e., matching overall size and shape). Therefore, only very severe and obvious pathologies on the macroscopic level (i.e., tumors and arteriovenous malformations) would lead to systematic misregistration. The presence of such atypical tissue types would additionally lead to misclassification during the segmentation step, which relies on a priori tissue probability maps for gray matter, white matter, and cerebrospinal fluid obtained from brain scans of healthy participants. With respect to developmental dyslexia, no evidence for such macroscopic brain malformations exists, although it is frequently reported that dyslexic readers exhibit overall smaller brain volume compared with typical readers (Ramus et al., 2017). There is, however, no known association between brain volume and cognitive function. As suggested by Ramus et al. (2017), smaller brain volume may be a general risk factor for developmental disorders, but clear-cut evidence is missing so far. Likewise, smaller brain volume could be a mere by-product of other disorders of early brain development.

7.5 Methodological Issues of VBM Studies on Dyslexia

Even in the absence of severe macroscopic brain pathologies in developmental dyslexia, there is the possibility of applying an additional processing step during VBM in order to compensate for subtle volumetric changes introduced by the normalization step (e.g., artificial enlargement of smaller regions). This step is referred to as "modulation", and is basically a multiplication of the spatially normalized image by its relative volume before and after normalization. In so doing, the absolute volume of the normalized image is preserved. This has an effect on the interpretation of VBM results: modulated VBM can be thought of as a measure of absolute volume of a tissue class in a region, whereas unmodulated VBM can be thought of as a measure of relative concentration of a tissue class (in relation to the other classes) in a region.

A further critique of the VBM method concerns its volume-based registration approach. As mentioned previously, it uses a relatively simple warping method attempting to match the overall size and shape of brains. It was shown that a surface-based registration approach, which attempts to match cortical gyral and sulcal folding patterns, can lead to improved inter-subject registration (e.g., Fischl et al., 2008). Another advantage of the surface-based approach is that it allows the measurement of more specific properties of gray matter architecture, such as cortical thickness, sulcal depth, and cortical folding complexity, as opposed to VBM, which provides a more general measure of gray matter volume. Studies on these more fine-grained attributes of cortical anatomy are only beginning to emerge in the field of developmental dyslexia. Promising results point to an atypical pattern of sulcal basin area in left temporo-parietal and occipito-temporal regions in children with developmental dyslexia compared with typically reading children (Im, Raschle, Smith, Ellen Grant, & Gaab, 2016). Sulcal pattern is a particularly interesting measure, because it is thought to relate to optimal organization and connections of cortical functional areas. Even more important is the fact that it is determined during prenatal development and may reflect early, genetically influenced brain development. Therefore, one would consider abnormalities in the sulcal pattern to be a cause rather than a consequence of later reading problems. Consequently, the sulcal pattern abnormalities identified in dyslexic children should also play a crucial role in adult dyslexia, although definite empirical evidence for this hypothesis is missing so far.

7.6 Structural Connectivity and the Use of Diffusion Tensor Imaging (DTI) to Study White Matter Abnormalities in Dyslexia

Two of the VBM studies – in addition to gray matter abnormalities – investigated white matter abnormalities in dyslexic readers (Eckert et al., 2005; Silani et al., 2005). Specifically, Eckert et al. (2005) reported white matter reduction in a right temporo-parietal region in dyslexic children, whereas Silani et al. (2005) reported white matter reduction in three left hemisphere regions (underneath inferior frontal, postcentral, and supramarginal gyri, respectively) in dyslexic adults. A more advanced method for the investigation of white abnormalities became available with diffusion tensor imaging (DTI) techniques, allowing examination of the integrity of white matter fiber tracts (e.g., Basser, Mattiello, & Lebihan, 1994). The emergence of this technique was paralleled by a conceptual focus on functional integration among different brain regions in contrast to a focus on functional specialization of discrete brain regions.

Several neuroimaging studies investigated dyslexic abnormalities in structural connectivity by means of DTI (Beaulieu et al., 2005; Carter et al., 2009; Deutsch et al., 2005; Dougherty et al., 2007; Frye et al., 2008, 2011; Jäncke, Siegenthaler, Preis, & Steinmetz, 2007; Keller & Just, 2009; Klingberg et al., 2000; Nagy, Westerberg, & Klingberg, 2004; Niogi & McCandliss, 2006; Odegard, Farris, Ring, McColl, & Black, 2009; Qiu, Tan, Zhou, & Khong, 2008; Richards et al., 2008; Rimrodt, Peterson, Denckla, Kaufmann, & Cutting, 2010; Rollins et al., 2009; Steinbrink et al., 2008; Vandermosten et al., 2015; Vandermosten, Boets, Wouters, & Ghesquière, 2012). Although the abnormalities identified in these structural connectivity studies are frequently not reported in terms of 3D coordinates in a standard stereotactic space, there is some systematic agreement across studies (for a comprehensive review and meta-analysis, see Vandermosten et al., 2012). The DTI studies frequently reported impaired integrity of white matter fiber tracts underlying left temporal and left temporo-parietal cortical regions. Unfortunately, due to the crossing of several large white matter tracts in this area, there is still little agreement on which fiber tracts within the white matter are specifically affected (Ben-Shachar, Dougherty, & Wandell, 2007). Possible candidates include the corpus callosum (running in the left-right direction and connecting the two cerebral hemispheres), the corona radiata (running in the inferior-superior direction and connecting the cerebellum, thalamus, and brain stem with cortical motor and somatosensory regions), and the main fiber tracts running in the posterior-anterior direction. These are the superior longitudinal fasciculus (SLF, connecting occipito-temporal, temporo-parietal, and inferior frontal language regions), the inferior longitudinal fasciculus (ILF, connecting occipital and temporal regions), and the inferior fronto-occipital fasciculus (IFOF, connecting occipital, parietal, and prefrontal regions).

Among these prime candidates for dyslexic abnormalities, the SLF received the most convincing support. Due to its unique location and architecture, the left SLF is of specific interest because it connects the occipito-temporal, temporo-parietal, and inferior frontal regions identified as major components of the left hemisphere reading network in numerous functional neuroimaging studies (Richlan, 2012). A recent DTI study with pre-reading children with and without a family risk for dyslexia found that phonological predictors of reading (i.e., phonological awareness) are sustained bilaterally by both ventral IFOF and dorsal arcuate fasciculus tracts (part of the SLF) (Vandermosten et al., 2015). In addition, children with a family risk for dyslexia exhibited white matter abnormalities mainly in the left ventral IFOF tract compared with children without a family risk for dyslexia. Again, similar to the previously described gray matter reductions, this difference in brain anatomy before the onset of formal reading instruction may be indicative of a cause rather than a consequence of reading problems. Follow-up analyses will show whether these early abnormalities lead to a full-blown clinical diagnosis of dyslexia and how these white matter fiber tract abnormalities develop through the school years and into adulthood.

7.7 The Relation Between Brain Structure and Brain Function

Whereas DTI studies inform about the structural connectivity of white matter anatomy, neuroimaging studies using functional magnetic resonance imaging (fMRI) have the potential to reveal the functional connectivity patterns underlying skilled reading and developmental dyslexia. Specifically, fMRI may be used to investigate which brain regions are engaged during particular tasks and how these brain regions interact with each other to yield behavior. Brain regions structurally connected by the SLF have been shown to be activated and functionally coupled in response to the demands of reading in skilled readers.

In dyslexic readers, activation and functional coupling are often impaired during reading or reading-related tasks (e.g., Boets et al., 2013; Cao, Bitan, & Booth, 2008; Finn et al., 2014; Richlan et al., 2010; Schurz et al., 2015; Shaywitz et al., 2003; van der Mark et al., 2011). For example, Schurz et al. (2015) analyzed differences between typically reading and dyslexic adults in both resting-state and task-based functional connectivity by means of seed voxel correlation mapping. Functional connectivity during the resting state can be thought of as an indicator of a history of consistent and repeated co-activation among regions. Methodologically, resting-state functional connectivity has the advantage that the data are obtained without any explicit task requirement, and therefore, group differences in resting-state data cannot be attributed to differences in task performance or processing strategies. Schurz et al. (2015) found reduced coupling in dyslexic readers between left posterior temporal regions and the left inferior frontal gyrus in both resting-state and task-based (i.e., reading-related) functional connectivity. This finding was interpreted as reflecting a permanent functional disruption between these regions in dyslexic adults, which is even present in the absence of the explicit demands of cognitive processes supporting skilled reading.

The relationship between gray matter, white matter, and functional activation as measured by fMRI in typical readers, however, is still very obscure. Even more difficult to answer are the questions of how abnormalities in these domains in developmental dyslexia might be related to each other, and how they might exert influence over each other during the school years and into adulthood.

Nevertheless, the last two decades brought significant advances in the functional neurobiological understanding of developmental dyslexia. This progress was substantially driven by advances in the fields of cognitive neuroscience and, more recently, of educational neuroscience. These interdisciplinary research areas integrate psychology, linguistics, pedagogy, neurobiology, genetics, medicine, bioengineering, and computer science. Another important factor for the progress in the understanding of brain-based disorders was the refinement of acquisition and analysis techniques of functional neuroimaging methods such as functional magnetic resonance imaging (fMRI), electroencephalography (EEG), and magnetoencephalography (MEG).

7.8 Multiple Perspectives on Dyslexia

It has become evident from numerous studies that developmental dyslexia may not be viewed as a simple, single-trait disorder. Genetic research has identified multiple candidate genes – most of them involved in prenatal neuronal migration and axon guidance – to be associated with dyslexia (e.g., Mascheretti et al., 2017; Peterson & Pennington, 2012, 2015; Scerri & Schulte-Körne, 2010). Likewise, no single behavioral phenotype can be considered a "typical" manifestation of dyslexia. There are problems in diverse aspects, including reading fluency, accuracy, comprehension, and spelling, and people affected by dyslexia often present a mixture of different severities of these literacy problems (e.g., Lyon, Shaywitz, & Shaywitz, 2003; Nation, Cocksey, Taylor, & Bishop, 2010). In addition, problems in learning to read are often comorbid with atypical or delayed oral language development (e.g., Catts, Bridges, Little, & Tomblin, 2008; Peterson, Pennington, Shriberg, & Boada, 2009), writing disabilities, attention deficit–hyperactivity disorder (ADHD), and math disabilities/dyscalculia (e.g., Landerl & Moll, 2010; Willcutt et al., 2010).

From this complex, multi-trait view of developmental dyslexia, it is clear that no single neurocognitive explanation can account for all of the associated dysfunctions. A number of competing hypotheses on the underlying cognitive deficits were postulated and empirically tested. The most prominent explanation posits a problem in phonological processing (e.g., Shaywitz & Shaywitz, 2005; Snowling, 2000; Vellutino & Fletcher, 2005), but alternative/complementary hypotheses include deficits in visual-verbal processing speed (e.g., Wolf & Bowers, 1999), visual attention (e.g., Bosse, Tainturier, & Valdois, 2007; Vidyasagar & Pammer, 2010), verbal short-term memory (e.g., Ahissar, 2007), low-level auditory (e.g., Goswami, 2011; Tallal, 1980) or visual processing (e.g., Eden, VanMeter, Rumsey, Maisog, & Zeffiro, 1996), magnocellular function (e.g., Stein & Walsh, 1997), and cerebellar automatization (e.g., Nicolson & Fawcett, 2007). Consequently, a variety of functional brain systems were assumed to be related to the cognitive processes associated with developmental dyslexia.

7.9 Functional Neuroimaging Studies on Dyslexia and the Phonological Deficit: Explanation of Dyslexia

Across many languages and writing systems, studies using functional neuroimaging methods have identified brain regions critically involved in typical and dyslexic reading using fMRI (e.g., Blau et al., 2010; Blau, Van Atteveldt, Ekkebus, Goebel, & Blomert, 2009; Eden et al., 1996; Gaab, Gabrieli, Deutsch, Tallal, & Temple, 2007; Heim et al., 2010; Heim, Wehnelt, Grande, Huber, & Amunts, 2013; Hoeft et al., 2006, 2007, 2011; Hu et al., 2010; Kronbichler et al., 2006; Richlan et al., 2010; Shaywitz et al., 1998, 2002; Siok, Perfetti, Jin, & Tan, 2004; Temple et al., 2000, 2001, 2003; van der Mark et al., 2009, 2011; Wimmer et al., 2010), EEG (e.g., Banaschewski & Brandeis, 2007; Brandeis, Vitacco, & Steinhause, 1994; Duffy, Denckla, Bartels, & Sandini, 1980; Klimesch et al., 2001a, 2001b; Maurer et al., 2007; Maurer, Bucher, Brem, & Brandeis, 2003), MEG (e.g., Cavalli et al., 2017; Helenius, Tarkiainen, Cornelissen, Hansen, & Salmelin, 1999; Salmelin, 2007; Simos et al., 2000b; Simos, Breier, Fletcher, Bergman, & Papanicolaou, 2000a), and PET (e.g.,

Brunswick, McCrory, Price, Frith, & Frith, 1999; Horwitz, Rumsey, & Bonohue, 1998; Paulesu et al., 1996, 2001; Rumsey et al., 1997).

Qualitative narrative reviews (e.g., Démonet, Taylor, & Chaix, 2004; Heim & Keil, 2004; McCandliss & Noble, 2003; Norton, Beach, & Gabrieli, 2015; Peterson & Pennington, 2012, 2015; Pugh et al., 2000; Richlan, 2012, 2014, 2020; Schlaggar & McCandliss, 2007; Shaywitz & Shaywitz, 2005) and quantitative meta-analyses of these studies (Linkersdörfer, Lonnemann, Lindberg, Hasselhorn, & Fiebach, 2012; Maisog, Einbinder, Flowers, Turkeltaub, & Eden, 2008; Martin, Kronbichler, & Richlan, 2016; Richlan et al., 2013; Richlan, Kronbichler, & Wimmer, 2009, 2011) have converged on a "standard" functional neuroanatomical model of dyslexia. Specifically, altered brain activation in dyslexic readers was consistently reported in left posterior temporo-parietal (middle and superior temporal, supramarginal, and angular gyri), left occipito-temporal (inferior temporal and fusiform gyri), and left frontal regions (inferior frontal and precentral gyri). For the posterior brain regions, the dominant finding is dyslexic underactivation, while the picture is less clear for the anterior regions. Objective meta-analytic evidence speaks for dyslexic overactivation in the left precentral gyrus and underactivation in the left inferior frontal gyrus (Richlan et al., 2009, 2011). In addition, there are occasional reports on other bilateral cortical, subcortical, and cerebellar dyslexic activation abnormalities, but consistency across studies is scarce.

The classical phonological deficit explanation served as a theoretical framework for the first functional neuroimaging studies of developmental dyslexia. These early studies culminated in a neurobiological model positing three left hemisphere regions with abnormal function in dyslexic readers (Démonet et al., 2004; McCandliss & Noble, 2003; Pugh et al., 2000; Sandak, Mencl, Frost, & Pugh, 2004; Schlaggar & McCandliss, 2007; Shaywitz & Shaywitz, 2005). In this model, the primary phonological word decoding difficulty in developmental dyslexia is seen as resulting from a dysfunction of a left dorsal temporo-parietal (TP) region, including the posterior aspect of the superior temporal gyrus and adjacent parietal regions. The secondary difficulty with fast word recognition in developmental dyslexia – based on stored orthographic word representations – is seen as resulting from a dysfunction of a left ventral occipito-temporal (OT) region including lateral extrastriate, fusiform, and inferior temporal regions. A third abnormality – presumably reflecting compensatory reliance on effortful articulatory processes in dyslexic readers – is overactivation of the left inferior frontal gyrus (IFG).

7.10 Meta-analyses of Functional Neuroimaging Studies on Dyslexia

A great leap forward in functional neuroimaging research on developmental dyslexia was gained from quantitative coordinate-based meta-analysis of published fMRI and PET studies. Richlan et al. (2009) used this approach in order to extend and spatially specify narrative reviews of functional dyslexic brain abnormalities. Their meta-analysis included 17 studies reporting foci of under- or overactivation (in relation to non-impaired readers) in reading or reading-related tasks. The coordinate-based meta-analytic approach relies on the fact that these foci are commonly reported in terms of 3D (x, y, z) coordinates in standard stereotaxic space. Each of the foci of brain activation of the original studies was modeled as the center of a Gaussian probability distribution in order to account for various sources of spatial error across studies. These probability distributions were then combined in order to create a whole-brain statistical map that estimates the likelihood of activation for each voxel.

The results of this meta-analysis supported the central role of left hemisphere TP and OT dysfunctions in developmental dyslexia. Specifically, convergent dyslexic underactivation across studies was found in the left inferior parietal lobule (IPL), superior temporal, middle temporal, inferior temporal, and fusiform regions. A novel finding was underactivation in a left IFG region associated with access to lexical and sublexical phonological output representations. Dyslexic overactivation was identified in the primary motor cortex and in the anterior insula, presumably reflecting compensatory reliance on articulatory-based phonological processes (Hancock, Richlan, & Hoeft, 2017).

7.11 The Roles of the Left Occipito-temporal (OT) and Temporo-parietal (TP) Cortex in Dyslexia and the Question of Development

The meta-analysis included original studies from quite different age levels, with beginning readers around 7 years of age to elderly readers of over 60 years of age. This feature of the meta-analysis is important in relation to the classical neurocognitive model of developmental dyslexia (e.g., Pugh et al., 2000). This model posits an early dysfunction of the left TP reading circuit, resulting in an additional secondary dysfunction of the left OT reading circuit. Therefore, one would expect to find dominance of left TP underactivation in children's studies and dominance of left OT underactivation in adult studies.

A second meta-analysis (Richlan et al., 2011) investigated exactly this expectation. The original studies were divided into nine studies with dyslexic children (age means: 9–11 years) and nine studies with dyslexic adults (age means: 18–30 years). Studies with adolescents were excluded. The meta-analysis allowed the identification of both age-related differences and commonalities of dyslexic brain dysfunctions. Contrary to expectation, the left TP dysfunction was identified in the adult studies but not in the children's studies. With respect to the left OT dysfunction, widespread underactivation extending in the posterior direction was found for the adult dyslexic readers. In contrast, for dyslexic children, left OT underactivation was limited to an anterior portion of the left ventral OT cortex. The left OT underactivation was markedly more pronounced in the adult studies compared with the children's studies. This finding is in agreement with the notion of an important role of the left OT region in skilled, efficient reading. For example, Shaywitz et al. (2007) found that normal reading development, but not dyslexic reading development, was associated with increasing engagement of the left lateral OT cortex. The finding of left OT underactivation in children is compatible with evidence from German-based studies in favor of early left OT engagement in typical reading development (e.g., Brem et al., 2010), and early failure of such engagement in developmental dyslexia (e.g., Maurer et al., 2007). In summary, the findings of the second meta-analysis raised serious doubts about the validity of the standard functional neuroanatomical dyslexia model. Specifically, there was no support for the critical developmental assumption that the primary and early emerging dysfunction resides in the left TP cortex. Rather, the findings suggest that an early small left OT dysfunction becomes increasingly extended in the posterior and superior directions and is later accompanied by a left TP dysfunction in dyslexic adults.

7.12 The Roles of the Left Frontal Cortex in Dyslexia

The identification of left IFG underactivation in the two meta-analyses was a novel finding and stood in contrast to overactivation in a close-by left precentral region. This finding was of specific importance, as in dominant formulations of the standard neurocognitive model (e.g., Pugh et al., 2000, it is assumed that a reading circuit in anterior frontal language regions exhibits overactivation in dyslexic readers in order to compensate for the dysfunction in posterior language regions. Obviously, the meta-analytic findings speak for a marked distinction within left frontal regions, that is, between a left IFG opercular region and a left precentral region, with dyslexic underactivation in the former and dyslexic overactivation in the latter. The former presumably is engaged by access to lexical and sublexical phonological representations, and the latter presumably by silent articulatory reading processes.

The second interpretation was recently confirmed by a systematic investigation applying large-scale reverse inference focusing exclusively on dyslexic overactivation (Hancock et al., 2017). There were several competing hypotheses about this overactivation. One hypothesis was that left precentral overactivation reflects higher neural engagement related to articulatory processing in order to compensate for reading-related underactivation in other regions. Alternatively, left precentral overactivation was hypothesized to reflect a more direct impairment in reading-related processes themselves, such as phonological processing or implicit sequence learning. Functional activation patterns related to these hypotheses were calculated from a large-scale database of over ten thousand fMRI studies (Yarkoni, Poldrack, Nichols, Van Essen, & Wager,

2011) and compared with the overactivation pattern of dyslexic readers identified by meta-analysis (Hancock et al., 2017). The pattern identified with dyslexic overactivation showed clearly highest neuroanatomical convergence with a fronto-striatal brain circuit supporting articulation. Less convergence with the dyslexic overactivation pattern was found for the networks supporting phonological processing and implicit sequence learning, respectively. Therefore, left precentral overactivation in dyslexic readers is most likely to reflect greater reliance on articulatory processing in order to compensate for reading-related underactivation in left TP and OT regions.

7.13 The Impaired Left Hemisphere Reading Network in Dyslexia: A Hypothetical Model

Based on the findings described above, we can assume a hypothetical model of the impaired (i.e., underactivated) left hemisphere reading network in developmental dyslexia (Figure 7.1), including at least four components, namely TP (including superior and middle temporal gyri), OT (including inferior temporal gyrus and occipito-temporal cortex), IFG (including opercular and

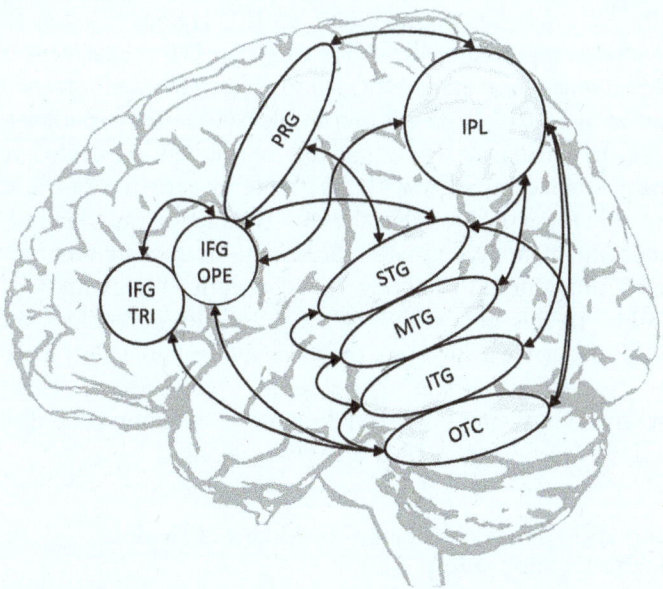

FIGURE 7.1 Schematic illustration of the presumably impaired left hemisphere reading network in developmental dyslexia. IFG = inferior frontal gyrus, IPL = inferior parietal lobule, ITG = inferior temporal gyrus, MTG = middle temporal gyrus, OPE = opercular, OTC = occipito-temporal cortex, PRG = precentral gyrus, STG = superior temporal gyrus, TRI = triangular.

triangular parts), and IPL regions. While there is evidence for strong connectivity (both functional and structural, see Ben-Shachar et al., 2007) between left TP, OT, and IFG regions, the connectivity of the left IPL region is less clear. With respect to the left IPL dysfunction, we can only speculate about possible underlying mechanisms. Assumedly, the function of the left IPL was not specifically related to reading or phonological decoding (Longo, Braun, Hutzler, & Richlan, 2022; Richlan et al., 2010). Rather, it was supposed to be associated with more general attention-related mechanisms. As put forward by Shaywitz and Shaywitz (2008), the left IPL may be part of a fronto-parietal attention network, which interacts with reading processes via top-down connections. The exact mechanisms of this interaction, however, are still unclear and may be targeted in future studies using functional and effective connectivity analysis.

An interesting question with respect to the model illustrated in Figure 7.1 is a developmental one. In accordance with the phonological deficit explanation of developmental dyslexia, one may reason that a dysfunction of the left TP and IFG components may be specifically critical in the early phase of learning to read, as these components are engaged by access to phonemes and other sublexical phonological representations (Richlan, 2019). To our knowledge, no evidence for such an early dysfunction of left IFG regions exists. Rather, developmental studies reported evidence for early left OT engagement in normal reading development and early left OT dysfunction in developmental dyslexia (e.g., Brem et al., 2010, 2020; Maurer et al., 2007). These findings raise the question of the particular functional role of the left OT region in reading development. Quite compatible with the idea of an early role of the left OT for learning to read is the position that the left OT functions as a kind of interface area connecting high-level visual representations (or representations from other sensory modalities) to language and conceptual representations (Price & Devlin, 2011). In this perspective, the aforementioned findings on reduced early left OT engagement in young dyslexic readers may reflect a kind of disconnection between visual and phonological representations. This would be consistent with Geschwind's classical account of developmental dyslexia as a disconnection syndrome (Geschwind, 1965a, 1965b).

7.14 Interaction of Brain Processes by Means of Flexible Functional Integration

Although we have convincing evidence that the functioning of the above-mentioned cortical regions is somehow altered in dyslexia during reading and reading-related tasks, it is still an open question how presumable impairments in these regions might interact with each other and lead to the severe reading problems of dyslexic readers often persisting into adulthood. For example, dyslexic brain dysfunctions related to auditory language processing and spelling are investigated relatively sparsely. In order to obtain a complete picture of the neurocognitive dysfunctions underlying dyslexia, however, an understanding of these proximal functions is a must. Only the integration of visual and auditory reading- and spelling-related brain processes and their development through the school years and into adulthood will lead to substantial progress in the field, with corresponding implications for diagnosis, prognosis, and treatment of the disorder.

As detailed above, it is most probable that skilled reading is supported by a network of inter-regionally coupled mainly left hemisphere brain regions and that dyslexia results from a dysfunction of this complex brain system (Figure 7.1). The dysfunction can affect the nodes per se (i.e., local brain regions) – expressed by dysfunctional activation or gray matter anatomical alterations – as well as the edges (i.e., connections) – expressed by dysfunctional coupling between brain regions and defectiveness of underlying white matter fiber tracts. We propose a flexible functional integration account, in the sense that different parts of the overall network interact in flexible ways depending on the required cognitive processes for a given task (Braun et al., 2019; Gagl et al., 2018, 2020, 2022). In order to investigate this complex brain system, future brain imaging studies will use functional and structural MRI (and other brain imaging techniques) with state-of-the-art analysis methods such as multivariate pattern analysis, effective connectivity, and graph theoretical analysis. Although relatively new, these methods are already well-established in other fields of research, but investigations of developmental dyslexia are missing (with few exceptions).

7.15 Natural Reading and the Use of Ecologically More Valid Experimental Settings

In addition to novel developments regarding data analysis, future neurocognitive studies on developmental dyslexia will make use of ecologically more valid experimental settings. That is, they will focus on self-paced, silent sentence reading and integrate fMRI with eye tracking. Critically, dyslexic brain dysfunctions were predominantly assessed in the context of single-word studies (i.e., studies presenting unrelated words in a serial one-by-one fashion) utilizing more or less artificial reading-related tasks (e.g., lexical decision, semantic judgment, rhyme judgment, etc.). Undoubtedly, these studies have contributed tremendously to our understanding of the neural mechanisms during visual word recognition in typical and dyslexic readers (for a recent overview, see Mascheretti et al., 2017). To what extent these findings generalize to natural reading, however, is an open issue. Comparatively few studies investigated brain responses of dyslexic readers in relation to whole sentences or paragraphs (e.g., Kronbichler et al., 2006; Meyler et al., 2007; Meyler, Keller, Cherkassky, Gabrieli, & Just, 2008; Rimrodt et al., 2009; Schulz et al., 2008,

2009; Seki et al., 2001) and even fewer did so in relation to words within sentences or paragraphs.

Recent fMRI studies addressed the gap between the limited ecological validity of contemporary functional neuroimaging paradigms and natural viewing behavior (Henderson, Choi, Luke, & Desai, 2015; Marsman, Renken, Velichkovsky, Hooymans, & Cornelissen, 2012; Richlan et al., 2014; Schuster et al., 2021; Schuster, Hawelka, Himmelstoss, Richlan, & Hutzler, 2020; Schuster, Hawelka, Hutzler, Kronbichler, & Richlan, 2016; Schuster, Hawelka, Richlan, Ludersdorfer, & Hutzler, 2015). In brief, the fixation-related fMRI approach allows researchers to analyze effects on the word-level while participants read whole texts at their own speed. It will be interesting to see how the previously identified abnormalities in the left hemisphere reading network in developmental dyslexia are related to natural reading, including parafoveal preprocessing of upcoming words (Cui, Richlan, & Zhou, 2022; Hutzler et al., 2013; Rayner, 2009; Vignali, Hawelka, Hutzler, & Richlan, 2019a, 2019b). Future studies will assess brain dysfunctions in dyslexic readers during self-paced, silent sentence reading using a combined analysis of eye movement (i.e., fixation durations, word skippings, re-fixations) and brain activation data (i.e., fixation-related fMRI). The investigation of functional brain abnormalities in developmental dyslexia under ecologically valid reading situations will hopefully pave the way to new impetus in the field, with important implications for early detection, accurate prognosis, and effective treatment of reading problems.

7.16 Clinical Perspectives and Neurological Markers of Adult Dyslexia

Up to now, the clinical implications of the above-described neuroscientific evidence on developmental dyslexia remain limited. Many of the studies suffer from small sample sizes, differing diagnostic criteria for inclusion in the dyslexia group, and unclear comorbidities. As a result, there is considerable heterogeneity of findings across studies. Furthermore, there is a recent general debate on the issue of low statistical power in neuroscience. In order to account for these problems, future studies will have to rely on larger samples and careful cognitive behavioral characterization of typically reading and dyslexic participants. Such a thorough behavioral characterization is the prerequisite for the analysis of neurological function and dysfunction in developmental dyslexia.

Even with the impressive progress in the study of the functional neuroanatomy of reading and dyslexia over the past decades in mind, one should be aware that most studies report statistically significant differences between groups of participants. Whether and how these statistically significant group differences translate into clinically and/or practically significant results relevant to individuals remains unclear (Braid & Richlan, 2022; Perdue et al.,

2022). Here, interdisciplinary research integrating brain imaging, genetic analysis, and computational approaches in order to examine diverse aspects of learning, socio-emotional processing, motivation, and resilience comes into play. Ultimately, this may lead to early identification of potential learning disorders and personalized education, including individual learning profiles. Taken together, one of the primary goals of reading and dyslexia research is to develop scientifically grounded models of diagnosis, prevention, therapy, and rehabilitation. Identification and characterization of the functional neuroanatomical networks involved in reading and dyslexia will facilitate progress toward these goals.

References

Ahissar, M. (2007). Dyslexia and the anchoring-deficit hypothesis. *Trends in Cognitive Neurosciences, 11*, 458–465.

Ashburner, J., & Friston, K. J. (2000). Voxel-based morphometry—The methods. *NeuroImage, 11*, 805–821.

Ashburner, J., & Friston, K. J. (2001). Why voxel-based morphometry should be used. *NeuroImage, 14*, 1238–1243.

Banaschewski, T., & Brandeis, D. (2007). Annotation: What electrical brain activity tells us about brain function that other techniques cannot tell us – A child psychiatric perspective. *The Journal of Child Psychology and Psychiatry, 48*, 415–435.

Basser, P. J., Mattiello, J., & Lebihan, D. (1994). MR diffusion tensor spectroscopy and imaging. *Biophysical Journal, 66*, 259–267.

Beaulieu, C., Plewes, C., Paulson, L. A., Roy, D., Snook, L., Concha, L., & Phillips, L. (2005). Imaging brain connectivity in children with diverse reading ability. *NeuroImage, 25*, 1266–1271.

Ben-Shachar, M., Dougherty, R. F., & Wandell, B. A. (2007). White matter pathways in reading. *Current Opinion in Neurobiology, 17*, 258–270.

Black, J. M., Tanaka, H., Stanley, L., Nagamine, M., Zakerani, N., Thurston, A., Kesler, S., Hulme, C., Lyytinen, H., Glover, G. H., Serrone, C., Raman, M. M., Reiss, A. L., & Hoeft, F. (2012). Maternal history of reading difficulty is associated with reduced language-related gray matter in beginning readers. *NeuroImage, 59*, 3021–3032.

Blau, V., Reithler, J., van Atteveldt, N., Seitz, J., Gerretsen, P., Goebel, R., & Blomert, L. (2010). Deviant processing of letters and speech sounds as proximate cause of reading failure: A functional magnetic resonance imaging study of dyslexic children. *Brain, 133*, 868–879.

Blau, V., Van Atteveldt, N., Ekkebus, M., Goebel, R., & Blomert, L. (2009). Reduced neural integration of letters and speech sounds links phonological and reading deficits in adult dyslexia. *Current Biology, 19*, 503–508.

Boets, B., Op de Beeck, H. P., Vandermosten, M., Scott, S. K., Gillebert, C. R., Mantini, D., Bulthé, J., Sunaert, S., Wouters, J., & Ghesquière, P. (2013). Intact but less accessible phonetic representations in adults with dyslexia. *Science, 342*, 1251–1254.

Bookstein, F. L. (2001). "Voxel-based morphometry" should not be used with imperfectly registered images. *NeuroImage, 14*, 1454–1462.

Bosse, M. L., Tainturier, M. J., & Valdois, S. (2007). Developmental dyslexia: The visual attention span hypothesis. *Cognition, 104*, 198–230.

Braid, J., & Richlan, F. (2022). The functional neuroanatomy of reading intervention. *Frontiers in Neuroscience, 16*, 921931.

Brambati, S. M., Termine, C., Ruffino, M., Stella, G., Fazio, F., Cappa, S. F., & Perani, D. (2004). Regional reductions of gray matter volume in familial dyslexia. *Neurology*, *63*, 742–745.

Brandeis, D., Vitacco, D., & Steinhause, H. C. (1994). Mapping brain electric microstates in dyslexic children during reading. *Acta Paedopsychiatrica*, *56*, 239–247.

Braun, M., Kronbichler, M., Richlan, F., Hawelka, S., Hutzler, F., & Jacobs, A. M. (2019). A model-guided dissociation between subcortical and cortical contributions to word recognition. *Scientific Reports*, *9*, 4506.

Brem, S., Bach, S., Kucian, K., Guttorm, T. K., Martin, E., Lyytinen, H., Brandeis, D., & Richardson, U. (2010). Brain sensitivity to print emerges when children learn letter-speech sound correspondences. *Proceedings of the National Academy of Sciences of the United States of America*, *107*, 7939–7944.

Brem, S., Maurer, U., Kronbichler, M., Schurz, M., Richlan, F., Blau, V., & Brandeis, D. (2020). Visual word form processing deficits driven by severity of reading impairments in children with developmental dyslexia. *Scientific Reports*, *10*, 18728.

Brown, W. E., Eliez, S., Menon, V., Rumsey, J. M., White, C. D., & Reiss, A. L. (2001). Preliminary evidence of widespread morphological variations of the brain in dyslexia. *Neurology*, *56*, 781–783.

Brunswick, N., McCrory, E., Price, C., Frith, C. D., & Frith, U. (1999). Explicit and implicit processing of words and pseudowords by adult developmental dyslexics: A search for Wernicke's Wortschatz? *Brain*, *122*, 1901–1917.

Cao, F., Bitan, T., & Booth, J. R. (2008). Effective brain connectivity in children with reading difficulties during phonological processing. *Brain and Language*, *107*, 91–101.

Carreiras, M., Seghier, M. L., Baquero, S., Estévez, A., Lozano, A., Devlin, J. T., & Price, C. J. (2009). An anatomical signature for literacy. *Nature*, *461*, 983–986.

Carter, J. C., Lanham, D. C., Cutting, L. E., Clements-Stephens, A. M., Chen, X., Hadzipasic, M., Kim, J., Denckla, M. B., & Kaufmann, W. E. (2009). A dual DTI approach to analyzing white matter in children with dyslexia. *Psychiatry Research*, *172*, 215–219.

Catts, H. W., Bridges, M. S., Little, T. D., & Tomblin, J. B. (2008). Reading achievement growth in children with language impairments. *Journal of Speech, Language, and Hearing Research*, *51*, 1569–1579.

Cavalli, E., Colé, P., Pattamadilok, C., Badier, J. M., Zielinski, C., Chanoine, V., & Ziegler, J. C. (2017). Spatiotemporal reorganization of the reading network in adult dyslexia. *Cortex*, *92*, 204–221.

Cui, X., Richlan, F., & Zhou, W. (2022). Fixation-related fMRI analysis reveals the neural basis of parafoveal processing in self-paced reading of Chinese words. *Brain Structure and Function*, *227*, 2609–2621.

Dejerine, J. (1891). Sur un cas de cecité verbale avec agraphie, suivi d'autopsie. *Memoires Societé Biologique*, *3*, 197–201.

Dejerine, J. (1892). Contribution of l'étude anatomo-pathologique et clinique des differentes varietiés de cecité verbale. *Memoires Societé Biologique*, *4*, 61–90.

Démonet, J. F., Taylor, M. J., & Chaix, Y. (2004). Developmental dyslexia. *Lancet*, *363*, 1451–1460.

Deutsch, G. K., Dougherty, R. F., Bammer, R., Siok, W. T., Gabrieli, J. D., & Wandell, B. (2005). Children's reading performance is correlated with white matter structure measured by diffusion tensor imaging. *Cortex*, *41*, 354–363.

Dougherty, R. F., Ben-Shachar, M., Deutsch, G. K., Hernandez, A., Fox, G. R., & Wandell, B. A. (2007). Temporal-callosal pathway diffusivity predicts phonological skills in children. *Proceedings of the National Academy of Sciences of the United States of America*, *104*, 8556–8561.

Duffy, F. H., Denckla, M. B., Bartels, P. H., & Sandini, G. (1980). Dyslexia: Regional differences in brain electrical activity by topographic mapping. *Annals of Neurology*, *7*, 412–420.

Eckert, M. A., Berninger, V. W., Vaden, K. I. Jr., Gebregziabher, M., & Tsu, L. (2016). Gray matter features of reading disability: A combined meta-analytic and direct analysis approach (1,2,3,4). *eNeuro*, *3*, ii. ENEURO.0103-15.2015.

Eckert, M. A., Leonard, C. M., Wilke, M., Eckert, M., Richards, T., Richards, A., & Berninger, V. (2005). Anatomical signatures of dyslexia in children: Unique information from manual and voxel based morphometry brain measures. *Cortex*, *41*, 304–315.

Eden, G. F., VanMeter, J. W., Rumsey, J. W., Maisog, J., & Zeffiro, T. A. (1996). Abnormal processing of visual motion in dyslexia revealed by functional brain imaging. *Nature*, *348*, 66–69.

Eliez, S., Rumsey, J. M., Giedd, J. N., Schmitt, J. E., Patwardhan, A. J., & Reiss, A. L. (2000). Morphological alteration of temporal lobe gray matter in dyslexia: An MRI study. *Journal of Child Psychology and Psychiatry*, *41*, 637–644.

Finn, E. S., Shen, X., Holahan, J. M., Scheinost, D., Lacadie, C., Papademetris, X., Shaywitz, S. E., Shaywitz, B. A., & Constable, R. T. (2014). Disruption of functional networks in dyslexia: A whole-brain, data-driven analysis of connectivity. *Biological Psychiatry*, *76*, 397–404.

Fischl, B., Rajendran, N., Busa, E., Augustinack, J., Hinds, O., Yeo, B. T., Mohlberg, H., Amunts, K., & Zilles, K. (2008). Cortical folding patterns and predicting cytoarchitecture. *Cerebral Cortex*, *18*, 1973–1980.

Friston, K. J., Frith, C. D., Liddle, P. F., Dolan, R. J., Lammertsma, A. A., & Frackowiak, R. S. J. (1990). The relationship between global and local changes in PET scans. *Journal of Cerebral Blood Flow and Metabolism*, *10*, 458–466.

Frye, R. E., Hasan, K., Xue, L., Strickland, D., Malmberg, B., Liederman, J., & Papanicolaou, A. (2008). Splenium microstructure is related to two dimensions of reading skill. *Neuroreport*, *19*, 1627–1631.

Frye, R. E., Liederman, J., Hasan, K. M., Lincoln, A., Malmberg, B., McLean, J., 3rd, & Papanicolaou, A. (2011). Diffusion tensor quantification of the relations between microstructural and macrostructural indices of white matter and reading. *Human Brain Mapping*, *32*, 1220–1235.

Gaab, N., Gabrieli, J. D., Deutsch, G. K., Tallal, P., & Temple, E. (2007). Neural correlates of rapid auditory processing are disrupted in children with developmental dyslexia and ameliorated with training: An fMRI study. *Restorative Neurology and Neuroscience*, *25*, 295–310.

Gagl, B., Richlan, F., Ludersdorfer, P., Sassenhagen, J., Eisenhauer, S., Gregorova, K., & Fiebach, C. J. (2022). The lexical categorization model: A computational model of left ventral occipito-temporal cortex activation in visual word recognition. *PLoS Computational Biology*, *18*, e1009995.

Gagl, B., Sassenhagen, J., Haan, S., Gregorova, K., Richlan, F., & Fiebach, C. J. (2018). Visual word recognition relies on an orthographic prediction error signal. *BioRxiv*, *431726*.

Gagl, B., Sassenhagen, J., Haan, S., Gregorova, K., Richlan, F., & Fiebach, C. J. (2020). An orthographic prediction error as the basis for efficient visual word recognition. *NeuroImage*, *214*, 116727.

Galaburda, A. M., & Kemper, T. L. (1979). Cytoarchitectonic abnormalities in developmental dyslexia: A case study. *Annals of Neurology*, *6*, 94–100.

Galaburda, A. M., Sherman, G. F., Rosen, G. D., Aboitiz, F., & Geschwind, N. (1985). Developmental dyslexia: Four consecutive patients with cortical anomalies. *Annals of Neurology*, *18*, 222–233.

Geschwind, N. (1965a). Disconnexion syndromes in animals and man. I. *Brain, 88*, 237–294.
Geschwind, N. (1965b). Disconnexion syndromes in animals and man. II. *Brain, 88*, 585–644.
Goswami, U. (2011). A temporal sampling framework for developmental dyslexia. *Trends in Cognitive Neurosciences, 15*, 3–10.
Hancock, R., Richlan, F., & Hoeft, F. (2017). Possible roles for fronto-striatal circuits in reading disorder. *Neuroscience and Biobehavioral Reviews, 72*, 243–260.
Heim, S., Grande, M., Pape-Neumann, J., van Ermingen, M., Meffert, E., Grabowska, A., Huber, W., & Amunts, K. (2010). Interaction of phonological awareness and 'magnocellular' processing during normal and dyslexic reading: Behavioural and fMRI investigations. *Dyslexia, 16*, 258–282.
Heim, S., & Keil, A. (2004). Large-scale neural correlates of developmental dyslexia. *European Child & Adolescent Psychiatry, 13*, 125–140.
Heim, S., Wehnelt, A., Grande, M., Huber, W., & Amunts, K. (2013). Effects of lexicality and word frequency on brain activation in dyslexic readers. *Brain and Language, 125*, 194–202.
Helenius, P., Tarkiainen, A., Cornelissen, P., Hansen, P. C., & Salmelin, R. (1999). Dissociation of normal feature analysis and deficient processing of letter- strings in dyslexic adults. *Cerebral Cortex, 9*, 476–483.
Henderson, J. M., Choi, W., Luke, S. G., & Desai, R. H. (2015). Neural correlates of fixation duration in natural reading: Evidence from fixation-related fMRI. *NeuroImage, 119*, 390–397.
Hickok, G., & Poeppel, D. (2007). The cortical organization of speech processing. *Nature Reviews. Neuroscience, 8*, 393–402.
Hoeft, F., Hernandez, A., McMillon, G., Taylor-Hill, H., Martindale, J. L., Meyler, A., Keller, T. A., Siok, W. T., Deutsch, G. K., Just, M. A., Whitfield-Gabrieli, S., & Gabrieli, J. D. (2006). Neural basis of dyslexia: A comparison between dyslexic and nondyslexic children equated for reading ability. *Journal of Neuroscience, 26*, 10700–10708.
Hoeft, F., McCandliss, B. D., Black, J. M., Gantman, A., Zakerani, N., Hulme, C., Lyytinen, H., Whitfield-Gabrieli, S., Glover, G. H., Reiss, A. L., & Gabrieli, J. D. (2011). Neural systems predicting long-term outcome in dyslexia. *Proceedings of the National Academy of Sciences, USA, 108*, 361–366.
Hoeft, F., Meyler, A., Hernandez, A., Juel, C., Taylor-Hill, H., Martindale, J. L., McMillon, G., Kolchugina, G., Black, J. M., Faizi, A., Deutsch, G. K., Siok, W. T., Reiss, A. L., Whitfield-Gabrieli, S., & Gabrieli, J. D. (2007). Functional and morphometric brain dissociation between dyslexia and reading ability. *Proceedings of the National Academy of Sciences, USA, 104*, 4234–4239.
Holloway, I. D., van Atteveldt, N., Blomert, L., & Ansari, D. (2015). Orthographic dependency in the neural correlates of reading: Evidence from audiovisual integration in English readers. *Cerebral Cortex, 25*, 1544–1553.
Horwitz, B., Rumsey, J. M., & Bonohue, B. C. (1998). Functional connectivity of the angular gyrus in normal reading and dyslexia. *Proceedings of the National Academy of Sciences, USA, 95*, 8939–8944.
Hu, W., Lee, H. L., Zhang, Q., Liu, T., Geng, L. B., Seghier, M. L., Shakeshaft, C., Twomey, T., Green, D. W., Yang, Y. M., & Price, C. J. (2010). Developmental dyslexia in Chinese and English populations: Dissociating the effect of dyslexia from language differences. *Brain, 133*, 1694–1706.
Humphreys, P., Kaufmann, W. E., & Galaburda, A. M. (1990). Developmental dyslexia in women: Neuropathological findings in three patients. *Annals of Neurology, 28*, 727–738.

Hutton, C., Draganski, B., Ashburner, J., & Weiskopf, N. (2009). A comparison between voxel-based cortical thickness and voxelbased morphometry in normal aging. *NeuroImage, 48*, 371–380.

Hutzler, F., Fuchs, I., Gagl, B., Schuster, S., Richlan, F., Braun, M., & Hawelka, S. (2013). Parafoveal X-masks interfere with foveal word recognition: Evidence from fixation-related brain potentials. *Frontiers in Systems Neuroscience, 7*, 33.

Im, K., Raschle, N. M., Smith, S. A., Ellen Grant, P., & Gaab, N. (2016). Atypical Sulcal pattern in children with developmental dyslexia and at-risk kindergarteners. *Cerebral Cortex, 26*, 1138–1148.

Jäncke, L., Siegenthaler, T., Preis, S., & Steinmetz, H. (2007). Decreased white-matter density in a left-sided fronto-temporal network in children with developmental language disorder: Evidence for anatomical anomalies in a motor-language network. *Brain and Language, 102*, 91–98.

Jednoróg, K., Marchewka, A., Altarelli, I., Monzalvo Lopez, A. K., van Ermingen-Marbach, M., Grande, M., Grabowska, A., Heim, S., & Ramus, F. (2015). How reliable are gray matter disruptions in specific reading disability across multiple countries and languages? Insights from a large-scale voxel-based morphometry study. *Human Brain Mapping, 36*, 1741–1754.

Keller, T. A., & Just, M. A. (2009). Altering cortical connectivity: Remediation-induced changes in the white matter of poor readers. *Neuron, 64*, 624–631.

Klimesch, W., Doppelmayr, M., Wimmer, H., Gruber, W., Röhm, D., Schwiager, J., & Hutzler, F. (2001a). Alpha and beta band power changes in normal and dyslectic children. *Clinical Neurophysiology, 112*, 1186–1195.

Klimesch, W., Doppelmayr, M., Wimmer, H., Schwaiger, J., Röhm, D., Gruber, W., & Hutzler, F. (2001b). Theta band power changes in normal and dyslectic children. *Clinical Neurophysiology, 112*, 1174–1185.

Klingberg, T., Hedehus, M., Temple, E., Salz, T., Gabrieli, J. D., Moseley, M. E., & Poldrack, R. A. (2000). Microstructure of temporo-parietal white matter as a basis for reading ability: Evidence from diffusion tensor magnetic resonance imaging. *Neuron, 25*, 493–500.

Krafnick, A. J., Flowers, D. L., Luetje, M. M., Napoliello, E. M., & Eden, G. F. (2014). An investigation into the origin of anatomical differences in dyslexia. *The Journal of Neuroscience, 34*, 901–908.

Kronbichler, M., Hutzler, F., Staffen, W., Mair, A., Ladurner, G., & Wimmer, H. (2006). Evidence for a dysfunction of left posterior reading areas in German dyslexic readers. *Neuropsychologia, 44*, 1822–1832.

Kronbichler, M., Wimmer, H., Staffen, W., Hutzler, F., Mair, A., & Ladurner, G. (2008). Developmental dyslexia: Gray matter abnormalities in the occipitotemporal cortex. *Human Brain Mapping, 29*, 613–625.

Landerl, K., & Moll, K. (2010). Comorbidity of learning disorders: Prevalence and familial transmission. *The Journal of Child Psychology and Psychiatry, 51*, 287–294.

Linkersdörfer, J., Lonnemann, J., Lindberg, S., Hasselhorn, M., & Fiebach, C. J. (2012). Grey matter alterations co-localize with functional abnormalities in developmental dyslexia: An ALE meta-analysis. *PLoS One, 7*, e43122.

Longo, F., Braun, M., Hutzler, F., & Richlan, F. (2022). Impaired semantic categorization during transcranial direct current stimulation of the left and right inferior parietal lobule. *Journal of Neurolinguistics, 62*, 101058.

Lyon, R. G., Shaywitz, S. E., & Shaywitz, B. A. (2003). A definition of dyslexia. *Annals of Dyslexia, 53*, 1–14.

Maisog, J. M., Einbinder, E. R., Flowers, D. L., Turkeltaub, P. E., & Eden, G. F. (2008). A meta-analysis of functional neuroimaging studies of dyslexia. *Annals of the New York Academy of Sciences, 1145*, 237–259.

Marsman, J. B., Renken, R., Velichkovsky, B. M., Hooymans, J. M., & Cornelissen, F. W. (2012). Fixation based event-related fMRI analysis: Using eye fixations as events in functional magnetic resonance imaging to reveal cortical processing during the free exploration of visual images. *Human Brain Mapping, 33*, 307–318.

Martin, A., Kronbichler, M., & Richlan, F. (2016). Dyslexic brain activation abnormalities in deep and shallow orthographies: A meta-analysis of 28 functional neuroimaging studies. *Human Brain Mapping, 37*, 2676–2699.

Mascheretti, S., De Luca, A., Trezzi, V., Peruzzo, D., Nordio, A., Marino, C., & Arrigoni, F. (2017). Neurogenetics of developmental dyslexia: From genes to behavior through brain neuroimaging and cognitive and sensorial mechanisms. *Translational Psychiatry, 7*, e987.

Maurer, U., Brem, S., Bucher, K., Kranz, F., Benz, R., Steinhausen, H. C., & Brandeis, D. (2007). Impaired tuning of a fast occipito-temporal response for print in dyslexic children learning to read. *Brain, 130*, 3200–3210.

Maurer, U., Bucher, K., Brem, S., & Brandeis, D. (2003). Altered responses to tone and phoneme mismatch in kindergartners at familial dyslexia-risk. *Neuroreport, 14*, 2245–2250.

McCandliss, B. D., & Noble, K. G. (2003). The development of reading impairment: A cognitive neuroscience model. *Mental Retardation and Developmental Disabilities Research Reviews, 9*, 196–204.

Mechelli, A., Price, C. J., Friston, K. J., & Ashburner, J. (2005). Voxel-based morphometry of the human brain: Methods and applications. *Current Medical Imaging Reviews, 1*, 105–113.

Menghini, D., Hagberg, G. E., Petrosini, L., Bozzali, M., Macaluso, E., Caltagirone, C., & Vicari, S. (2008). Structural correlates of implicit learning deficits in subjects with developmental dyslexia. *Annals of the New York Academy of Sciences, 1145*, 212–221.

Meyler, A., Keller, T. A., Cherkassky, V. L., Gabrieli, J. D., & Just, M. A. (2008). Modifying the brain activation of poor readers during sentence comprehension with extended remedial instruction: A longitudinal study of neuroplasticity. *Neuropsychologia, 46*, 2580–2592.

Meyler, A., Keller, T. A., Cherkassky, V. L., Lee, D., Hoeft, F., Whitfield-Gabrieli, S., Gabrieli, J. D., & Just, M. A. (2007). Brain activation during sentence comprehension among good and poor readers. *Cerebral Cortex, 17*, 2780–2787.

Nagy, Z., Westerberg, H., & Klingberg, T. (2004). Maturation of white matter is associated with the development of cognitive functions during childhood. *Journal of Cognitive Neuroscience, 16*, 1227–1233.

Nation, K., Cocksey, J., Taylor, J. S., & Bishop, D. V. (2010). A longitudinal investigation of early reading and language skills in children with poor reading comprehension. *Journal of Child Psychology and Psychiatry, 51*, 1031–1039.

Nicolson, R. I., & Fawcett, A. J. (2007). Procedural learning difficulties: Reuniting the developmental disorders? *Trends in Neuroscience, 30*, 135–141.

Niogi, S. N., & McCandliss, B. D. (2006). Left lateralized white matter microstructure accounts for individual differences in reading ability and disability. *Neuropsychologia, 44*, 2178–2188.

Norton, E. S., Beach, S. D., & Gabrieli, J. D. (2015). Neurobiology of dyslexia. *Current Opinion in Neurobiology, 30*, 73–78.

Odegard, T. N., Farris, E. A., Ring, J., McColl, R., & Black, J. (2009). Brain connectivity in non-reading impaired children and children diagnosed with developmental dyslexia. *Neuropsychologia, 47*, 1972–1977.

Paulesu, E., Démonet, J. F., Fazio, F., McCrory, E., Chanoine, V., & Brunswick, N. (2001). Dyslexia: Cultural diversity and biological unity. *Science, 291*, 2165–2167.

Paulesu, E., Frith, U., Snowling, M., Gallagher, A., Morton, J., Frackowiak, R. S., & Frith, C. D. (1996). Is developmental dyslexia a disconnection syndrome? Evidence from PET scanning. *Brain, 119,* 143–157.

Perdue, M. V., Mahaffy, K., Vlahcevic, K., Wolfman, E., Erbeli, F., Richlan, F., & Landi, N. (2022). Reading intervention and neuroplasticity: A systematic review and meta-analysis of brain changes associated with reading intervention. *Neuroscience & Biobehavioral Reviews, 132,* 465–494.

Pernet, C., Andersson, J., Paulesu, E., & Demonet, J. F. (2009a). When all hypotheses are right: A multifocal account of dyslexia. *Human Brain Mapping, 30,* 2278–2292.

Pernet, C. R., Poline, J. B., Demonet, J. F., & Rousselet, G. A. (2009b). Brain classification reveals the right cerebellum as the best biomarker of dyslexia. *BMC Neuroscience, 10,* 67.

Peterson, R. L., & Pennington, B. F. (2012). Developmental dyslexia. *The Lancet, 379,* 1997–2007.

Peterson, R. L., & Pennington, B. F. (2015). Developmental dyslexia. *Annual Review of Clinical Psychology, 11,* 283–307.

Peterson, R. L., Pennington, B. F., Shriberg, L. D., & Boada, R. (2009). What influences literacy outcome in children with speech sound disorder? *Journal of Speech, Language, and Hearing Research, 52,* 1175–1188.

Price, C. J., & Devlin, J. T. (2011). The interactive account of ventral occipitotemporal contributions to reading. *Trends in Cognitive Sciences, 15,* 246–253.

Pugh, K. R., Mencl, W. E., Jenner, A. R., Katz, L., Frost, S. J., Lee, J. R., Shaywitz, S. E., & Shaywitz, B. A. (2000). Functional neuroimaging studies of reading and reading disability (developmental dyslexia). *Mental Retardation and Developmental Disabilities Research Reviews, 6,* 207–213.

Qiu, D., Tan, L. H., Zhou, K., & Khong, P. L. (2008). Diffusion tensor imaging of normal white matter maturation from late childhood to young adulthood: Voxel-wise evaluation of mean diffusivity, fractional anisotropy, radial and axial diffusivities, and correlation with reading development. *NeuroImage, 41,* 223–232.

Ramus, F., Altarelli, I., Jednoróg, K., Zhao, J., & Scotto di Covella, L. (2017). Neuroanatomy of developmental dyslexia: Pitfalls and promise. *Neuroscience and Biobehavioral Reviews, 84,* 434–452.

Raschle, N. M., Becker, B. L., Smith, S., Fehlbaum, L. V., Wang, Y., & Gaab, N. (2017). Investigating the influences of language delay and/or familial risk for dyslexia on brain structure in 5-year-olds. *Cerebral Cortex, 27,* 764–776.

Raschle, N. M., Chang, M., & Gaab, N. (2011). Structural brain alterations associated with dyslexia predate reading onset. *NeuroImage, 57,* 742–749.

Rayner, K. (2009). Eye movements and attention in reading, scene perception, and visual search. *Quarterly Journal of Experimental Psychology, 62,* 1457–1506.

Richards, T., Stevenson, J., Crouch, J., Johnson, L. C., Maravilla, K., Stock, P., Abbott, R., & Berninger, V. (2008). Tract-based spatial statistics of diffusion tensor imaging in adults with dyslexia. *AJNR. American Journal of Neuroradiology, 29,* 1134–1139.

Richlan, F. (2012). Developmental dyslexia: Dysfunction of a left hemisphere reading network. *Frontiers in Human Neuroscience, 6,* 120.

Richlan, F. (2014). Functional neuroanatomy of developmental dyslexia: The role of orthographic depth. *Frontiers in Human Neuroscience, 8,* 347.

Richlan, F. (2019). The functional neuroanatomy of letter-speech sound integration and its relation to brain abnormalities in developmental dyslexia. *Frontiers in Human Neuroscience, 13,* 21.

Richlan, F. (2020). The functional neuroanatomy of developmental dyslexia across languages and writing systems. *Frontiers in Psychology, 11,* 493771.

Richlan, F., Gagl, B., Hawelka, S., Braun, M., Schurz, M., Kronbichler, M., & Hutzler, F. (2014). Fixation-related fMRI analysis in the domain of reading research: Using self-paced eye movements as markers for hemodynamic brain responses during visual letter string processing. *Cerebral Cortex*, *24*, 2647–2656.

Richlan, F., Kronbichler, M., & Wimmer, H. (2009). Functional abnormalities in the dyslexic brain: A quantitative meta-analysis of neuroimaging studies. *Human Brain Mapping*, *30*, 3299–3308.

Richlan, F., Kronbichler, M., & Wimmer, H. (2011). Meta-analyzing brain dysfunctions in dyslexic children and adults. *NeuroImage*, *56*, 1735–1742.

Richlan, F., Kronbichler, M., & Wimmer, H. (2013). Structural abnormalities in the dyslexic brain: A meta-analysis of voxel-based Morphometry studies. *Human Brain Mapping*, *34*, 3055–3065.

Richlan, F., Sturm, D., Schurz, M., Kronbichler, M., Ladurner, G., & Wimmer, H. (2010). A common left occipito-temporal dysfunction in developmental dyslexia and acquired letter-by-letter reading? *PLoS One*, *5*, e12073.

Rimrodt, S. L., Clements-Stephens, A. M., Pugh, K. R., Courtney, S. M., Gaur, P., Pekar, J. J., & Cutting, L. E. (2009). Functional MRI of sentence comprehension in children with dyslexia: Beyond word recognition. *Cerebral Cortex*, *19*, 402–413.

Rimrodt, S. L., Peterson, D. J., Denckla, M. B., Kaufmann, W. E., & Cutting, L. E. (2010). White matter microstructural differences linked to left perisylvian language network in children with dyslexia. *Cortex*, *46*, 739–749.

Rollins, N. K., Vachha, B., Srinivasan, P., Chia, J., Pickering, J., Hughes, C. W., & Gimi, B. (2009). Simple developmental dyslexia in children: Alterations in diffusion-tensor metrics of white matter tracts at. 3 T. *Radiology*, *251*, 882–891.

Rumsey, J. M., Nace, K., Bonohue, B., Wise, D., Maisog, J. M., & Andreason, P. A. (1997). A positron emission tomographic study of impaired word recognition and phonological processing in dyslexic men. *Archives of Neurology*, *54*, 562–573.

Salmelin, R. (2007). Clinical neurophysiology of language: The MEG approach. *Clinical Neurophysiology*, *118*, 237–254.

Sandak, R., Mencl, W. E., Frost, S. J., & Pugh, K. R. (2004). The neurobiological basis of skilled and impaired reading: Recent findings and new directions. *Scientific Studies of Reading*, *8*, 273–292.

Scerri, T. S., & Schulte-Körne, G. (2010). Genetics of developmental dyslexia. *European Child & Adolescent Psychiatry*, *19*, 179–197.

Schlaggar, B. L., & McCandliss, B. D. (2007). Development of neural systems for reading. *Annual Review of Neuroscience*, *30*, 475–503.

Schulz, E., Maurer, U., van der Mark, S., Bucher, K., Brem, S., Martin, E., & Brandeis, D. (2008). Impaired semantic processing during sentence reading in children with dyslexia: Combined fMRI and ERP evidence. *NeuroImage*, *41*, 153–168.

Schulz, E., Maurer, U., van der Mark, S., Bucher, K., Brem, S., Martin, E., & Brandeis, D. (2009). Reading for meaning in dyslexic and young children: Distinct neural pathways but common endpoints. *Neuropsychologia*, *47*, 2544–2557.

Schurz, M., Wimmer, H., Richlan, F., Ludersdorfer, P., Klackl, J., & Kronbichler, M. (2015). Resting-state and task-based functional brain connectivity in developmental dyslexia. *Cerebral Cortex*, *25*, 3502–3514.

Schuster, S., Hawelka, S., Himmelstoss, N. A., Richlan, F., & Hutzler, F. (2020). The neural correlates of word position and lexical predictability during sentence reading: Evidence from fixation-related fMRI. *Language, Cognition and Neuroscience*, *35*, 613–624.

Schuster, S., Hawelka, S., Hutzler, F., Kronbichler, M., & Richlan, F. (2016). Words in context: The effects of length, frequency, and predictability on brain responses during natural Reading. *Cerebral Cortex*, *26*, 3889–3904.

Schuster, S., Hawelka, S., Richlan, F., Ludersdorfer, P., & Hutzler, F. (2015). Eyes on words: A fixation-related fMRI study of the left occipito-temporal cortex during self-paced silent reading of words and pseudowords. *Scientific Reports, 5*, 12686.

Schuster, S., Himmelstoss, N. A., Hutzler, F., Richlan, F., Kronbichler, M., & Hawelka, S. (2021). Cloze enough? Hemodynamic effects of predictive processing during natural reading. *NeuroImage, 228*, 117687.

Seki, A., Koeda, T., Sugihara, S., Kamba, M., Hirata, Y., Ogawa, T., & Takeshita, K. (2001). A functional magnetic resonance imaging study during sentence reading in Japanese dyslexic children. *Brain and Development, 23*, 312–316.

Shaywitz, B. A., Shaywitz, S. E., Pugh, K. R., Mencl, W. E., Fulbright, R. K., Skudlarski, P., Constable, R. T., Marchione, K. E., Fletcher, J. M., Lyon, G. R., & Gore, J. C. (2002). Disruption of posterior brain systems for reading in children with developmental dyslexia. *Biological Psychiatry, 52*, 101–110.

Shaywitz, B. A., Skudlarski, P., Holahan, J. M., Marchione, K. E., Constable, R. T., Fulbright, R. K., Zelterman, D., Lacadie, C., & Shaywitz, S. E. (2007). Age-related changes in reading systems of dyslexic children. *Annals of Neurology, 61*m 363–370.

Shaywitz, S. E., & Shaywitz, B. A. (2005). Dyslexia (specific reading disability). *Biological Psychiatry, 57*, 1301–1309.

Shaywitz, S. E., & Shaywitz, B. A. (2008). Paying attention to reading: The neurobiology of reading and dyslexia. *Development and Psychopathology, 20*, 1329–1349.

Shaywitz, S. E., Shaywitz, B. A., Fulbright, R. K., Skudlarski, P., Mencl, W. E., Constable, R. T., Pugh, K. R., Holahan, J. M., Marchione, K. E., Fletcher, J. M., Lyon, G. R., & Gore, J. C. (2003). Neural systems for compensation and persistence: Young adult outcome of childhood reading disability. *Biological Psychiatry, 54*, 25–33.

Shaywitz, S. E., Shaywitz, B. A., Pugh, K. R., Fulbright, R. K., Constable, R. T., Mencl, W. E., Shankweiler, D. P., Diberman, A. M., Skudlarski, P., Fletcher, J. M., Katz, L., Marchione, K. E., Lacadie, C., Gatenby, C., & Gore, J. C. (1998). Functional disruption in the organization of the brain for reading in dyslexia. *Proceedings of the National Academy of Sciences, USA, 95*, 2636–2641.

Silani, G., Frith, U., Demonet, J. F., Fazio, F., Perani, D., Price, C., Frith, C. D., & Paulesu, E. (2005). Brain abnormalities underlying altered activation in dyslexia: A voxel based morphometry study. *Brain, 128*, 2453–2461.

Simos, P. G., Breier, J. I., Fletcher, J. M., Bergman, E., & Papanicolaou, A. C. (2000a). Cerebral mechanisms involved in word reading in dyslexic children: A magnetic source imaging approach. *Cerebral Cortex, 10*, 809–816.

Simos, P. G., Breier, J. I., Fletcher, J. M., Foorman, B. R., Bergman, E., Fishbeck, K., & Papanicolaou, A. C. (2000b). Brain activaton profiles in dyslexic children during nonword reading: A magnetic source imaging study. *Neuroscience Letters, 290*, 61–65.

Siok, W. T., Perfetti, C. A., Jin, Z., & Tan, L. H. (2004). Biological abnormality of impaired reading is constrained by culture. *Nature, 431*, 71–76.

Snowling, M. J. (2000). *Dyslexia*. Oxford, UK: Blackwell.

Stein, J., & Walsh, V. (1997). To see but not to read; the magnocellular theory of dyslexia. *Trends in Neurosciences, 20*, 147–152.

Steinbrink, C., Vogt, K., Kastrup, A., Müller, H. P., Juengling, F. D., Kassubek, J., & Riecker, A. (2008). The contribution of white and gray matter differences to developmental dyslexia: Insights from DTI and VBM at 3.0 T. *Neuropsychologia, 46*, 3170–3178.

Tallal, P. (1980). Language disabilities in children: A perceptual or linguistic deficit? *Journal of Pediatric Psychology, 5*, 127–140.

Temple, E., Deutsch, G. K., Poldrack, R. A., Miller, S. L., Tallal, P., Merzenich, M. M., & Gabrieli, J. D. (2003). Neural deficits in children with dyslexia ameliorated by behavioral remediation: Evidence from functional MRI. *Proceedings of the National Academy of Sciences, USA, 100*, 2860–2865.

Temple, E., Poldrack, R. A., Protopapas, A., Nagarajan, S., Salz, T., Tallal, P., Merzenich, M. M., & Gabrieli, J. D. (2000). Disruption of the neural response to rapid acoustic stimuli in dyslexia: Evidence from functional MRI. *Proceedings of the National Academy of Sciences, USA, 97*, 13907–13912.

Temple, E., Poldrack, R. A., Salidis, J., Deutsch, G. K., Tallal, P., Merzenich, M. M., & Gabrieli, J. D. (2001). Disrupted neural responses to phonological and orthographic processing in dyslexic children: An fMRI study. *Neuroreport, 12*, 299–307.

Van Atteveldt, N., Formisano, E., Goebel, R., & Blomert, L. (2004). Integration of letters and speech sounds in the human brain. *Neuron, 43*, 271–282.

Van der Mark, S., Bucher, K., Maurer, U., Schulz, E., Brem, S., Buckelmüller, J., Kronbichler, M., Loenneker, T., Klaver, P., Martin, E., & Brandeis, D. (2009). Children with dyslexia lack multiple specializations along the visual word-form (VWF) system. *NeuroImage, 47*, 1940–1949.

Van der Mark, S., Klaver, P., Bucher, K., Maurer, U., Schulz, E., Brem, S., Martin, E., & Brandeis, D. (2011). The left occipitotemporal system in reading: Disruption of focal fMRI connectivity to left inferior frontal and inferior parietal language areas in children with dyslexia. *NeuroImage, 54*, 2426–2436.

Vandermosten, M., Boets, B., Wouters, J., & Ghesquière, P. (2012). A qualitative and quantitative review of diffusion tensor imaging studies in reading and dyslexia. *Neuroscience and Biobehavioral Reviews, 36*, 1532–1552.

Vandermosten, M., Vanderauwera, J., Theys, C., De Vos, A., Vanvooren, S., Sunaert, S., Wouters, J., & Ghesquière, P. (2015). A DTI tractography study in pre-readers at risk for dyslexia. *Developmental Cognitive Neuroscience, 14*, 8–15.

Vellutino, F. R., & Fletcher, J. M. (2005). Developmental dyslexia. In M. J. Snowling & C. J. Hulme (Eds.), *The science of Reading: A handbook* (pp. 362–378). Oxford: Blackwell.

Vidyasagar, T. R., & Pammer, K. (2010). Dyslexia: A deficit in visuo-spatial attention, not in phonological processing. *Trends in Cognitive Sciences, 14*, 57–63.

Vignali, L., Hawelka, S., Hutzler, F., & Richlan, F. (2019a). No effect of cathodal tDCS of the posterior parietal cortex on parafoveal preprocessing of words. *Neuroscience Letters, 705*, 219–226.

Vignali, L., Hawelka, S., Hutzler, F., & Richlan, F. (2019b). Processing of parafoveally presented words. An fMRI study. *NeuroImage, 184*, 1–9.

Vinckenbosch, E., Robichon, F., & Eliez, S. (2005). Gray matter alteration in dyslexia: Converging evidence from volumetric and voxelby-voxel MRI analyses. *Neuropsychologia, 43*, 324–331.

Willcutt, E. G., Betjemann, R. S., McGrath, L. M., Chhabildas, N. A., Olson, R. K., DeFries, J. C., & Pennington, B. F. (2010). Etiology and neuropsychology of comorbidity between RD and ADHD: The case for multiple-deficit models. *Cortex, 46*, 1345–1361.

Wimmer, H., Schurz, M., Sturm, D., Richlan, F., Klackl, J., Kronbichler, M., & Ladurner, G. (2010). A dual-route perspective on poor reading in a regular orthography: An fMRI study. *Cortex, 46*, 1284–1298.

Wolf, M., & Bowers, P. (1999). The double-deficit hypothesis for the developmental dyslexias. *Journal of Education & Psychology, 91*, 415–438.

Yarkoni, T., Poldrack, R. A., Nichols, T. E., Van Essen, D. C., & Wager, T. D. (2011). Large-scale automated synthesis of human functional neuroimaging data. *Nature Methods, 8*, 665–670.

8
SCREENING AND DIAGNOSIS OF DYSLEXIA IN HIGHER EDUCATION

Wim Tops and Marc Brysbaert

8.1 Introduction

Developmental dyslexia, also referred to as a specific learning disorder in reading, writing, or both (5th ed.; DSM–5; American Psychiatric Association, 2013), is an impairment characterized by persistent problems in learning to read or write words, or in the automatization of reading or writing (Stichting Dyslexie Nederland, 2016).

To see whether an individual has dyslexia or not, two types of investigation can be distinguished. First, a screening for dyslexia can determine if enough arguments for dyslexia are present and help to decide if a more comprehensive dyslexia assessment is desirable. Such a comprehensive assessment is called a diagnostic assessment. Whereas (remedial) teachers or other paraprofessionals are competent to do screenings, diagnostic assessments can only be done by trained diagnosticians (e.g., psychologists with a special psychodiagnostic admission). Screenings for dyslexia are mostly done at school, and diagnostic assessments are done in private reading clinics.

It is also important to note that screening tools differ from diagnostic tools. When screening and diagnosis used the same tools, children would show a learning effect and perform better the second time they did a test. Evidently, this has a negative effect on the reliability of the test results. Although we focus on a diagnostic protocol in this study, we want to mention some excellent screening tools that are available for adults with a suspicion of dyslexia, for instance, the Adult Reading History Questionnaire[1] (ARHQ; Lefly & Penningtion, 2000) or the Dyslexia Adult Screening Test (DAST; Nicolson & Fawcett, 1997).

A diagnosis of dyslexia, which includes a more comprehensive assessment than a screening, involves three aspects. The first aspect is the so-called *categorical diagnosis*. At this level, one wants to decide if a participant has dyslexia or not by looking for typical symptoms and exclusion criteria. To come to a categorical diagnosis of dyslexia, three criteria must be fulfilled. First, the level of reading or writing (or both) must be significantly lower than what can be expected based on the educational level and age of the individual. In Belgium and the Netherlands, scientists and clinicians agree upon percentile 10 as a cutoff point (SDN, 2016). Second, the lack of response to instruction has to be confirmed by looking at the outcome of remedial help. Remedial help is considered adequate when it meets the requirements as stated in the "response to instruction" model (RTI; Vaughn & Fuchs, 2003) or the "response to intervention' model (Haager, Klinger, & Vaughn, 2007). Starting with high-quality classroom instruction, RTI allows for the identification and support of students with (special) educational needs. Struggling learners will receive additional instruction and/or individual remediation while progress is continuously monitored to isolate low or non-responders. Finally, a categorical diagnosis of dyslexia requires that the reading and writing impairment cannot be attributed to external or individual factors such as socio-economic status, cultural background, or sensory problems.

The criterion of a significantly impaired reading or writing level implies a need for age-appropriate reading and spelling tests for (young) adults with dyslexia. These are not always easily available, especially not for non-English speakers. As a consequence, it has been difficult to reliably assess adults with reading and writing problems in the past. Most common diagnostic instruments, like word reading tests (where participants are asked to read as many words aloud in one minute, for instance) or pseudo-word reading tests (pseudo-words are non-existing words without meaning that can be read according to the grapheme-to-phoneme correspondence rules of a specific language), have up until now only been available for primary school children. Recently, new diagnostic tools for adults or adjustments of old tests especially for adults have been developed in different languages, among them the test for advanced reading and writing (GL&SCHR; Depessemier & Andries, 2009) and the test for automatized spelling (TASP; Mostaert et al., 2016) in Dutch, the Alouette test (Cavalli et al., 2017;Lefavrais, 1967) and a standardized screening procedure based on conditional inference trees from a subset of seven tests (Cavalli et al., 2024) in French, a computerized assessment battery in Spanish called Bateria de Evaluacion de Dyslexia in Adultos (BEDA; Mejía, Diaz, Jimenez, & Fabregat, 2012), a one-minute reading test for college students in Portuguese (Fernandes, Araujo, Sucena, Reis, & Castro, 2017), and the York Adult Assessment Battery Revised in English (YAA-R; Warmington, Stothard, & Snowling, 2012). Previous research has shown that literacy skills depend on the education level. It is therefore important not only to use age-appropriate norms but also to take into account the education level of the participants.

The second aspect of dyslexia assessment is often referred to as the *explanatory diagnosis*. It involves identifying the cognitive origins of dyslexia, such as problems with phonological awareness or verbal short-term memory. This aspect of dyslexia assessment is the least developed, because the causes of dyslexia are not yet well known. It is still unclear which risk factors are (not) involved in dyslexia and how they play a role. The most studied risk factor is phonological awareness. In general, a deficient phonological awareness refers to the observation that the sound structure of words is not properly processed and that sounds in words are not (all) identified correctly (Ziegler & Goswami, 2005). This hypothesis is known as the phonological deficit hypothesis. Individuals with dyslexia can also have problems with other phonological skills, like verbal short-term memory. Individuals with dyslexia and a deficient verbal short-term memory have problems with phonological representations or access to these representations (Vellutino, Fletcher, Snowling, & Scanlon, 2004). However, not all researchers agree that verbal short-term memory is phonological in nature. According to Wolf and Bowers (1999), founders of the double deficit hypothesis, rapid automatized naming (RAN) is independent of phonological processing. The double deficit hypothesis argues that dyslexia can stem from an additional deficit in fluency apart from the phonological deficit. Accounts for dyslexia are, however, not limited to the cognitive-linguistic domain but also target more basal perceptual mechanisms, for instance, temporal information processing (Livingstone, Rosen, Drislane, & Galaburda, 1991). This account, also called the magnocellular theory, states that dyslexia is caused by a processing deficit of rapidly changing sensorial (visual or auditory) stimuli. Phonological problems are a direct consequence of this deficit, impeding the development of age-appropriate phonological skills in individuals with dyslexia. Subsequently, these reduced phonological skills impede in their turn the automatization of reading and/or spelling (Ghesquière, Boets, Gadeyne, & Vandewalle, 2011; McBride-Chang, 1995). Although impairments in one or more of these cognitive functions are common in adults with dyslexia, only one in two individuals with the categorical diagnosis has a dyslexia specific cognitive profile (i.e., fit the explanatory diagnosis). Therefore, more recently, dyslexia is considered to be a multifactorial problem because scientists have failed to isolate a single determining cause (Pennington, 2006). Instead, several probabilistic risk factors seem to play a role. An explanatory diagnosis is nevertheless informative in an assessment. First, it strengthens the evidence for an eventual diagnosis of dyslexia. Second, it contributes to better or more personal advice when strengths and weaknesses are taken into account. This is fundamental in developing customized treatment.

This brings us to the third aspect of the diagnostic cycle, which is called the *action-oriented diagnosis*. At this level, clinicians strive to formulate thoughtful and evidence-based advice tailored to the participant's needs. In this diagnosis, external factors like intelligence, motivation, memory skills, executive functions, but also double diagnosis or comorbidities are taken into account. Since dyslexia is a multifactorial problem, there is a considerable overlap in the risk factors of different (developmental) disorders. Actually, comorbidity is the rule rather than the exception in developmental disorders (Pennington, 2006). To our knowledge, this is another shortcoming of the prevailing diagnosis: To what extent should the treatment of dyslexia differ as a function of known comorbidities? This question applies more to the assessment of primary school children than of students in higher education, however.

A good diagnosis of dyslexia involves the three aspects outlined above and results in a clear report summarizing the findings. It mentions which standardized instruments or tests were used, including raw scores, standard scores, reference group, authors, and publication year of the test. Further, it contains a (brief) description of the remedial help and, alternatively, therapy that was given to the participant. For adults with dyslexia, it can be difficult to remember this kind of information accurately, and it is not always easy to retrieve this information from original sources such as schools or therapists. Being an adult, one has had a lifelong exposure to print and definitely enough opportunities for practice. Even if the history of extra remedial help cannot be retraced (in detail), a diagnosis of dyslexia is not automatically excluded in adults. If the (young) adult is still in (higher) education, a good assessment report should also include compensatory means, as well as exam facilities that help the student to overcome his or her reading or spelling problems (Desoete et al., 2010).

8.2 Evidence-based Diagnostic Protocol for Students with Dyslexia in Higher Education

There are a number of reasons why students with dyslexia may require a (new) diagnostic assessment when they enter higher education. The most frequent reason is that their previous diagnosis is no longer available (or has never been properly documented). Another reason is that the student never had a formal diagnostic assessment and managed to cope nevertheless, but is now confronted with a much higher working load. At the same time, authorities must learn not to needlessly retest well-documented cases. Indeed, all too often, students find themselves confronted with new requirements for testing whenever they change school, despite the fact that the reading and/or writing problems are stable within individuals.

Despite pleas for evidence-based practice in the diagnosis of dyslexia (Geudens et al., 2012; Levant & Hasan, 2008), scientific evidence is still scarce, especially for (young) adults. The little evidence that is available (Hatcher, Snowling, & Griffiths, 2002; Swanson & Hsieh, 2009; Tops, Callens, Lammertyn, Van Hees, & Brysbaert, 2012), pleads for assessments with a limited number of tests focusing strongly on word reading and word spelling (where speed is also taken into account) rather than the use of elaborate and time-consuming test batteries for general cognitive skills like intelligence and memory. Previous (English) studies suggest that a small number of tests are enough to reliably discriminate individuals with and without dyslexia (Hatcher et al., 2002; Nicolson & Fawcett, 1997; Swanson & Hsieh, 2009). Hatcher et al. (2002) developed a postdiction model categorizing 95% of the participants correctly as having dyslexia based on only four tests: (1) spelling, (2) word reading, (3) verbal short-term memory, and (4) writing speed. As we will see below, a similar finding was obtained in Dutch, suggesting that the data can be generalized to French as well.

8.2.1 Empirical Study with Undergraduate Students with Dyslexia

Studies suggest that a small number of tests suffice to reliably assess dyslexia in English-speaking adults with dyslexia (Hatcher et al., 2002; Nicolson & Fawcett, 1997; Swanson & Hsieh, 2009). To know to what extent the English data can be generalized to other languages (and educational contexts), Callens, Tops, and Brysbaert (2012) set up a study in which they examined the situation for the Dutch language (one of the three national languages spoken in Belgium).

To measure the cognitive profile of students entering higher education with a diagnosis of dyslexia, Callens et al. (2012) compared a group of 100 students with dyslexia with 100 control students. All students were Dutch speakers and in their first year of higher education, following a university or university college bachelor's program. Students with dyslexia were diagnosed prior to the study according to the criteria of the SDN (2016). If they did not meet these criteria, reading and spelling skills were re-evaluated by clinicians who worked within local student support offices and who were experienced in assessing (adult) dyslexia. For every student with dyslexia, a control student was found with the same age, gender, and within the same field of study, but evidently without any neurobiological or psychiatric disorder(s).

All students were assessed on a battery of 52 tests, consisting of an intelligence test, a memory test, and tests for vocabulary, processing speed, phonological awareness, rapid naming, and arithmetic skills. To evaluate reading, word reading, pseudo-word reading (silently and aloud), text reading, and text comprehension were assessed. For writing, the authors presented a word and sentence dictation task (both in Dutch and English as a second language).

The results of Callens et al. (2012) showed selective deficits in reading and writing (effect sizes between $d = 1$ and $d = 2$), arithmetic ($d \approx 1$), and phonological processing ($d \approx 1$). Except for spelling, these deficits were larger for processing speed than for accuracy. No significant differences were observed in the fluid intelligence of both groups. The profile the authors obtained agreed with a meta-analysis of English findings (Swanson & Hsieh, 2009), suggesting that it generalizes to all alphabetic languages. These findings served as a starting point to search for the minimum number of tests needed to validly and efficiently diagnose dyslexia in young adults entering higher education.

8.2.2 Discriminating Variables

Table 8.1 shows the 10 variables that yielded the largest differences between the groups with and without dyslexia in the study of Callens et al. (2012). Results are presented in terms of standardized effect sizes. A positive number indicates a better performance of the control students. An effect size of 0.8 or higher indicates a large and clinically relevant difference between students with and without dyslexia (which is the case for all the variables in Table 8.1), whereas effect sizes smaller than 0.4 are too small to have practical consequences (see Table 8.2 below).

Seven of the variables in Table 8.1 are related to reading and spelling at the word level. Adults with dyslexia who enter higher education thus continue to have problems with reading and spelling at the word level. Next, they need more time to complete advanced tasks for phonological awareness, like

TABLE 8.1 Ten Variables with the Largest Difference between Students with and Without Dyslexia

Word spelling (GL&SCHR; Depessemier & Andries, 2009)	
Correctly spelled words	2.05
Word reading (EMT; Brus & Voeten, 1991)	
Correctly read words in one minute	1.97
Sentence dictation (AT-GSN; Ghesquière, not published)	
Number of errors	2.10
Pseudo-word reading (De Klepel; van den Bos, Spelberg, Scheepsma, & de Vries, 1999)	
Correctly read pseudo-words in two minutes	1.59
Word spelling English L2 (WRAT; Wilkinson, 1993)	
Correctly spelled words	1.50
Phonological awareness (GL&SCHR; Depessemier & Andries, 2009)	
Spoonerisms (time in seconds)	1.42
Reversals (time in seconds)	1.30
Word reading English L2 (OMT; Kleijnen & Loets, 2006)	
Correctly read words in one minute	1.40
Text reading aloud (GL&SCHR; Depessemier & Andries, 2009)	
Reading time (in seconds)	1.29
Arithmetic (TTR; De Vos, 1992)	
Mixed operations (+, −, ×, :)	1.13

Note. Results are expressed as effect sizes. A positive number indicates a better performance of the control group. An effect size higher than 0.8 is large, between 0.8 and 0.4 medium, and smaller than 0.4 small.

TABLE 8.2 Five Variables with the Smallest Difference between Students with and without Dyslexia

Block patterns (KAIT; Dekker, Dekker, & Mulder, 2004)	0.03
Symbol learning (KAIT; Dekker et al., 2004)	0.07
Auditory comprehension (KAIT; Dekker et al., 2004)	0.09
Logical reasoning (KAIT; Dekker et al., 2004)	0.12
Fluid intelligence (KAIT; Dekker et al., 2004)	0.13

Note. Results are expressed as effect sizes. A positive number indicates a better performance of the control group. An effect size higher than 0.8 is large, between 0.8 and 0.4 medium, and smaller than 0.4 small.

spoonerisms (e.g., *Harry Potter* becomes *Parry Hotter*) or reversals (e.g., *spot* becomes *tops*). They also have serious problems doing timed arithmetic tasks. These findings confirm that dyslexia is more of a speed problem than an accuracy problem in adults, apart from spelling in where accuracy is the issue (e.g., Conlon, Sanders, & Zapart, 2004; Swanson & Hsieh, 2009).

In Table 8.2, an overview of the five tasks that yielded the smallest differences between both the groups with and without dyslexia in Callens et al. (2012) is provided. Again, the results are expressed as standardized effect sizes.

Four of the variables in Table 8.2 are measures of fluid intelligence, assessing analytic thinking and problem solving. In Callens et al. (2012), these skills were measured with the Dutch adaptation of the Kaufman Adolescent and Adult Intelligence Test (KAIT; Dekker et al., 2004). Similar findings were reported in the meta-analysis of Swanson and Hsieh (2009), including other tests of fluid intelligence. So, we can conclude that students with dyslexia do not differ from their non-dyslexic peers when it comes to logical reasoning and fluid intelligence. In other words, they show a pattern of results that is in line with the classical definition of dyslexia: they have comparable intelligence to their peers, but experience serious problems with word spelling, word reading, and phonological awareness.

8.2.3 Prediction Model

Tops et al. (2012) ran a prediction model on the data of Table 8.1 to see which tests were needed to predict the presence of dyslexia in students entering higher education. Unlike Hatcher et al. (2002), the authors used cross-validation to ensure that the findings were not limited to the participants tested but also generalized to newly tested participants. The model yields a combination of variables that has the best discriminating power not only for the sample tested but also for future, comparable samples of young adults with dyslexia.

Of all models built, a model with three predictors came out as the most powerful. It included word reading (correctly read words within one minute), word spelling (number of correctly spelled words), and a timed, advanced

TABLE 8.3 Classification Table Based on the Best Prediction Model

Reference Group	Prediction	
	Dyslexia	Control
Dyslexia	91	8
Control	10	90

phonological awareness task (time in seconds to do 20 reversals).[2] Table 8.3 shows the classification outcome for the participants based on the predictions. Of the students with dyslexia, 91 were correctly classified on the basis of three tests. Only 8 were not correctly classified (one student with dyslexia was not included in the analysis because of missing data). In the control group, 90 students were correctly classified as not having dyslexia, and 10 were wrongly classified as having dyslexia without actually having a diagnosis. No further gains in terms of prediction were to be expected if more tests were included.

In addition, Tops et al. (2012) discuss how the results of the cross-validation classification analysis can be used to predict the probability of dyslexia in new participants. Because the results are limited to the Dutch tests used, we do not discuss them here, although the procedure can easily be extended to a new study involving another language (for a technical description of this procedure, see Tops et al., 2012).[3]

8.3 Discussion

An elaborate or time-consuming assessment is not necessary to determine whether a student has dyslexia or not. A short test protocol containing three simple tests is enough to identify higher education students whose literacy skills are significantly below expectations regarding age and education level. These tests involve word reading, word spelling, and phonological awareness (as assessed with a word reversal test, in which participants have to decide whether two words are each other's reversal). The fact that two of the three tests were literacy tests, confirms that undergraduate students with dyslexia continue having serious problems with reading and writing in adulthood, as was shown in previous research with the English language (Erskine & Seymour, 2005; Everatt, Bradshaw, Hibbard, et al., 1997; Hatcher et al., 2002; Swanson & Hsieh, 2009). Next, two out of three tests were speed-related (word reading and reversals). So, in assessments of students with dyslexia, it is important to take speed into account. Finally, assessing at the word level is sufficient, even in high-functioning students. Sentence dictation was not a better predictor than word dictation (rather the contrary). With respect to the French language, results seem a bit different. Recently, Cavalli et al. (2024)

conducted a similar study to ours with French university students. Instead of cross-validation, the authors used conditional inference trees. Spelling was not selected in the final screening protocol, and text reading was a more discriminatory factor than word reading. Cavalli et al.'s screening procedure consisted of a combination of four tests (ARHQ, text reading fluency, phonemic awareness, pseudo-word reading) with an overall classification accuracy of approximately 90%.

Although the short protocol meets the first criterion of a categorical assessment, a history of a delay in (early) language and literacy development and resistance to remedial help/therapy is necessary to judge the other two criteria, that of the resistance to instruction and of exclusion. It is therefore advisable to comprehensively question the socio-medical history before the start of the assessment. This socio-medical history (also called anamnesis) should be focused on the course of pregnancy and the delivery, concerns in early childhood behavior (e.g., eating, sleeping), language and motor development (milestones like first words, sitting, first steps, etc.), school career, medical history (e.g., vision or hearing problems, autoimmune diseases, etc.[4]).

Next to the classification diagnosis, a clinician should also pay attention to the explanatory and action-oriented part of the diagnosis, and stay focused on the initial expectations of students signing up for an assessment. An action-oriented approach consists primarily of efficiently questioning and sharpening the needs of an individual student rather than blindly using long-lasting and expensive test batteries. Having said that, it has been convincingly demonstrated that objective, evidence-based test results are a necessary completion of clinical interpretations. Several studies have shown that well-founded tests have a larger predictive power than impressions based on clinical conversations (for references, see Brysbaert & Rastle, 2013). Currently, students with dyslexia (and also those with other developmental disorders) are often submitted to extensive test batteries without a clear indication or action-oriented advice. The results from such assessments are not always translated into an action plan tailored to the individual needs of a student. These kinds of assessments are not only very stressful for students, but they are also very time-consuming and expensive. Often, they do not even offer useful suggestions for future guidance of a student or for efficient exam facilities. Shorter protocols not only make it possible to assess a larger number of students but also allow to invest the extra time and financial resources in the guidance of students with dyslexia, which positively impacts the academic success of this group.

One extra test practitioners may want to include is a test of fluid intelligence (that is not primarily based on time pressure). These include symbol learning, logical reasoning, or symbol memory (block patterns) from the KAIT or other tests covered in the meta-analysis of Swanson and Hsieh (2009). On these subtests, students with dyslexia do not perform differently from their non-dyslexic peers. Therefore, scores can be interpreted equally for both groups (Callens et al., 2012). If the results on one or more such tests are good, the student is reassured of their mental capacity, and the information can be forwarded to lecturers, questioning the intellectual capabilities of the student. At the same time, the use of an extra fluid intelligence may have the advantage of identifying simulators or students who cannot validly estimate their level of performance. A complaint sometimes heard from students without learning disabilities is that students with dyslexia have unfair benefits, increasing their chances of success. As a result, students may be tempted to fake dyslexia "symptoms" in order to be eligible for exam facilities and the use of compensatory means (Harrison, Edwards, & Parker, 2008; Lindstrom, Coleman, Thomassin, Southall, & Lindstrom, 2011). Harrison et al. (2008) and Lindstrom et al. (2011) asked students to feign dyslexia during an assessment. Simulators seemed less effective in feigning processing deficits like phonological awareness and rapid automatized naming. Moreover, Harrison et al. (2008) developed a Dyslexia Assessment of Simulation or Honesty (DASH) consisting of texts with scrambled words with increasing difficulty. Easy letter manipulations were shown to be as easy to decode for dyslexic students as for control students (e.g., *Mnoday instead of Monday), whereas more difficult manipulations were harder for students with dyslexia than for controls (*Manody instead of Monday). Simulating students, however, seemed unaware of this difference and performed (far) below average on both versions of the test. Harrison also developed an eight-point Feigning Index to discriminate between students with dyslexia and simulators. Although very valuable, adding such tasks to a dyslexia assessment makes it more time-consuming (and more expensive). Adding a short test for fluid intelligence is an easier way to identify possible simulators. These students are indeed likely to perform badly on all tests, including the fluid intelligence test. Next, a more elaborate feigning protocol, like the DASH or Feigning Index, can still be done if a clinician feels the need to exclude fraud. Adding a test for fluid intelligence has a second advantage. A bad performance on the fluid intelligence test is also true for students with a low level of fluid intelligence, who may be better advised to go for a less demanding degree.

Higher education students are a selective group of young adults. Higher education differs from primary and secondary education because it is no longer compulsory. In addition, students with dyslexia entering higher education have been successful in both primary and secondary school, and are likely to have developed strategies that compensate to some extent for their problems. This seems particularly true for accuracy in reading and phonological processing (at the expense of speed). Still, we saw quite some variability in the students we tested (also because entrance to higher education is free in Belgium, and not limited to students who passed entry exams). So, for students with dyslexia, it is interesting to receive information about their strengths and challenges, so that they can prepare better.

As for compensatory measures, we think there is good evidence for three allowances. First, students with dyslexia are extra penalized under time pressure. So, if time pressure is not an inherent property of what the exam wants to test, students with dyslexia should be given extra time. One quarter to one third would seem reasonable, although examiners may want to ask themselves whether the exam would not be more valid if all students were given enough time to complete it.

A second compensatory measure is the use of reading software. We found that students with dyslexia were less handicapped on the understanding of a test that was read aloud than when they had to read it themselves (under time pressure). Given the ease with which computers with reading software can be made available nowadays, this is a very reasonable compensation. Kirby, Silvestri, Allingham, Parrila, and La Fave (2008) found a negative correlation between reading and the use of aids like software. The authors interpreted this as a compensation strategy following the difficulties students with dyslexia have in word reading.

A third compensatory measure involves access to a calculator. Given the extra time students with dyslexia need for simple arithmetic operations, it would seem sensible to give them access to a calculator if many of these operations must be done for an exam (e.g., in a class on statistics). Again, the examiner should ask themselves whether such an allowance should not be given to all students, certainly if being able to do arithmetic by hand is not the primary goal of the course.

Finally, we would like to stress that in the study we discussed, we selected a large number of skills based on existing test batteries. It cannot be ruled out that other variables turn out to be important, but were not included among the predictors we selected. This is the challenge for future research. We believe that our results form a firm basis, to which other researchers can add new or understudied variables.

Notes

1 The ARHQ is freely available at https://dyslexiaida.org/screening-for-dyslexia/dyslexia-screener-for-adults/
2 More specifically, the first test is the Dutch One Minute (EMT; Brus & Voeten, 1991). The second test is the word dictation task of a test battery for advanced reading and writing in Dutch (GL&SCHR; Depessemier & Andries, 2009). It contains many irregular spellings and foreign borrowings (e.g., barbecue [barbecue], hockeyen [to hockey], and fusilleren [to shoot]). The third test is the timed reversal task, also coming from the GL&SCHR (Depessemier & Andries, 2009).
3 This article is freely available and can be downloaded via http://crr.ugent.be/archives/862
4 Autoimmune diseases (like childhood rheumatism) are considered a risk factor for learning disorders like dyslexia. The prevalence of dyslexia is significantly higher in this population. See Hugdahl, Synnevag, and Satz (1990) for more information.

References

American Psychiatric Association. (2013). *Diagnostic and statistical manual of mental disorders* (5th ed.). https://doi.org/10.1176/appi.books.9780890425596

Brus, B., & Voeten, M. (1991). *Eén-minuut-test vorm A en B, schoolvorderingstest voor de technische leesvaardigheid bestemd voor groep 4 tot en met 8 van het basisonderwijs. Verantwoording en handleiding.* Lisse, Nederland: Swets & Zeitlinger.

Brysbaert, M., & Rastle, K. (2013). *Historical and conceptual issues in psychology* (2nd ed.). Harlow: Pearson Education.

Callens, M., Tops, W., & Brysbaert, M. (2012). Cognitive profile of students who enter higher education with an indication of dyslexia. *PLoS One, 7,* e38081. https://doi.org/10.1371/journal.pone.0038081

Cavalli, E., Brèthes, H., Lefèvre, E., El Ahmadi, A., Duncan, L. G., Bianco, M., Melmi, J.-B., Denis-Noël, A., & Colé, P. (2024). Screening for dyslexia in university students: A standardized procedure based on conditional inference trees. *Archives of Clinical Neuropsychology, 39*(1), 1–18. https://doi.org/10.1093/arclin/acad103

Cavalli, E., Colé, P., Leloup, G., Poracchia-George, F., Sprenger-Charolles, L., & El Ahmadi, A. (2017). Screening for dyslexia in French-speaking university students: An evaluation of the detection accuracy of the Alouette test. *Journal of Learning Disabilities.* https://doi.org/10.1177/0022219417704637

Conlon, E., Sanders, M., & Zapart, S. (2004). Temporal processing in poor adult readers. *Neuropsychologia, 42,* 142–157. https://doi.org/10.1016/j.neuropsychologia.2003.07.004

de Vos, T. (1992). *Tempo test Rekenen.* Amsterdam, Nederland: Pearson Education.

Dekker, R., Dekker, P. H., & Mulder, J. L. (2004). *Kaufman adolescent and adult intelligence test – Nederlandstalige Versie: Handleiding.* Leiden, Nederland: PITS.

Depessemier, P., & Andries, C. (2009). *Test voor Gevorderd Lezen en Schrijven.* Antwerpen, België –Apeldoorn, Nederland: Garant.

Desoete, A., Brysbaert, M., Tops, W., Callens, M., De Lange, C., & Van Hees, V. (2010). *Studeren met dyslexie. Cel Diversiteit en Gender.* Universiteit Gent. www.dyslexie.ugent.be

Erskine, J. M., & Seymour, P. H. K. (2005). Proximal analysis of developmental dyslexia in adulthood: The cognitive mosaic model. *Journal of Educational Psychology, 97,* 406–424. https://doi.org/10.1037/0022-0663.97.3.406

Everatt, J., Bradshaw, M. F., Hibbard, P. B., et al. (1997). Visual processing deficits and dyslexia. *Perception, 26,* 1330–1330.

Fernandes, T., Araujo, S., Sucena, A., Reis, A., & Castro, S. L. (2017). The 1-min screening test for reading problems in college students: Psychometric properties of the 1-min TIL. *Dyslexia, 23,* 66–87.

Geudens, A., Baeyens, D., Schraeyen, K., Maetens, K., De Brauwer, J., & Loncke, M. (2012). *Jongvolwassenen met dyslexie: Diagnostiek en begeleiding in wetenschap en praktijk.* Leuven, België: Acco.

Ghesquière, P., Boets, B., Gadeyne, E., & Vandewalle, E. (2011). Dyslexie: Een beknopt wetenschappelijk overzicht. In A. Geudens, D. Baeyens, K. Schraeyen, K. Maetens, J. De Brauwer, & M. Loncke (Eds.), *Jongvolwassenen met dyslexie: Diagnostiek en begeleiding in wetenschap en praktijk.* Acco: Leuven, België.

Haager, D., Klinger, J., & Vaughn, S. (2007). *Evidence-based reading practices for response to intervention.* Baltimore, MD: Brookes.

Harrison, A. G., Edwards, M. J., & Parker, K. C. H. (2008). Identifying students feigning dyslexia: Preliminary findings and strategies for detection. *Dyslexia, 14*(3), 228–244.

Hatcher, J., Snowling, M. J., & Griffiths, Y. M. (2002). Cognitive assessment of dyslexic students in higher education. *British Journal of Educational Psychology, 72,* 119–133. https://doi.org/10.1348/000709902158801

Hugdahl, K., Synnevag, B., & Satz, P. (1990). Immune and autoimmune diseases in dyslexic children. *Neuropsychologia, 28*, 673–679.

Kirby, J. R., Silvestri, R., Allingham, B. H., Parrila, R., & La Fave, C. B. (2008). Learning strategies and study approaches of postsecondary students with dyslexia. *Journal of Learning Disabilities, 41*, 85–96.

Kleijnen, R., & Loets, M. (2006). *Protocol Dyslexie Hoger Onderwijs*. Apeldoorn, Nederland: Garant Uitgeverij.

Lefavrais, P. (1967). *Test de l'Alouette* (2éme ed.). Paris: Editions du Centre de Psychologie Appliquée.

Lefly, D. L., & Penningtion, B. F. (2000). Reliability and validity of the adult reading history questionnaire. *Journal of Learning Disabilities, 33*, 286–296.

Levant, R. F., & Hasan, N. T. (2008). Evidence-based practice in psychology. *Professional Psychology: Research and Practice, 39*, 658–662. https://doi.org/10.1037/0003-066X.61.4.271

Lindstrom, W., Coleman, C., Thomassin, K., Southall, C. M., & Lindstrom, J. H. (2011). Simulated dyslexia in postsecondary students: Description and detection using embedded validity indicators. *The Clinical Neuropsychologist, 25*(2), 302–322.

Livingstone, M. S., Rosen, G. D., Drislane, F. W., & Galaburda, A. M. (1991). Physiological and anatomical evidence for a magnocellular deficit in developmental dyslexia. *Proceedings of the National Academy of Sciences, 88*, 7943–7947.

McBride-Chang, C. (1995). Phonological processing, speech perception and reading disability: An integrative review. *Educational Psychologist, 30*, 109–121. https://doi.org/10.1207/s15326985ep3003_2

Mejía, C., Diaz, A., Jimenez, J. E., & Fabregat, R. (2012). BEDA: A computerized assessment battery for dyslexia in adults. *Procedia - Social and Behavioral Sciences, 46*, 1795–1800.

Mostaert, C., Smits, I., Tops, W., De Kerf, L., Liekens, E., & Schraeyen, K. (2016). *TASP – Test geautomatiseerd spellen voor jongvolwassenen. Handleiding en verantwoording*. Leuven: Acco.

Nicolson, R. I., & Fawcett, J. A. (1997). Development of objective procedures for screening and assessment of dyslexic students in higher education. *Journal of Research in Reading, 20*, 77–83. https://doi.org/10.1111/1467-9817.00022

Pennington, B. F. (2006). From single to multiple deficit models of developmental disorders. *Cognition, 10*, 385–413.

SDN, De Jong, P. F., De Bree, E. H., Henneman, K., Kleijnen, R., Loykens, E. H. M., Rolak, M., Struiksma, A. J. C., Verhoeven, L., & Wijnen, F. N. K. (2016). *Dyslexie: Diagnostiek en behandeling* (p. 2016). Geheel herziene versie: Brochure van de Stichting Dyslexie Nederland.

Swanson, H. L., & Hsieh, C. J. (2009). Reading Disabilities in adults: A selective meta-analysis of the literature. *Review of Educational Research, 79*, 1362–1390. https://doi.org/10.1348/000712603321661859

Tops, W., Callens, M., Lammertyn, J., Van Hees, V., & Brysbaert, M. (2012). Identifying students with dyslexia in higher education. *Annals of Dyslexia, 62*, 186–203. https://doi.org/10.1007/s11881-012-0072-6

van den Bos, K., Spelberg, H., Scheepsma, A., & de Vries, J. (1999). De klepel vorm A en B, een test voor leesvaardigheid van pseudowoorden. In *Verantwoording, handleiding, diagnostiek en behandeling*. Lisse, Nederland: Swets & Zeitlinger.

Vaughn, S., & Fuchs, L. S. (2003). Redefining learning disabilities as inadequate response to instruction: The promise and potential problems. *Learning Disabilities Research & Practice, 18*, 137–146.

Vellutino, F. R., Fletcher, J. M., Snowling, M. J., & Scanlon, D. M. (2004). Specific reading disability (dyslexia): What have we learned in the past four decades? *Journal of Child Psychology and Psychiatry, 45*, 2–40. https://doi.org/10.1046/j.0021-9630.2003.00305.x

Warmington, M., Stothard, S. E., & Snowling, M. J. (2012). *York Adult Assessment Battery – Revised (YAA-R)*. York, UK: University of York

Wilkinson, G. S. (1993). *Wide range achievement test*. Wilmington, DE: Jastak Assessment.

Wolf, M., & Bowers, P. G. (1999). The double-deficit hypothesis for the developmental dyslexias. *Journal of Educational Psychology, 91*, 415–438.

Ziegler, J. C., & Goswami, U. C. (2005). Reading acquisition, developmental dyslexia and skilled reading across languages: A psycholinguistic grain size theory. *Psychological Bulletin, 131*, 3–29.

9
LEARNING STRATEGIES AND METACOGNITION IN ADULTS WITH DYSLEXIA

Rauno Parrila, Bradley W. Bergey and S. Helene Deacon

9.1 Introduction

As successful inclusion practices are being implemented in elementary and secondary education, the number of students in colleges and universities who experience significant learning challenges has increased in all developed countries where such numbers are available (e.g., Canadian University Survey Consortium, 2011; Mortimore & Crozier, 2006; Sanford et al., 2011). Warmington, Stothard, and Snowling (2013) estimated that as many as 3.2% of students in post-secondary education have a diagnosis of dyslexia, or of a specific reading disability.[1] In addition, many college and university students have reading skills similar to their peers with diagnosed learning disabilities (LD), but they either have never received a formal diagnosis or they choose not to disclose their diagnosis upon entry to the university (e.g., Deacon, Cook, & Parrila, 2012; Deacon, Parrila, & Kirby, 2006; Jackson & Doellinger, 2002; Parrila, Georgiou, & Corkett, 2007). Several studies have shown that, as a group, university students who self-report difficulty learning to read as children have reading skills similar to students with a diagnosis of reading disabilities and lower than those of university students who report no history of reading difficulty (e.g., Corkett, Parrila, & Hein, 2006; Deacon et al., 2006; Deacon et al., 2012; Parrila et al., 2007). For example, Deacon et al. (2012) found that university students who self-reported a history of reading difficulty had word identification and timed reading comprehension scores close to four grade levels below their peers with no history of reading difficulty. In this chapter, we will review the existing literature on learning and study strategies of college and university students with reading disabilities. In doing so, we mostly treat students who self-report reading disabilities and students with diagnosed

DOI: 10.4324/9781003491125-10

reading disabilities/dyslexia as representing the same population; we refer to both groups as students with a history of reading difficulties (HRD). Further, we assume that learning and study strategies are important compensatory mechanisms for these students if they experience academic challenges (e.g., Parrila & McQuarrie, 2015).

Perhaps not surprisingly, university students with HRD indeed do encounter academic challenges more than students without such a history. For example, Bergey, Deacon, and Parrila (2017) followed a large sample of first-year university students and found that students with HRD obtained a significantly lower first-year cumulative grade point average (GPA; a cumulative average of student's final course grades over time) than students who reported no such history (see also Chevalier, Parrila, Ritchie, & Deacon, 2017). Further, one in every three students with a HRD failed or withdrew from a course in their first year, whereas only a handful of students without a HRD did so (Bergey et al., 2017). Interestingly, the results of this study were LD somewhat different than what earlier research has reported for students with diagnosed (studies that focus specifically on diagnosed reading disabilities are not available). Students with diagnosed LD have been reported to progress through their studies more slowly but to earn GPAs similar to those of university students without LD (Heiman & Precel, 2003; Hen & Goroshit, 2014; but see Witte, Philips, & Kakela, 1998). The observed parity in GPAs is often attributed to the accommodations and services universities offer to students with diagnosed LD. Despite below average reading abilities, students with HRD who do not have a diagnosis must tackle the academic challenges of university without any accommodations and access to targeted supports; given that the majority of students with HRD in Bergey et al. study did not have a diagnosis, we suspect that lack of accommodations and supports impeded their academic performance, both in terms of grades achieved as well as in terms of the number of courses completed.

Whether diagnosed or not, the majority of university students who report a significant HRD are somehow able to compensate for their persistent literacy difficulties sufficiently to have their academic performance meet the university expectations. The form that this compensation takes is of great interest to reading researchers for both practical and theoretical reasons. Theoretically, for example, individuals with significant decoding problems should not be able to read words fluently enough to comprehend complex texts at the level of their peers, yet clearly many are able to do so (e.g., Deacon et al., 2012; Parrila et al., 2007), and sometimes despite substantial errors in oral reading (e.g., Pedersen, Fusaroli, Lauridsen, & Parrila, 2016). Existing theories of word reading and reading comprehension development have difficulties accommodating these performance patterns, as they generally assume that comprehension relies on accurate and automatic word recognition. From a practical standpoint, understanding the pathways to academic success and the protective and risk factors impacting the path taken can inform the design of programmes and interventions for younger students with dyslexia. Undoubtedly, the search for protective and risk factors is going to take various research groups in different directions, as evidenced by this book. In this chapter, we will focus on one set of possible protective factors: learning and study strategies. Somewhat surprisingly, not much is known about the learning and study strategies that students with HRD employ in post-secondary education. We will discuss briefly the theoretical models that have guided our research into risk and protective factors, including study and learning strategies, and then we will go on to define the concepts of interest and review the existing studies.

9.2 Models of Dyslexia and Compensation

Figure 9.1 presents what we call "the simple model of dyslexia" that guided many reading studies in the 1980s and 1990s. The figure is naturally a simplification and does not do full justice to early complications put forth by many researchers, including Frith (1999) and Ramus (2003). However, we believe that Figure 9.1 is a relatively accurate representation of what many of us (including the first author of this chapter) believed to capture the pathway to dyslexia.

According to this model, brain anomalies (possibly preceded by atypical genetic endowment) result in poor phonological awareness that then has cascading effects all the way through to reading comprehension. Without going into details that are beyond the scope of this paper, we believe this model adequately summarizes the observed performance patterns of many adolescents and adults we have assessed in two different countries and four different universities (e.g., Deacon et al., 2012; Parrila et al., 2007; Pedersen et al., 2016). However, the model fails to explain why many other students read words

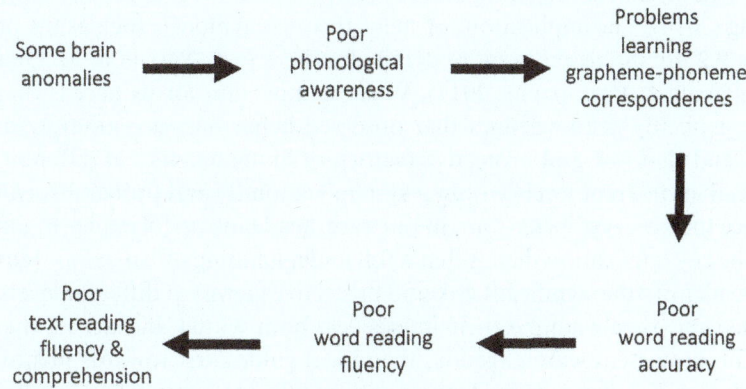

FIGURE 9.1 Simple model of dyslexia.

accurately, and sometimes also fluently, despite poor phonological awareness. It also cannot explain why individuals with poor word and text reading fluency, and sometimes even poor accuracy, can comprehend the texts they read at the university level. In terms of compensation, all models of this kind guide the research towards looking for alternative word reading and reading comprehension mechanisms (e.g., Deacon et al., 2006; Kemp, Parrila, & Kirby, 2008), but not towards other psychological and social factors that may support the resilience of students with reading disabilities (Haft, Myers, & Hoeft, 2016).

One somewhat surprising initial observation was that some students with a history of reading problems participating in our studies (e.g., Corkett et al., 2006; Parrila et al., 2007) struggled with all levels of reading tasks, including reading comprehension, yet they were passing their courses and graduating from the university. A distinction that is important here is between timed and untimed reading comprehension tasks – most of our participants seemed to struggle with timed tasks but not always with untimed tasks (e.g., Parrila et al., 2007). However, in our research, we also encountered individuals whose reading comprehension and writing skills were substantially below those of their peers, but these literacy deficits seemed to have little impact on their academic performance (e.g., Pedersen et al., 2016). In interviews, these students reported compensation mechanisms that we termed socio-cognitive or psychological rather than cognitive, and varied ways of coping with everyday demands of university life (e.g., Corkett et al., 2006). These observations lead us towards broader and more interactive theoretical models (Parrila, 2008; Parrila & McQuarrie, 2015; Parrila & Protopapas, 2017), the latest version of which is depicted in Figure 9.2.

The model in Figure 9.2, termed the *multiple systems model of reading* (Parrila, 2008; Parrila & McQuarrie, 2015), is substantially indebted to the developmental systems theories and, more specifically, to the theoretical propositions put forth by Gottlieb (1983, 2002, Gottlieb, Wahlsten & Lickliter, 2006), Pennington (2006), and, more recently, by van Bergen, van der Leij, and de Jong (2014). The implications of meta-theoretical models such as the one in Figure 9.2 are discussed in more detail elsewhere (e.g., Parrila & McQuarrie, 2015; Parrila & Protopapas, 2017). What is important for us here is that the model explicitly acknowledges that observed behaviours are multiply determined and that risk and protective factors, or "interactants," at different systems and at different levels within a system act jointly and probabilistically to produce the observed behaviour, in our case, academic performance in university. The key implication then is that a full understanding of behaviour requires that we identify the significant risk and protective factors at different levels and systems, and then examine their interaction both within and across the systems. In terms of research agenda, the model guides first towards identifying individual risk and protective factors within different systems (e.g., within the individual, or environment), and then to examining their interactions both

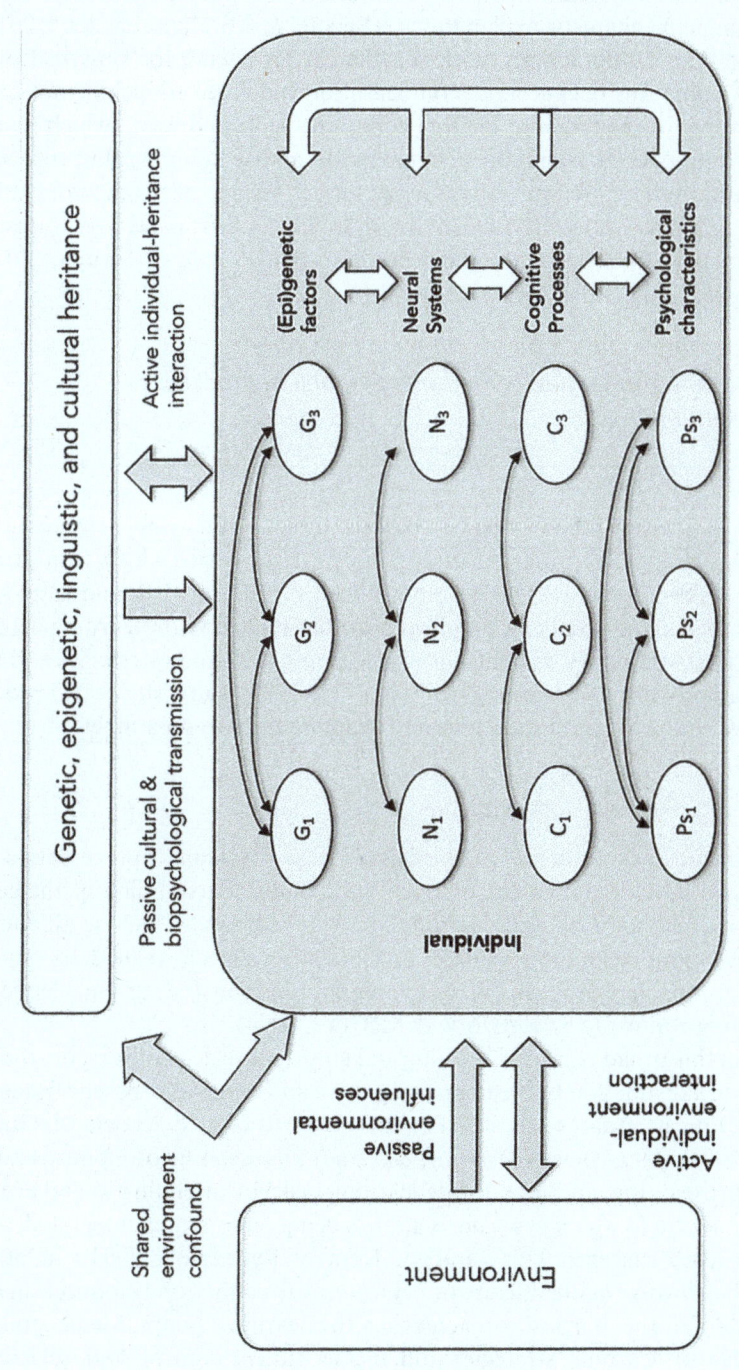

FIGURE 9.2 Multiple systems model of reading.

across and within systems. Implicitly, then, the model guides towards developing "dynamic mechanistic explanations" (Bechtel & Abrahamsen, 2005, 2010) of how different interactants work together in producing the observed outcomes. Against this background, compensation is defined to include not only alternative word reading and reading comprehension pathways (which themselves are influenced by multiple interactants across systems), but also the interactants across different systems in the model, such as environmental influences (e.g., Stack-Cutler, Parrila, Jokisaari & Nurmi, 2015) and psychological characteristics (Corkett et al., 2006; Stack-Cutler, Parrila & Torppa, 2015), including learning and study strategies.

9.2.1 Learning Strategies, Study Strategies, and Approaches to Learning

9.2.1.1 Terminology

As in many fields of human sciences, the terminology and assessment methods used in research on learning and study strategies have varied widely from study to study, making comparisons between studies difficult. Entwistle and Waterson (1988) classified the broader theoretical positions related to the learning behaviours of post-secondary students into (1) learning and study strategies and (2) student approaches to learning (Biggs, 1979, 1987; Entwistle & Ramsden, 1983). We will use this division here and examine the two separately.

9.2.1.2 Learning and Study Strategies

Learning and study strategies can be defined as any systematic process used by a learner to develop a memory representation and understanding of the content. From this point of view, learning and study strategies include all cognitive, metacognitive, socio-cognitive, and affective aspects related to how a student approaches the tasks of obtaining and demonstrating knowledge in the learning context (e.g., Entwistle & McCune, 2004).

Within this broad rubric of learning and study strategies, some prior studies have made a distinction between metacognitive and behaviour-based strategies (Proctor, Prevatt, Adams, Hurst, & Petscher, 2006; Ruban, McCoach, McGuire, & Reis, 2003). *Metacognitive learning and study strategies* involve purposefully planning, executing, and monitoring learning tasks by attending to and evaluating the degree to which new information is being understood, integrated, and retained (e.g., Flavell, 1979; Taraban, Kerr, & Rynearson, 2004); in other words, they involve deliberate use of behaviours, thoughts, and emotions in the individual for the purpose of achieving the learning goals. Metacognitive knowledge of learning strategies and metacognitive control over selecting, monitoring, and modifying them are considered hallmarks of self-regulated learning (Zimmerman, 2002). Typical metacognitive learning and study strategies include the management of time, effort, attention, and emotions; approaches to processing information (e.g., elaboration, comprehension monitoring); and the deliberate use of social and informational supports.

A commonly used tool to identify metacognitive learning and study strategies used by college and university students is the Learning and Study Strategies Inventory (LASSI; Weinstein, 1987; Weinstein, Palmer, & Shulte, 2002; Weinstein, Palmer, & Acee, 2016). LASSI was developed to assess trainable thoughts, behaviours, attitudes, motivations, and beliefs related to academic success (Weinstein et al., 2002) and consists of ten scales: Anxiety (e.g., *When I am studying, worrying about doing poorly in a course interferes with my concentration*), Attitude (e.g., *I only study the subjects I like*), Concentration (e.g., *My mind wanders a lot when I study*), Information Processing (e.g., *I try to find relationships between what I am learning and what I already know*), Motivation (e.g., *When work is difficult I either give up or study only the easy parts*), Self-Testing (e.g., *I stop periodically while reading and mentally go over or review what was said*), Study Aids (e.g., *I try to find a study partner or study group for each of my classes*), Selecting Main Ideas (e.g., *I have difficulty identifying the important points in my reading* [reverse scored]), Test Strategies (e.g., *I have difficulty adapting my studying to different types of courses*), and Time Management (e.g., *I set aside more time to study the subjects that are difficulty for me*).

Metacognitive reading strategies are a specific subset of metacognitive learning and study strategies involving activities designed to control, monitor, and evaluate the reading process (Pressley, 2000; Pressley, Brown, El-Dinary, & Allferbach, 1995). These may include planning reading tasks, monitoring that information is understood, and integrating new information with background knowledge (Wade, Trathen, & Schraw, 1990). A commonly used tool for assessing these is the analytic scale of the Metacognitive Reading Strategies Questionnaire (MRSQ) that measures "cognitions aimed at reading comprehension" (Taraban et al., 2004, p. 67); the actual questions cover various comprehension monitoring, inferencing, and elaboration strategies students may use while reading a text.

Behavioural, or behaviour based, learning and study strategies involve concrete behaviours or actions designed to facilitate information acquisition and storage. These can include highlighting or underlining text, reviewing notes, organizing activities (Lawson, 2009; Reis, McGuire, & Neu, 2000), or actively seeking help from others (Corkett et al., 2006; Corkett & Parrila, 2008; Reis et al., 2000; Ruban et al., 2003; Trainin & Swanson, 2005). Behavioural learning and study strategies may also include the use of academic support services, such as academic advising (Vogel & Adelman, 1992), study skills and writing centres (Deacon, Tucker, Bergey, Laroche, & Parrila, 2017), or test-taking accommodations (Alster, 1997). Both LASSI and the pragmatic scale of MRSQ assess some of these behaviours. For example, the MRSQ pragmatic scale includes questions about taking notes, highlighting, underlining, and re-reading.

9.2.1.3 Approaches to Learning

The concept of approaches to learning focuses on the interaction between a student and the learning context (Biggs, 1987; Marton & Saljo, 1976). Approaches to learning refer to students' understanding of the nature and purpose of learning as well as the use of learning strategies that support their learning goals (for a review, see Asikainen & Gijbels, 2017). More specifically, it refers to the predispositions and beliefs that students have about learning, along with the cognitive strategies used during learning. Whereas research on the learning and study strategies focuses primarily on tactics or strategies that students report themselves as employing, studies of approaches to learning examine a pattern of learning motives as well as strategies as these relate to motives and learning contexts.

Students' approaches to learning are frequently assessed with the Study Process Questionnaire (SPQ; Biggs, Kember, & Leung, 2001), which classifies them into two dimensions: deep and surface. A deep approach is characterized by intrinsic motivation and the use of strategies that support comprehension of the underlying meanings of content and connections within and between learning tasks. In the context of reading, students who adopt a deep approach to learning are intrinsically motivated and focus on identifying and understanding main ideas and relating ideas to prior knowledge. As a result, we would expect these students also to use metacognitive learning and study strategies while studying. A meta-analysis by Richardson, Abraham, and Bond (2012) reported that a deep approach to learning was positively associated with academic performance in university. By contrast, a surface approach to learning is characterized by extrinsic motivation, the desire to meet minimum requirements of the learning task, and the use of information processing strategies that rely on reproduction and repetition. As a result, students adopting a surface approach may use learning and study strategies that are more behavioural in nature. Studies with university students typically find a negative correlation between a surface approach and academic performance (Richardson et al., 2012). While deep and surface approaches to learning represent opposite ends of a conceptual spectrum of motives and strategies, in practice, students may be influenced by a variety of motives and draw on a range of strategies. As a result, deep and surface approaches are not seen as orthogonal, and it is possible for a student to report high levels of both.

9.2.2 Review of Research

A significant body of research spanning over 30 years has indicated a relationship between learning and study skills and academic performance in general populations of university students (e.g., Biggs, 1987; Entwistle & Ramsden, 1983). For example, a meta-analysis by Robbins et al. (2004) concluded that self-reported use of study strategies is a robust predictor of both academic performance and retention. Performance on LASSI has also been found to differentiate academically successful and unsuccessful university students (Marrs, Sigler, & Hayes, 2009), and many of the LASSI scales and associated latent constructs have been found to predict academic performance (Cano, 2006; Daffner, DuPaul, Anastopoulos, & Weyandt, 2022; Marrs et al., 2009; Ning & Downing, 2010; Proctor et al., 2006). Similarly, MRSQ scores have been shown to correlate with academic achievement in typical university populations (Taraban et al., 2004).

Studies of learning and study strategies of university students with dyslexia or other forms of reading disabilities are rare, and we review first what studies with students with learning difficulties have found before focusing on reading difficulties (RD). Studies with students with diagnosed LD point to the importance of learning and study strategies. Research with younger participants has indicated that students with LD are less likely than their peers to develop and employ effective learning strategies (e.g., Wong, 1994). In some studies, college students with LD have also been shown to use fewer learning and study strategies (Wang & Chung, 2022) and to lack effective learning and study strategies (Bursuck & Jayanthi, 1993; Deschler, Schumaker, Alley, Warner, & Clark, 1982; Policastro, 1993), whereas other studies have highlighted differences in selected strategies between students with and without LD. Heiman and Precel (2003), for example, reported that university students with LD were less likely to use study strategies that relied on writing (e.g., writing summaries) to enhance information retention than university students without LD. Instead, the students with LD preferred to use other mnemonics, such as singing the text or making diagrams. In terms of understanding material, students with LD also preferred oral or visual explanations, whereas students without LD preferred written examples. Other studies point similarly to the use of alternative strategies that rely less on reading and writing, and to note-taking in particular, as a challenge for post-secondary students. Across different studies, challenges with note taking include problems with handwriting, keeping up with lecture content while taking notes, writing fast enough, knowing what information is important to record, and making sense of notes after the class (e.g., Bireley, Landers, Vernooy, & Schlaerth, 1986; Cowen, 1988; Hughes, 1991; Hughes & Smith, 1990).

In terms of the LASSI scales, students with LD have been reported to perform below students with no LD (e.g., Proctor et al., 2006). For example, compared to non-learning-disabled students, those with LD have been found to have lower LASSI scores on motivation (Proctor et al., 2006; Reaser, Prevatt, Petscher, & Proctor, 2007), selecting main ideas (Kovach & Wilgosh, 1999; Proctor et al., 2006), test strategies (Kovach & Wilgosh, 1999; Proctor et al., 2006), concentration (Proctor et al., 2006), information processing (Proctor et al., 2006), and self-testing (Kovach & Wilgosh, 1999), and higher scores on anxiety (Kovach & Wilgosh, 1999; Proctor et al., 2006). Other studies have suggested self-reported problems with academic motivation, planning, and organization (Kovach, 1992; Kovach, Whyte, & Vosahlo, 1990). In contrast, students with LD have self-reported higher use of study aids (Proctor et al., 2006; Reaser et al., 2007) and have a better attitude and stronger motivation to succeed (Kovach & Wilgosh, 1999). Furthermore, there is evidence, mainly from qualitative studies, that awareness and reported use of learning and study strategies may help students with LD to compensate for learning difficulties (e.g., Reis et al., 2000). Thus, prior research on learning and study strategies conducted mostly with students with LD (as opposed to RD alone) has identified a somewhat inconsistent pattern of areas of relative strengths and weaknesses.

9.2.2.1 Review of RD/Dyslexia Studies

As the LD population in universities can be very diverse (see e.g., Heiman & Precel, 2003; Proctor et al., 2006), it is not clear that studies of students with LD can identify significant risk and protective factors for students with reading disabilities. Generalizability of findings is further complicated by both significant comorbidity of RD in many samples with other learning, behavioural, and psychological conditions (e.g., Stack-Cutler et al., 2016) and by variable legislative and support frameworks across countries and universities. Thus, all conclusions have to be tentative at best while we wait for studies with better-defined populations. That said, as a starting point, it may be useful to review in more detail the handful of studies that (1) examined learning and study strategies or approaches to learning, and (2) specifically focused on students with diagnosed or self-reported reading disabilities (albeit without controlling for comorbidity). Given that individuals with a HRD report and exhibit significant reading and writing issues in university (e.g., Deacon et al., 2012), it seems important to examine whether individuals with RD in higher education use different strategies and approaches to learning than their normally reading peers, and whether any of these strategies are associated with better academic outcomes.

Trainin and Swanson's (2005) study is the first we were able to locate that focused on individuals with RD; although the authors described their sample as LD, their selection criteria screened specifically for RD. Trainin and Swanson examined both cognitive compensation and metacognitive compensation (Baltes & Baltes, 1990) and included tasks assessing what the authors described as "metacognitive learning strategies." In this study, the RD group scored higher than the comparison group on some self-regulated learning strategies (management of resources and time, effort regulation, working with peers, and help-seeking), with similar performance across a wide variety of metacognitive measures. The RD group also showed poorer performance in most cognitive tasks, and the results did not provide any evidence for cognitive compensation.

Similarly, Corkett et al. (2006) found that students with and without HRD reported comparable levels of use of a range of learning and study strategies; the only significant difference was the more frequent reported use of organizational strategies by students with HRD. Corkett et al. also noted an interesting null finding. We would expect that the residual reading problems exhibited by students with HRD could lead them to use learning and study strategies that rely on writing and reading to a lesser degree than the participants without HRD (see e.g., Heiman & Precel, 2003, above). However, the participants with HRD in Corkett et al. reported substantial use of reading and writing-based learning and study strategies and little use of possible alternative strategies, such as visualization.

Turning to approaches to learning, we identified only one relevant study. Kirby, Silvestri, Allingham, Parrila, and La Fave (2008) reported that university students with reading disabilities were significantly more likely to report a deep approach to learning than their normally reading peers. However, the remaining results were not entirely consistent with a deep approach to learning, as students with reading disabilities reported significantly greater use of both some behavioural strategies (e.g., study aids) and the metacognitive strategy of time management, but lesser use of other metacognitive strategies, such as selecting main ideas and test-taking strategies. Kirby et al. interpreted the results to indicate that, while aspiring towards a deep approach, students with dyslexia compensated for their RD by using approaches and strategies available to them in spite of the word-reading problems. To support this, Tops, Glatz, Premchand, Callens, and Brysbaert (2020) found that the first-year undergraduate students with dyslexia showed less knowledge of one metacognitive strategy, test taking, and a higher fear of failure than their non-dyslexic peers. It is conceivable that fear of failure could prevent students with dyslexia from experimenting with more effective learning and study strategies.

Chevalier et al. (2017) found that students with and without a HRD reported similar levels of learning and study strategy use on most LASSI scales and on the pragmatic scale of MRSQ. Intriguingly, there were two exceptions: Students with HRD had lower scores on the MRSQ analytic scale and, similar to Kirby et al. (2008), on the selecting main ideas scale of LASSI.

Chevalier et al. (2017) also examined whether the reported use of learning and study strategies was associated with academic achievement as measured by first-year GPA. They found that for students with HRD, the self-reported use of metacognitive reading and self-testing strategies and study aids was associated positively with GPA; all reported strategies accounted for 17% of the variance in GPA for students with HRD, but only 6% for the control students. To our knowledge, this is the first study that directly tied learning and study strategy use to academic achievement in a sample specifically selected for RD. Perhaps not surprisingly, the results indicate that strategy use is more important for success for the students with HRD than for the students who report no RD.

Bergey et al. (2017) attempted to replicate and extend Chevalier et al.'s results with a larger sample of first-year students. Bergey et al.'s sample included over 100 students with HRD, far more than in prior studies, and a control group of 375 students with no HRD. Analyses indicated that students with HRD performed more poorly than the control group in the analytic scale of MRSQ and in all but three LASSI scales – self-testing, time management, and using study aids – where no differences were observed. Further, neither the MRSQ nor the LASSI scales were significantly associated with academic achievement for students with HRD, but were for students without HRD, thus contradicting the findings by Chevalier et al.

Finally, two studies have examined self-reported study strategies. Howard-Gosse, Bergey, and Deacon (2023) used a questionnaire to assess first-year university students' reading challenges, strategies, and habits. Their results showed that compared to students with no history of reading problems, students with a history of RD spend more time reading, use alternative study materials more often if those were available, and find concentrating on and comprehending the assigned reading more difficult. For both groups, higher reported difficulty with reading load and fewer completed assigned readings were associated with poorer GPA.

Andreassen, Jensen, and Bråten (2017) compared self-reported study strategy use of first-year students with (n = 17) and without (n = 17) dyslexia by asking them to respond to a web-based diary over 12 consecutive days instead of a one-time questionnaire (as in all the above studies) or interview (see below). Due to the novel nature of this methodology, we will describe the study in more detail here. In the diaries, students responded to specific questions separately for three study contexts: attending lectures, studying alone, and studying with others. If students had attended lectures the previous day, they were asked whether they had taken notes on paper or on a computer, asked the lecturer questions, audio-recorded the lectures, discussed the lectures with other students, and constructed summaries of the lectures. In terms of studying alone, students were asked to report on the presence of note-taking, summarising, underlining or highlighting, searching for additional information, making drawings or figures, listening to audio books, listening to audio-recorded lectures, and using text-to-speech software. For the studying with others, the participants were asked to report whether they participated in groups organized by students and/or in groups organized by instructors, consulted fellow students and/or family and friends, and used social media for academic purposes. All of the above questions involved simple yes/no responses, but because they were repeated 12 times, the results allow examination of both the number of individuals reporting a specific strategy and the frequency of its use. Finally, students were asked whether the strategies they reported using were beneficial to them on a Likert scale varying from 1 (not at all helpful) to 5 (very helpful).

The results indicated that, in the context of lectures, the two groups reported similarly widespread and frequent notetaking, asking questions, discussing with peers, and summarizing lectures, and very infrequent audio-recording of lectures. When studying alone, note-taking and summarizing were also used by most students. In studying alone, two-thirds of students also reported underlining or highlighting the text, with dyslexic students reporting slightly lower frequency of use of these strategies. Interestingly, six students in each group reported making drawings or figures, with dyslexic students reporting a slightly higher frequency of this strategy. Only three students with dyslexia listened to audiobooks, two listened to recorded lectures, and none used text-to-speech software. Studying with others was frequently reported in both groups; a few more students with dyslexia than without dyslexia reported participating in groups organized by students and consulting other students slightly more frequently. No between-group differences were observed for consulting instructors or family and friends, or using social media for academic purposes. The students with dyslexia, however, reported benefitting substantially more from consulting family and friends, although the small sample size did not allow for establishing whether any of the differences were reliable. Finally, Andreassen et al. reported that strategy use was positively correlated with self-reported academic performance for students with dyslexia, but not for students without dyslexia.

We should also note that some interview studies with college or university students with dyslexia have also touched upon learning and study strategies. For example, in their review of interview studies, Pino and Mortari (2014) noted that students identified both text-based and alternative (visual and oral) strategies, time management, as well as support from family, friends, and student peers as useful. Students with dyslexia interviewed by Olofsson, Ahl, and Taube (2012) described many reading and writing-based strategies (e.g., taking notes, underlining, use of sticky notes, writing summaries, checking Google or Wikipedia for additional information). These students also indicated that they used audiobooks, recorded lectures, and drew pictures, as well as got help from family and friends with written assignments. Some of the Stampoltzis and Polychronopoulou's (2009) informants with dyslexia acknowledged relying on assistive technology; however, many indicated using no specific strategies to cope with dyslexia. University students with HRD interviewed by Corkett et al. (2006) also identified seeking assistance from peers, family, and instructors as useful strategies. In the most recent interview study, MacCullagh, Bosanquet, and Badcock's (2017) informants with dyslexia reported both text-based as well as visual and oral strategies. In this study, many students with dyslexia described reading very strategically and selectively, and a third of them mentioned looking for online videos to replace or supplement prescribed readings. MacCullagh et al. interpreted their results to be consistent with a deep approach to learning by the students with dyslexia.

In sum, both quantitative and qualitative studies have produced a highly varied picture of the learning and study strategies of students with dyslexia, but we also have some replicated findings across the studies. For example, in all three studies that used LASSI, students with reading disabilities consistently reported poorer ability to select main ideas when reading, and in both studies that used MRSQ, they reported poorer metacognitive reading strategies. The existence of continuing reading challenges suggests that students with dyslexia would likely benefit from having the content available in alternative formats, including summaries, videotaped lectures, and audiobooks. Test-taking strategies also emerged as a problem area in two studies, suggesting that students with dyslexia may also require alternative assessments to show their learning fully. Several studies have also indicated that students with reading disabilities make widespread use of both text-based and alternative strategies and often rely on a network of friends, family, and peers for support. One key clinical implication of these results is the importance of understanding each student's individual risk and protective factors broadly across multiple systems (see 9.2 above) before advising them on the best course of action.

9.3 Discussion

Reviewing the research literature on learning and study strategies used by post-secondary students with reading disabilities is a challenging and, at times, disappointing exercise for educators and researchers interested in compensation. The most common result in quantitative studies is that students with RD are not different from their peers with no RD in *most* learning and study strategies assessed. Even in large-scale studies with no apparent problems with statistical power, the differences are often limited to a few scales; when differences are observed, they are as frequently negative as positive and possibly compensatory. We will discuss below two problem areas – how we measure learning and study strategies, and how we sample the students with RD – as possibly responsible for this state of affairs, and suggest some potential solutions.

9.3.1 *What Do Current Measures of Learning and Study Strategies Assess?*

First, it seems that different measures frequently produce different results, and sometimes even the same measures used with seemingly similar samples of students (e.g., Bergey et al., 2017; Chevalier et al., 2017) fail to produce converging results. This suggests significant shortcomings with the current measures. As an example, the underlying structure of the most commonly used measure, LASSI, has not withstood empirical examination. LASSI was initially developed to assess the impact of a study skills training programme (Entwistle & McCune, 2004). Later, Weinstein and colleagues grouped the scales into *skill, will,* and *self-regulation* categories (Weinstein et al., 2002; Weinstein et al., 2016). However, studies of the factor structure have not supported the intended factor structure (Bergey et al., 2017; Cano, 2006; Murphy & Alexander, 1998; Olaussen & Bråten, 1998; Olivárez Jr. & Tallent-Runnels, 1994; Prevatt, Petscher, Proctor, Hurst, & Adams, 2006; see Fong et al., 2023, for recent meta-analytic structural equation modelling). Empirical data suggest that the factor structure is influenced by the frequent negatively worded items within some scales, which subsequently are more likely to assess perceived difficulty than perceived ability. Because the latent constructs are defined variably across the studies, their nature is ambiguous, and LASSI cannot be used to address theoretical questions. Further, as the scales are often correlated, minor variations in correlations between the scales and the dependent variables can result in widely different predictive relationships due to multicollinearity. For this reason, we avoided focusing on results from regression analyses in this review, but more generally, the current measures all but guarantee that two studies using the same measures will produce at least partly conflicting results.

Second, most measures of study and learning strategies are outdated and often do not sample study and learning strategies we now know to be the most effective (see e.g., Dunlosky, Rawson, Marsh, Nathan, & Willingham, 2013). It is therefore possible that the null effects are explained by our sampling behaviours that cannot be expected to produce consistent positive effects. We know that very short interventions that focus at least partly on effective study and learning strategies can improve student outcomes (e.g., Bergey, Parrila, Laroche, & Deacon, 2019) and we can only assume that focusing our teaching on the study and learning strategies with most evidence would further enhance the impact (e.g., Weinstein, Madan, & Sumeracki, 2018).

A third explanation for the mixed and null results may lie in the widespread use of self-reports on the generalized and somewhat abstract strategies and approaches across different learning tasks and contexts. While this may be less of a problem for approaches to learning, we question the extent to which the decontextualized report of strategies reflects actual behaviours in real learning tasks completed in everyday learning settings. Andreassen et al. (2017) note that both questionnaires and interviews are offline measures of strategy use; there is substantial evidence that offline self-reports of strategy use may not correspond to actual behaviours observed in learning situations (see overview in Veenman, 2011). Because off-line measures assess recollection of past experiences, they are open to memory reconstruction failures and distortions. Thus, both self-report questionnaires and interview data may fail to accurately capture the learning and study strategies used by university students with dyslexia.

Research on study strategies in general populations has placed greater emphasis on the context (e.g., differences in academic domain and types of learning tasks) and processes (Winne, 2010; Zimmerman, 2008). For example, microanalytic studies that examine learners' beliefs and decisions during a learning activity (e.g., Cleary, Callan, & Zimmerman, 2012; Strømsø, Bråten, & Samuelstuen, 2003) or studies that analyse trace data of learning behaviours in computer-based environments (e.g., Azevedo, 2007) have moved the field forward. Using similar online approaches in studies of adults with reading disabilities would likely illuminate how individuals develop, select, and apply learning and study strategies across different learning tasks to compensate for their residual RD. Andreassen et al. (2017) moved the field towards this goal, but the diary format they used was still offline and included limited response options, possibly creating a prompting bias. To move the field forward both theoretically and practically, we clearly need studies that employ online measures of learning and study strategies across a wide variety of learning tasks. Such studies are likely to produce better information than offline studies on how different individual and task characteristics interact in everyday learning environments. This kind of information is critical for understanding the different pathways to successful learning that individuals with dyslexia can take in different contexts, as well as for designing accessible and equitable learning and assessment materials.

9.3.2 Who Are the Students with RD?

The second significant confounding issue lies in the differences in the samples of students with RD studied. The level of remaining RD likely impacts the availability and willingness to employ some strategies over others. For example, Andreassen et al. (2017) suggested that oral, social, and visual strategies may be relied on more by individuals who continue to display poor decoding and spelling, whereas those who do not may rely more on text-based strategies. In other words, some level of successful cognitive compensation may be necessary to access at least some of the metacognitive compensation strategies. The granularity of the reported data in available qualitative and quantitative studies alike does not allow examination of these propositions; the vast majority of the studies simply do not have adequate sample sizes and/or measures of reading skills to evaluate how current reading skills interact with learning and study strategies. It is, for example, possible that students with more significant remaining RD may require a deep approach and strong motivation to succeed, whereas students with more limited current reading problems can manage their reading and writing load with only better time management and a few more hours of work. How cognitive compensation impacts the choice and effectiveness of metacognitive learning and study strategies is an important focus for future studies with significant potential to inform services for students with dyslexia. The diary method, albeit still offline, introduced by Andreassen et al., could allow us to tap into some of these interactions better than questionnaires if implemented with large enough samples.

An additional issue with sampling lies in the students' prior experiences with learning and disability support services. Studies recruiting participants via these services will end up with a sample that has a diagnosis and has likely received training in at least some learning and study strategies, such as time management and using study aids. Further, participants' responses in questionnaire and interview studies may partly reflect what was best understood and subsequently remembered from such training (Kirby et al., 2008), rather than what strategies are actually used in learning tasks. In contrast, if participants who self-report a significant HRD (such as the Adult Reading History Questionnaire – Revised used in Chevalier et al., 2017, and Bergey et al., 2017, studies) are recruited, the sample will include both individuals with a diagnosis and those who have never received a diagnosis. While the levels of current reading performance of these two groups are likely comparable (e.g., Deacon et al., 2012; Parrila et al., 2007), their educational histories are likely to be very different, as only those with a diagnosis have likely had access to remedial or special education classes and therefore also training on study and learning strategies. Deacon et al. (2012) observed some interesting differences between the two groups in terms of approaches to a reading comprehension task, and it is conceivable that differences also exist in approaches to learning and in preferred learning and study strategies. Results of multiple studies reporting on interviews of students with dyslexia indicate that receiving a diagnosis significantly impacts awareness of learning challenges, and therefore likely also motivation to identify and implement alternative learning and study strategies. Being regarded as having dyslexia, as opposed to being lazy and dumb, impacts one's desire to learn (Stampoltzis & Polychronopoulou, 2009), as well as access to services and accommodations that can change the learning and study strategies required for success.

The final sampling issue that may explain variable results across studies is the prevalent comorbidity of different learning and behavioural conditions. We know that individuals with dyslexia are more likely than their peers to experience other issues that can affect learning, such as dyscalculia and attention problems (e.g., Landerl & Moll, 2010; Pennington, 2006). From a purely research perspective, it would be desirable to have samples of "pure dyslexics"; in reality, such samples are all but impossible to locate, and they are not representative of students with reading disabilities in post-secondary education (see e.g., Stack-Cutler et al., 2016). Nevertheless, comorbidity should be reported on and, as much as possible, taken into account when analysing and interpreting findings. To give an example, comorbid memory problems (and not only phonological memory problems) could lead to a preference for a deep approach to learning that deemphasizes the importance of remembering details (Kirby et al., 2008). No quantitative study reviewed above reported on possible comorbidity; as such, we have no way to establish whether the variability in the reported results reflects different levels or kinds of comorbidity in the samples included. Again, we clearly need better information on who the participants we study are.

9.4 Conclusion

All students employ a broad range of cognitive, metacognitive, and socio-cognitive mechanisms to make the best of their study opportunities. Metacognitive and behavioural learning and study strategies have been suggested as a possible compensatory mechanism for students with RD who successfully manage the complex literacy environments of post-secondary education. Learning and study strategies may be particularly important for students who continue to struggle with reading, as they may constitute behavioural and psychological means for coping with difficulties with word reading and reading comprehension (Parrila & McQuarrie, 2015). And yet, the evidence in support of these suggestions is far from consistent. In this chapter, we have identified some gaps in existing knowledge, and the remaining chapters in this book undoubtedly will identify many others. We have also suggested some small steps forward, specifically pointing to the need for much more research to better understand how university students with significant RD differ from those without RD in their paths to success. While the task ahead may seem daunting, the end goal of improving the educational outcomes of all students with RD and the theories that explain their functioning is worthy of all the necessary efforts.

Note

1 In many jurisdictions in North America, students are not likely to receive a diagnosis of dyslexia. If their difficulties are limited to reading, they may receive a diagnosis of a specific reading disability or of a learning disability. However, the latter category includes a wide variety of students with diverse learning issues (and normal intelligence).

References

Alster, E. H. (1997). The effects of extended time on algebra test scores for college students with and without learning disabilities. *Journal of Learning Disabilities, 30*(2), 222–227. https://doi.org/10.1177/002221949703000210

Andreassen, R., Jensen, M. S., & Bråten, I. (2017). Investigating self-regulated study strategies among postsecondary students with and without dyslexia: A diary method study. *Reading and Writing, 30*, 1891–1916. https://doi.org/10.1007/s11145-017-9758-9

Asikainen, H., & Gijbels, D. (2017). Do students develop towards more deep approaches to learning during studies? A systematic review on the development of students' deep and surface approaches to learning in higher education. *Educational Psychology Review, 29*(2), 205–234. https://doi.org/10.1007/s10648-017-9406-6

Azevedo, R. (2007). Understanding the complex nature of self-regulatory processes in learning with computer-based learning environments: An introduction. *Metacognition and Learning, 2*(2–3), 57–65.

Baltes, P. B., & Baltes, M. M. (1990). Psychological perspectives on successful aging: The model of selective optimization with compensation. In P. B. Baltes & M. M. Baltes (Eds.), *Successful aging: Perspectives from the behavioral sciences* (pp. 1–34). New York: Cambridge University Press.

Bechtel, W., & Abrahamsen, A. (2005). Explanation: A mechanistic alternative. *Studies in History and Philosophy of Biological and Biomedical Sciences, 36*, 421–441.

Bechtel, W., & Abrahamsen, A. (2010). Dynamic mechanistic explanation: Computational modeling of circadian rhythms as an exemplar for cognitive science. *Studies in History and Philosophy of Science, 41*, 321–333.

Bergey, B. W., Deacon, H., & Parrila, R. (2017). Metacognitive reading and study strategies and academic achievement of university students with and without a history of reading difficulties. *Journal of Learning Disabilities, 50*(1), 81–94. https://doi.org/10.1177/0022219415597020

Bergey, B. W., Parrila, R. K., Laroche, A., & Deacon, S. H. (2019). Effects of peer-led training on academic self-efficacy, study strategies, and academic performance for first-year university students with and without reading difficulties. *Contemporary Educational Psychology, 56*, 25–39. https://doi.org/10.1016/j.cedpsych.2018.11.001

Biggs, J., Kember, D., & Leung, D. Y. P. (2001). The revised two factor study process questionnaire: R-SPQ-2F. *British Journal of Educational Psychology, 71*, 133–149.

Biggs, J. B. (1979). Individual differences in the study processes and the quality of learning outcomes. *Higher Education, 8*, 381–394.

Biggs, J. B. (1987). *Student approaches to learning and studying.* Melbourne, Australia: Australian Council for Educational Research.

Bireley, M. K., Landers, M. G., Vernooy, J. A., & Schlaerth, P. (1986). The Wright State University program: Implications of the first decade. *Reading, Writing, and Learning Disabilities, 2*, 349–357.

Bursuck, W. D., & Jayanthi, M. (1993). Strategy instruction: Programming for independent study skills usage. In S. A. Vogel & P. B. Adelman (Eds.), *Success for college students with learning disabilities* (pp. 177–205). New York: Springer-Verlag.

Canadian University Survey Consortium (2011). *Undergraduate University Student Survey – June 23, 2011.* Retrieved from http://www.cusc-ccreu.ca/publications/CUSC_2011_UG_MasterReport.pdf

Cano, F. (2006). An in-depth analysis of the learning and study strategies inventory (LASSI). *Educational and Psychological Measurement, 66*(6), 1023–1038. https://doi.org/10.1177/0013164406288167

Chevalier, T., Parrila, R., Ritchie, K., & Deacon, H. (2017). The role of metacognitive study and learning strategies, and behavioural study and learning strategies in predicting academic success in students with and without a history of reading difficulties. *Journal of Learning Disabilities, 50*(1), 34–48. https://doi.org/10.1177/0022219415588850

Cleary, T. J., Callan, G. L., & Zimmerman, B. J. (2012). Assessing self-regulation as a cyclical, context-specific phenomenon: Overview and analysis of SRL microanalytic protocols. *Education Research International, 2012.* https://doi.org/10.1155/2012/428639

Corkett, J. K., & Parrila, R. (2008). Use of context in the word recognition process by adults with a significant history of reading difficulties. *Annals of Dyslexia, 58*, 139–161. https://doi.org/10.1007/s11881-008-0018-1

Corkett, J. K., Parrila, R., & Hein, S. F. (2006). Learning and study strategies of university students who report a significant history of reading difficulties. *Developmental Disabilities Bulletin, 34*(1), 57–79.

Cowen, S. E. (1988). Coping strategies of university students with learning disabilities. *Journal of Learning Disabilities, 21*, 161–164.

Daffner, M. S., DuPaul, G. J., Anastopoulos, A. D., & Weyandt, L. L. (2022). From orientation to graduation: Predictors of academic success for freshmen with ADHD. *Journal of Postsecondary Education and Disability, 35*(2), 113–130.

Deacon, H. S., Tucker, R., Bergey, B. W., Laroche, A., & Parrila, R. (2017). Personalized outreach to university students with a history of reading difficulties: Early screening and outreach to support academically at-risk students. *Journal of College Student Development.* https://doi.org/10.1353/csd.2017.0032

Deacon, S. H., Cook, K., & Parrila, R. (2012). Identifying high-functioning dyslexics: Is self-report of early reading problems enough? *Annals of Dyslexia, 62,* 120–134. https://doi.org/10.1007/s11881-012-0068-2

Deacon, S. H., Parrila, R., & Kirby, J. R. (2006). Processing of derived forms in high-functioning dyslexics. *Annals of Dyslexia, 56*(1), 103–128. https://doi.org/10.1007/s11881-006-0005-3

Deschler, D. D., Schumaker, J. B., Alley, G. R., Warner, M. M., & Clark, F. L. (1982). Learning disabilities in adolescent and young adult populations: Research implications. *Focus on Exceptional Children, 15*(1), 1–12.

Dunlosky, J., Rawson, K. A., Marsh, E. J., Nathan, M. J., & Willingham, D. T. (2013). Improving students' learning with effective learning techniques: Promising directions from cognitive and educational psychology. *Psychological Science in the Public Interest, 14*(1), 4–58. https://doi.org/10.1177/1529100612453266

Entwistle, N., & McCune, V. (2004). The conceptual bases of study strategy inventories. *Educational Psychology Review, 16,* 325–345. https://doi.org/10.1007/s10648-004-0003-0

Entwistle, N. J., & Ramsden, P. (1983). *Understanding student learning.* London: Croom Helm.

Entwistle, N. J., & Waterson, S. (1988). Approaches to studying and levels of processing in university students. *British Journal of Educational Psychology, 58,* 258–265.

Flavell, J. H. (1979). Metacognition and cognitive monitoring: A new area of cognitive-developmental inquiry. *American Psychologist, 34*(10), 906–911. https://doi.org/10.1037//0003-066X.34.10.906

Fong, C. J., Lee, J., Krou, M. R., Hoff, M. A., Johnston-Ashton, K., Gonzales, C., & Beretvas, S. N. (2023). Meta-analyzing the factor structure of the learning and study strategies inventory. *Journal of Experimental Education, 91*(2), 380–400. https://doi.org/10.1080/00220973.2021.2021842

Frith, U. (1999). Figureof dyslexia. *Dyslexia, 5,* 192–214. https://doi.org/10.1002/(SICI)1099-0909(199912)5:4<192::AID-DYS144>3.0.CO;2-N

Gottlieb, G. (1983). The psychobiological approach to developmental issues. In M. M. Haith & J. J. Campos (Eds.), *Handbook of child psychology* (Vol. 2, 4th ed., pp. 1–26). New York: John Wiley & Sons.

Gottlieb, G. (2002). *Individual development and evolution.* Mahwah, NJ: Lawrence Erlbaum Associates.

Gottlieb, G., Wahlsten, D., & Lickliter, R. (2006). The significance of biology for human development: A developmental psychobiological systems view. In R. M. Lerner & W. Damon (Eds.), *Handbook of child psychology* (Vol. 1, 6th ed., pp. 210–257). Hoboken, NJ: John Wiley & Sons.

Haft, S. L., Myers, C. A., & Hoeft, F. (2016). Socio-emotional and cognitive resilience in children with reading disabilities. *Current Opinion in Behavioral Sciences, 10,* 133–141. https://doi.org/10.1016/j.cobeha.2016.06.005

Heiman, T., & Precel, K. (2003). Students with learning disabilities in higher education: Academic strategies profile. *Journal of Learning Disabilities, 36,* 248–258. https://doi.org/10.1177/002221940303600304

Hen, M., & Goroshit, M. (2014). Academic procrastination, emotional intelligence, academic self-efficacy, and GPA: A comparison between students with and without learning disabilities. *Journal of Learning Disabilities, 47,* 116–124. https://doi.org/10.1177/0022219412439325

Howard-Gosse, A., Bergey, B. W., & Deacon, S. H. (2023). The reading challenges, strategies, and habits of university students with a history of reading difficulties and their relations to academic achievement. *Journal of Learning Disabilities, 57*(2), 91–105. https://doi.org/10.1177/00222194231190678

Hughes, C. A. (1991). Studying for and taking tests: Self reported difficulties and strategies of university students with learning disabilities. *Learning Disabilities, 2,* 65–71.

Hughes, C. A., & Smith, J. O. (1990). Cognitive and academic performance of college students with learning disabilities: A synthesis of the literature. *Learning Disability Quarterly, 13*, 66–79.

Jackson, N. E., & Doellinger, H. L. (2002). Resilient readers? University students who are poor recoders but sometimes good text comprehenders. *Journal of Educational Psychology, 94*, 64–78. https://doi.org/10.1037/0022-0663.94.1.64

Kemp, N., Parrila, R. K., & Kirby, J. R. (2008). Phonological and orthographic spelling in high-functioning adult dyslexics. *Dyslexia, 15*, 105–128. https://doi.org/10.1002/dys.364

Kirby, J. R., Silvestri, R., Allingham, B. H., Parrila, R., & La Fave, C. B. (2008). Learning strategies and study approaches of postsecondary students with dyslexia. *Journal of Learning Disabilities, 41*(1), 85–96. https://doi.org/10.1177/0022219407311040

Kovach, K. (1992). *Perceptions of ability: Students with and without learning disabilities at postsecondary institutions.* Unpublished doctoral dissertation, University of Alberta, Edmonton, Alberta, Canada.

Kovach, K., Whyte, L., & Vosahlo, M. (1990). *A brief description of a sample of 42 university students with learning disabilities assisted from 1986 to 1989.* Unpublished manuscript, Office of Services for Students with Disabilities, University of Alberta, Canada.

Kovach, K., & Wilgosh, L. R. (1999). Learning and study strategies, and performance anxiety in postsecondary students with learning disabilities: A preliminary study. *Developmental Disabilities Bulletin, 27*, 47–57.

Landerl, K., & Moll, K. (2010). Comorbidity of learning disorders: Prevalence and familial transmission. *Journal of Child Psychology and Psychiatry, 51*(3), 287–294. https://doi.org/10.1111/j.1469-7610.2009.02164.x

Lawson, L. (2009). The learning and study strategies inventory as a predictive measure of 1st semester academic performance of at-risk students. Electronic Theses, Treatises and Dissertations, Paper 3223. Retrieved from http://diginole.lib.fsu.edu/etd/3223/

MacCullagh, L., Bosanquet, A., & Badcock, N. A. (2017). University students with dyslexia: A qualitative exploratory study of learning practices, challenges, and strategies. *Dyslexia, 23*, 3–23. https://doi.org/10.1002/dys.1544

Marrs, H., Sigler, E., & Hayes, K. (2009). Study strategy predictors of performance in introductory psychology. *Journal of Instructional Psychology, 36*, 125–133.

Marton, F., & Saljo, R. (1976). On qualitative differences in learning: Outcomes and process. *British Journal of Educational Psychology, 46*, 4–11.

Mortimore, T., & Crozier, W. R. (2006). Dyslexia and difficulties with study skills in higher education. *Studies in Higher Education, 31*, 235–251. https://doi.org/10.1080/03075070600572173

Murphy, P. K., & Alexander, P. A. (1998). Using the learning and study strategies inventory-high school version with Singaporean females: Examining psychometric properties. *Educational and Psychological Measurement, 58*(3), 493–510.

Ning, H. K., & Downing, K. (2010). Connections between learning experience, study behaviour and academic performance: A longitudinal study. *Educational Research, 52*, 457–468. https://doi.org/10.1080/00131881.2010.524754

Olaussen, B., & Bråten, I. (1998). Identifying latent variables measured by the learning and study strategies inventory (LASSI) in Norwegian college students. *Journal of Experimental Education, 67*, 82–96. https://doi.org/10.1080/00220979809598346

Olivárez, A., Jr., & Tallent-Runnels, M. K. (1994). Psychometric properties of the learning and study strategies inventory-high school version. *The Journal of Experimental Education, 62*(3), 243–257. https://doi.org/10.1080/00220973.1994.9943843

Olofsson, Å., Ahl, A., & Taube, K. (2012). Learning and study strategies in university students with dyslexia: Implications for teaching. *Procedia – Social and Behavioral Sciences, 47*, 1184–1193. https://doi.org/10.1016/j.sbspro.2012.06.798

Parrila, R. (2008). The multiple systems model of Reading: Understanding reading disabilities and their effect on academic achievement across individuals and orthographies (invited paper). *The Japanese Journal of Special Education, 45*, 383–404.

Parrila, R., Georgiou, G., & Corkett, J. (2007). University students with a significant history of reading difficulties: What is and is not compensated? *Exceptionality Education Canada, 17*(2), 195–220.

Parrila, R., & McQuarrie, L. (2015). Cognitive processes and academic achievement: Multiple systems model of academic achievement. In T. C. Papadopoulos, R. Parrila, & J. R. Kirby (Eds.), *Cognition, intelligence, and achievement: A tribute to J. P. Das* (pp. 79–100). San Diego: Elsevier.

Parrila, R., & Protopapas, A. (2017). Dyslexia and word reading problems. In K. Cain, D. Compton, & R. Parrila (Eds.), *Theories of reading development* (pp. 333–358). Amsterdam: Benjamins.

Pedersen, H. F., Fusaroli, R., Lauridsen, L. L., & Parrila, R. (2016). Reading processes of university students with dyslexia: An examination of the relationship between oral reading and reading comprehension. *Dyslexia, 22*, 305–321. https://doi.org/10.1002/dys.1542

Pennington, B. F. (2006). From single to multiple deficit models of developmental disorders. *Cognition, 101*, 385–413.

Pino, M., & Mortari, L. (2014). The inclusion of students with dyslexia in higher education: A systematic review using narrative synthesis. *Dyslexia, 20*, 346–369. https://doi.org/10.1002/dys.1484

Policastro, M. M. (1993). Assessing and developing metacognitive attributes in college students with learning disabilities. In S. A. Vogel & P. B. Adelman (Eds.), *Success for college students with learning disabilities* (pp. 151–176). New York: Springer-Verlag.

Pressley, M. (2000). Comprehension instruction in elementary school: A quarter-century of research progress. In B. Taylor, M. F. Graves, & P. van den Broek (Eds.), *Reading for meaning: Fostering comprehension in the middle grades* (pp. 32–51). New York: Teachers College Press.

Pressley, M., Brown, R., El-Dinary, P., & Allferbach, P. (1995). The comprehension instruction that students need: Instruction fostering constructively responsive reading. *Learning Disabilities Research & Practice, 41*(4), 215–224.

Prevatt, F., Petscher, Y., Proctor, B. E., Hurst, A., & Adams, K. (2006). The revised learning and study strategies inventory: An evaluation of competing models. *Educational and Psychological Measurement, 66*(3), 448–458. https://doi.org/10.1177/00131644405282454

Proctor, B. E., Prevatt, F. F., Adams, K., Hurst, A., & Petscher, Y. (2006). Study skills profiles of normal-achieving and academically-struggling college students. *Journal of College Student Development, 47*(1), 37–51. https://doi.org/10.1353/csd.2006.0011

Ramus, F. (2003). Developmental dyslexia: Specific phonological deficit or general sensorimotor dysfunction? *Current Opinion in Neurobiology, 13*, 212–218.

Reaser, A., Prevatt, F., Petscher, Y., & Proctor, B. (2007). The learning and study strategies of college students with ADHD. *Psychology in the Schools, 44*(6), 627–638. https://doi.org/10.1002/pits.20252

Reis, S. M., McGuire, J. M., & Neu, T. W. (2000). Compensation strategies used by high-ability students with learning disabilities who succeed in college. *Gifted Child Quarterly, 44*(2), 123–134.

Richardson, M., Abraham, C., & Bond, R. (2012). Psychological correlates of university students' academic performance: A systematic review and meta-analysis. *Psychological Bulletin, 138*(2), 353–387. https://doi.org/10.1037/a0026838

Robbins, S. B., Lauver, K., Le, H., Davis, D., Langley, R., & Carlstrom, A. (2004). Do psychosocial and study skill factors predict college outcomes? A meta-analysis. *Psychological Bulletin, 130,* 261–288. https://doi.org/10.1037/0033-2909.130.2.261

Ruban, L., McCoach, D., McGuire, M., & Reis, S. (2003). The differential impact of academic self-regulatory methods on academic achievement among university students with and without learning disabilities. *Journal of Learning Disabilities, 36*(3), 270–286.

Sanford, C., Newman, L., Wagner, M., Cameto, R., Knokey, A., & Shaver, D. (2011). The post–high school outcomes of young adults with disabilities up to 6 years after high school. *Key findings from the National Longitudinal Transition Study-2 (NLTS2).* Menlo Park, CA: National Center for Special Education Research. http://www.eric.ed.gov/ERICWebPortal/recordDetail?accno=ED524044

Stack-Cutler, H., Parrila, R., Jokisaari, M., & Nurmi, J.-E. (2015). How university students with reading difficulties are supported in achieving their goals. *Journal of Learning Disabilities, 48*(3), 323–334. https://doi.org/10.1177/0022219413505773

Stack-Cutler, H., Parrila, R., & Torppa, M. (2015). Using a multidimensional measure of resilience to explain life satisfaction and academic achievement of adults with reading disabilities. *Journal of Learning Disabilities, 48*(6), 646–657. https://doi.org/10.1177/0022219414522705

Stack-Cutler, H., Parrila, R., & Torppa, M. (2016). University students with reading difficulties: Do perceived supports and comorbid difficulties predict well-being and GPA? *Learning Disabilities Research & Practice, 31*(1), 45–55. https://doi.org/10.1111/ldrp.12092

Stampoltzis, A., & Polychronopoulou, S. (2009). Greek university students with dyslexia: An interview study. *European Journal of Special Needs Education, 24,* 307–321. https://doi.org/10.1080/08856250903020195

Strømsø, H. I., Bråten, I., & Samuelstuen, M. S. (2003). Students' strategic use of multiple sources during expository text reading. *Cognition and Instruction, 21,* 113–147. https://doi.org/10.1207/S1532690XCI2102_01

Taraban, R., Kerr, M., & Rynearson, K. (2004). Analytic and pragmatic factors in college students' metacognitive reading strategies. *Reading Psychology, 25*(2), 67–81. https://doi.org/10.1080/02702710490435547

Tops, W., Glatz, T., Premchand, A., Callens, M., & Brysbaert, M. (2020). Study strategies of first-year undergraduates with and without dyslexia and the effect of gender. *European Journal of Special Needs Education, 35*(3), 398–413. https://doi.org/10.1080/08856257.2019.1703580

Trainin, G., & Swanson, H. (2005). Cognition, metacognition, and achievement of college students with learning disabilities. *Learning Disability Quarterly, 28*(4), 261–272. https://doi.org/10.2307/4126965

van Bergen, E., van der Leij, A., & de Jong, P. F. (2014). The intergenerational multiple deficit model and the case of dyslexia. *Frontiers in Human Neuroscience, 8,* 346.

Veenman, M. V. J. (2011). Learning to self-monitor and self-regulate. In R. Mayer & P. Alexander (Eds.), *Handbook of research on learning and instruction* (pp. 197–218). New York: Routledge.

Vogel, S. A., & Adelman, P. B. (1992). The success of college students with learning disabilities: Factors related to educational attainment. *Journal of Learning Disabilities, 25*(7), 430–441. https://doi.org/10.1177/002221949202500703

Wade, S., Trathen, W., & Schraw, G. (1990). An analysis of spontaneous study strategies. *Reading Research Quarterly, 25*(2), 147–166. https://doi.org/10.2307/747599

Wang, L., & Chung, K. K. H. (2022). Do Taiwanese undergraduate students with SLD use different learning strategies than students without these disabilities? *Learning Disabilities Research & Practice, 37*(1), 6–17. https://doi.org/10.1111/ldrp.12269

Warmington, M., Stothard, S. E., & Snowling, M. J. (2013). Assessing dyslexia in higher education: The York Adult Assessment Battery–Revised. *Journal of Research in Special Educational Needs, 13*, 48–56.

Weinstein, C. E. (1987). *LASSI user's manual for those administering the learning and study strategies inventory.* Clearwater, FL: H & H.

Weinstein, C. E., Palmer, D. R., & Acee, T. W. (2016). *Learning and study strategies inventory* (3rd ed.). H & H Publishing.

Weinstein, C. E., Palmer, D. R., & Shulte, A. C. (2002). *LASSI user's manual* (2nd ed.). Clearwater, FL: H & H.

Weinstein, Y., Madan, C. R., & Sumeracki, M. A. (2018). Teaching the science of learning. *Cognitive Research: Principles and Implications, 3*, #2. https://doi.org/10.1186/s41235-017-0087-y

Winne, P. H. (2010). Improving measurements of self-regulated learning. *Educational Psychologist, 45*(4), 267–276.

Witte, R. H., Philips, L., & Kakela, M. (1998). Job satisfaction of college graduates with learning disabilities. *Journal of Learning Disabilities, 31*, 259–265. https://doi.org/10.1177/002221949803100305

Wong, B. Y. L. (1994). Instructional parameters promoting transfer of learning strategies in students with LD. *Learning Disability Quarterly, 17*, 110–120.

Zimmerman, B. J. (2002). Becoming a self-regulated learner: An overview. *Theory Into Practice, 41*(2), 64–70. https://doi.org/10.1207/s15430421tip4102_2

Zimmerman, B. J. (2008). Investigating self-regulation and motivation: Historical background, methodological developments, and future prospects. *American Educational Research Journal, 45*(1), 166–183. https://doi.org/10.3102/0002831207312909

10
COGNITIVE REMEDIATION AND NEURAL CHANGES IN ADULTS WITH DYSLEXIA

Floriana Costanzo, Stefano Vicari and Deny Menghini

10.1 Introduction

Cognitive remediation plays an important role in learning intervention by training and enhancing low-level processes underpinning high-order cognitive abilities such as attention, working memory, reasoning, visual and auditory processing, cognitive flexibility, processing speed, and learning.

Typical treatments for learning disorders consist of intensive explicit instruction intervention in phonological awareness and decoding strategies. Nevertheless, long-term effects are rarely verified and, when ascertained, persisted only in 50 percent of children (Gabrieli et al., 2009). Thus, there are still challenges in developing training that is long-lasting, effective for most people, and relevant at any age.

The present chapter focuses attention on cognitive remediation in adults with dyslexia, highlighting the most frequently used treatment in reading disorders. In addition, it discusses recent studies on neurobiological bases and on neural plasticity induced by cognitive remediation. Finally, the chapter presents non-invasive brain stimulation as a new perspective treatment in the remediation of reading disabilities, also in adults.

10.2 Cognitive Remediation

The persistence of reading deficits that continues into adulthood has been partly attributed to a reduction in brain plasticity beyond childhood. Research literature on children indicates that early intervention leads to better outcomes as it promotes greater automaticity in the targeted skills (Fletcher & Grigorenko, 2017). In line with this view, it has been suggested that remedial interventions would prove less effective in adults (Shaywitz & Shaywitz, 2008). Nevertheless, research suggests that neuroplasticity, including experience-dependent plasticity, extends well into adulthood, challenging the earlier notion that it was mainly confined to childhood. This has implications for adult learning and interventions aimed at skills like reading. Studies have shown that the brain's ability to reorganize and adapt continues through life, influenced by various factors such as sensory inputs and specific training (Draganski et al., 2004, 2006).

For instance, the concept of neuroplasticity has been expanded to include different regulators of plasticity across the lifespan, not just in early development. This is evident in how the brain's structure and function can still undergo changes in response to targeted interventions or training, even in adults. Evidence has demonstrated that with the right interventions, such as structured cognitive or motor skill training, adults can retain the capacity to learn new skills or recover lost abilities (Dayan & Cohen, 2011; Fattinger et al., 2017). Moreover, recent findings indicate that adult plasticity can be enhanced by altering inhibitory circuits or removing molecular "brakes" that restrict neuroplastic changes, especially in areas like the visual system (He et al., 2007; Morishita et al., 2010).

Thus, these recent findings support the idea that the adult brain remains highly plastic, and with proper interventions, adult learners can still achieve substantial cognitive and structural brain improvements. This is particularly relevant for remediation programs that aim to retrain skills like reading in adulthood.

Reading remediation training could develop different components of reading, as phonology, morphology, syntax, and semantics—as well as visual and orthographic processes, working memory, attention, and motor movements (see Table 10.1). However, the automaticity and reading fluency should lead to the ultimate objective of reading, which is higher-level comprehension or the reconstruction of meaning.

Although there are many theories attempting to explain neuropsychological deficits in dyslexia, the phonological deficit theory received major support (Ramus et al., 2003). Phonological deficit theory suggests that dyslexia emerges from problems in phonological processing: deficits in representation and access/manipulation of phonological information involving poor speech-sound awareness, slow lexical retrieval, and poor phonological short-term memory (see Goswami et al., 2000; Snowling et al., 2000). This theory may explain specific deficits in auditory-phonological perception, representation, and phonological memory. Based on phonological deficit theory, phonics trainings were developed to improve reading abilities, and nowadays they are the most frequently used treatment for reading disability. Phonics programs teach people to learn to read via letter-sound rules, and they improve performance on processes that are involved in letter-sound reading (such as letter identification, letter-sound knowledge, and phonological output) and that tax these processes simultaneously (such as nonword reading and regular word

TABLE 10.1 Different Reading Remediation Training Programs

Remediation Training	Brief Description	Examples
Phonics Training	Phonics training is structured exercises, which facilitate reading words, both isolated and integrated in a passage. Phonics training involves the teaching of letter-sound correspondences, of blending the sounds in order, and of segmenting words into phonemes to spell.	*Phonological and Graphological Processing*: uses groups of letters to represent words; says and writes the beginning and ending sounds of spoken words; identifies two or more letters that are the same in words; names and spells some letters in a given word; writes approximate letters for some sounds.
Fast ForWord	Fast ForWord is a suite of computer programs that contain language-based audiovisual games. It consists of a series of adaptive, interactive exercises that use acoustically processed speech and speech sounds.	*Phonic Match and Discrimination*: matches sounds represented by a grid of tiles by clicking on one tile and finding another tile with the identical word; phoneme discrimination. *Processing speed tasks*

(Continued)

TABLE 10.1 (Continued)

Remediation Training	Brief Description	Examples
Rhythmic Reading Training (RRT)	The Rhythmic Reading Training (RRT) is a training program specifically designed to enhance reading skills in individuals with developmental dyslexia (DD). This approach utilizes rhythm as a key element to facilitate reading learning. Participants in RRT are exposed to rhythmic stimuli integrated with reading activities, which may involve music or other methods incorporating regular and predictive rhythms to support text decoding and comprehension. The main goal is to improve word reading accuracy and reading speed, crucial components for effective reading skills.	During the Rhythmic Reading Training (RRT) session, the child starts with rhythmic exercises that help anticipate the flow of words while the teacher reads from a storybook. Subsequently, reading continues with the accompaniment of rhythmic music that guides reading pace and enhances fluency. The teacher provides continuous feedback and adjusts the difficulty level, enabling the child to improve word decoding and reading speed. By the end of the session, the child has developed improved reading skills thanks to the rhythmic support provided by RRT. 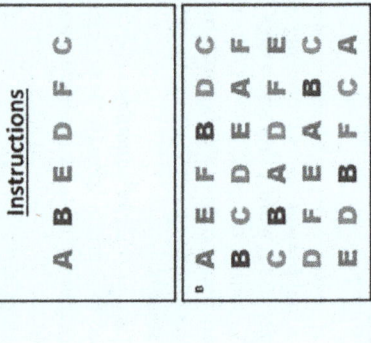

Cognitive Remediation and Neural Changes in Adults with Dyslexia 247

Reading acceleration program	A series of sentences is presented consecutively on the computer screen. The letters in each sentence disappear one after the other according to the mean reading rate (milliseconds per letter) recorded on a pre-test. Following the disappearance of the sentence from the computer screen, the participant is instructed to answer the question at a self-paced rate.	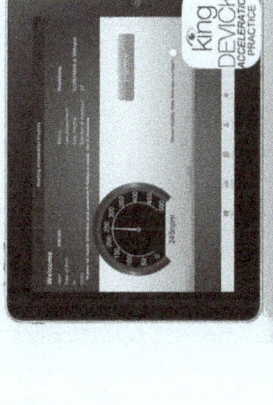 https://www.youtube.com/watch?v=1T-WPpwsx6o
The Rapid Automatized Naming Training (RANt)	The Rapid Automatized Naming Training (RANt) is a type of therapeutic intervention designed to improve rapid automatized naming skills.	This treatment is frequently used with children who have difficulties in reading acquisition, such as dyslexia, but it can also be applied to other related disorders. During RANt, participants engage in a series of exercises aimed at improving the speed and accuracy with which they can verbally name a set of visual stimuli such as letters, numbers, colors, or objects. The main goal is to increase the speed at which the brain processes and retrieves visual and verbal information, crucial skills for fluent reading and text comprehension. This type of training is based on the principle that increased rapid automatized naming correlates positively with reading abilities, as it helps improve the speed of word decoding and fluency in reading texts.

(*Continued*)

TABLE 10.1 (Continued)

Remediation Training	Brief Description	Examples
Action Video Games	Action Video Games present specific qualitative features. It includes extraordinary speed (both in terms of very transient events and in terms of the velocity of moving objects), a high degree of perceptual, cognitive, and motor load to plan a motor response (multiple items that need to be tracked and/or kept in memory, multiple action plans that need to be considered and quickly executed typically through precise and timely aiming at a target), unpredictability (both temporal and spatial), and an emphasis on peripheral processing (with important items most often appearing away from the center of the screen).	http://www.dpg.unipd.it/en/deconelab

reading). These gains in word reading should, in turn, have knock-on effects on more complex literacy skills that depend on word reading, such as reading comprehension and spelling.

One of the first letter-sound reading-focused interventions for adults with dyslexia was "The Project Success Summer Program for Adult Dyslexics", a 15-week intervention aimed at improving reading and spelling skills (Kitz & Nash, 1992). The program focused on direct instruction of sound-symbol relationships and blending sounds to form words. Participants showed significant improvements in reading isolated words, reading speed, text comprehension, and spelling. Afterward, the Cochrane[1] systematic review by McArthur et al. (2018) evaluated the effect of phonics training on the literacy skills of English-speaking populations, including studies on poor readers' adults. The review comprised studies that used a phonics program that trained reading via the letter-sound rules alone (phonics only) or with one other type of training (e.g., a program that combined phonics with phoneme awareness or irregular word reading). The authors concluded that phonics training was effective in enhancing literacy-related skills, particularly in improving word and non-word reading fluency, as well as the accuracy of reading irregular words. However, they noted that further studies were required to better refine outcomes related to reading accuracy and reading comprehension.

A meta-analysis by Galuschka et al. (2014) compared the effects of phonics training with other treatment approaches, to assess their impact on reading and spelling performance, aiming to identify the most effective method. Twenty-two randomized controlled trials in children and adolescents with dyslexia were included in the meta-analysis and classified into distinct categories based on treatment approaches: the phonics training, that systematically teaches letter-sound-correspondences; the phonemic awareness instruction, which includes interventions that promote the ability to recognize and manipulate phonemes in words with tasks presented orally; the reading fluency training, which includes interventions that contain repeated oral word reading practice or guided repeated word reading; the reading comprehension training, which includes interventions that extract textual information, summarize it, and relate it to existing knowledge; the auditory training, which includes interventions with non-linguistic auditory training; medical treatment, which includes interventions with drugs to enhance reading and spelling performance; the colored overlays training, with colored filters or colored overlays. The results revealed that phonics instruction is the only approach whose efficacy on reading and spelling performance in children and adolescents with dyslexia was statistically confirmed. The mean effect sizes of the remaining treatment approaches did not reach statistical significance.

The efficacy of phonics instruction programs has not only been documented in English-speaking countries, but also in other languages, such as Spanish, Finnish, Korean, and Italian (Brem et al., 2010; Ki-Ju, 2022; Kyle et al., 2013;

Saine et al., 2010, 2011). Nevertheless, there are many cross-linguistic studies showing that reading acquisition does not exactly develop in the same way and at the same speed as a function of the orthographic transparency (Landerl et al., 2013; Seymour et al., 2003; Ziegler et al., 2003). The issue of the generalization of the training efficacy in different languages is still debated, and further studies are needed to clarify this aspect.

In the context of cognitive remediation, a crucial challenge is the generalization beyond the training domain to untrained skills. Phonics training is structured exercises that teach to learn letter-sound rules, focus on letter identification, letter-sound knowledge, and phonological output, but also nonwords and regular word reading. A specific effect of phonics training on text comprehension is then unlikely. Conversely, a metacognitive training on text comprehension scarcely could affect reading speed and accuracy, since it is more focused on high-order processes required to understand the text, such as language, attention, and logical reasoning.

Some reading interventions targeting the effects of dyslexia-related deficits in adults have emphasized the enhancement of cognitive functions. These interventions involve teaching new strategies to manage situations where these deficits create challenges, training the use of assistive tools, and modifying the environment to minimize the impact of reading deficits (Jensen et al., 2000; Nukari et al., 2020). For example, Jensen et al. (2000) proposed a 5-month full-time educational program for 60 unemployed adults, aiming to improve skills like reading, writing, verbal memory, and self-esteem. The program included teacher-led instruction in reading, writing, and mathematics, along with personalized learning plans. Participants showed significant improvements in spelling, letter decoding, self-confidence, and cognitive flexibility compared to a control group. A recent study conducted by Nukari et al. (2020) investigated the effectiveness of a structured neuropsychological intervention on 120 young adults, including cognitive strategy learning, supporting self-esteem, and using psychoeducation. The results showed significant improvements in processing speed and attention, with sustained benefits even after a 5-month follow-up. Additionally, positive trends were observed in self-evaluations regarding reading and writing performance and speed, concentration, and memory.

However, it seems that populations with mild reading disabilities show more improvement in literacy than more severely impaired participants. Moreover, interventions with longer durations seem to have higher efficacy, and programs that were conducted by experts on reading disability tend to show higher effect sizes than interventions that were implemented by less experienced conductors.

A different approach to reading remediation involves low-level basic processes training. It has been argued (Harrar et al., 2014) that phonics training, being essentially a reading-based program, is analogous to treating the symptoms of dyslexia, whereas training the low-level basic processes may treat the underlying causes of reading deficits. An example of low-level programs developed from a theory that claims language and reading difficulties may arise from a rapid auditory temporal processing deficit. The rapid auditory temporal processing deficit found in adults with dyslexia can be described as the limited ability to process "acoustic elements of short duration", such as consonants with rapid formant transitions. Rapid formant transitions are rapid changes in formant frequency, crucial in identifying sound segments (e.g., \ba\-\pa\). Individuals with dyslexia appear to have difficulties in perceiving and distinguishing these sounds properly within the speech spectrum. Consequently, they would be unable to associate letters with their specific sounds even in adulthood (Cheema et al., 2023; Fitch et al., 1997; Habib, 2000; Tallal, 1980). A corollary of this theory is that, given neuroplasticity, appropriate training can lead to lasting improvements in underlying neural systems and concomitant improvements in language and reading skills (Merzenich & Jenkins, 1998). However, a systematic review (Strong et al., 2010) designed to verify the effectiveness of the so-called *Fast ForWord* computer-based intervention program, based on the auditory temporal processing activities, showed that there was no significant effect on any outcome measure in comparison to active or untreated control groups. No evidence that Fast ForWord is effective as a treatment for language or reading difficulties has been supported in children and adolescents. Subsequently, the temporal training using Fast ForWord was proposed to a group of participants between 65 and 75 years of age for an hour a day, 4 days a week, for 8 weeks (Szelag & Skolimowska, 2012). Significant benefits were documented on different aspects of cognitive function: after the training, the temporal training group improved temporal information processing on the tone task, some aspects of attention, and short-term memory. These results, showing an impact of temporal training on the senior population, could also have an effect on reading in adults with dyslexia, and, if verified, could open new perspectives for the application of temporal training in adults with reading disorders.

The potential of using rhythmic auditory interventions to address dyslexia-related difficulties has also been empirically explored in various studies, yielding encouraging results. These findings have inspired the design of a new rhythm-based intervention, Rhythmic Reading Training (RRT), specifically for students with dyslexia (Cancer et al., 2023). To measure the effectiveness of RRT, a controlled clinical trial was conducted. Specifically, RRT combined with musical games was compared to a customized multicomponent treatment for dyslexia known for its proven effectiveness, the *Abilmente* approach. Results revealed that, consistent with previous research, the RRT showed consistent effects on reading speed. These findings confirmed the effectiveness of a unimodal intervention based on rhythm in inducing overall reading effects comparable to those following a customized multicomponent intervention (Cancer et al., 2023).

Moreover, studies have promoted music training as a therapeutic tool for treating individuals with dyslexia (Bishop-Liebler et al., 2014; Cogo-Moreira et al., 2012, 2013; Weiss et al., 2014). Habib et al. (2016) tested the efficacy of a cognitive-musical program. Such a program encompasses a series of musical exercises emphasizing rhythmic perception and production to train various features of the musical auditory signals. Generally, the cognitive-musical method involves simultaneously visual, auditory, somatosensory, and motor systems. The method is founded on the music-language analogies, on the temporal and rhythmic features of music, and on cross-modal integration. The study (Habib et al., 2016) showed significant improvement in categorical and auditory perception of temporal components of speech in children with dyslexia. Authors revealed additional benefits also in auditory attention, phonological awareness (syllable fusion), reading abilities, and nonword repetition. Importantly, most beneficial effects persisted after an untrained period of 6 weeks. However, some limits of the study could be pointed out. In particular, the study was not a randomized controlled trial, and there was no control group with another training regimen for comparing effects. Improvement could be obtained by the specific music program, but it could also derive from ameliorating general attentional abilities. Some studies investigated the connection between rhythmic abilities and cognitive development. Specifically, Tierney and Kraus (2013) demonstrated correlations between synchronization with a metronome and both attentional and reading abilities in typically developing adolescents, based on the knowledge that rhythm perception is related to reading performance (Huss et al., 2011). Recently, Vonthron et al. (2024) developed a successful serious game called Mila-Learn, based on rhythmic training for children with dyslexia, which makes training remotely accessible and consistently reproducible. In sum, the literature on music training is still poor and exclusively directed to children. It is necessary to develop controlled trials concerning music as an effective intervention program, both for children and adults with dyslexia.

Another promising approach focusing on improving basic processing for greater fluency and accuracy included Rapid Automatized Naming (RAN). This program aims to enhance the speed at which people recognize and name letters and images, addressing one of the key cognitive deficits associated with dyslexia. After 3 months of intensive home exercises, 24 children with dyslexia showed significant improvements in reading speed and accuracy. These results suggest that RAN-based training, which avoids the direct use of alphanumeric stimuli, represents a promising strategy for children with severe reading difficulties or those at risk of developing them (Pecini et al., 2019). However, low-level function programs to improve reading in adults with dyslexia were also proposed in adults (Harrar et al., 2014), demonstrating that adults with dyslexia distribute attention asymmetrically between auditory and visual modalities, more than controls. For individuals with dyslexia, crossmodal shifts of attention only appear to be problematic for attention shifts from vision to audition—and, importantly, not vice versa—causing especially delayed responses to auditory stimuli that directly follow visual stimuli. The result that adults with dyslexia showed difficulties in disengaging their attention from visual stimuli and shifting it to auditory stimuli brings authors to the hypothesis—which needs to be tested—that adults with dyslexia might learn audiovisual phonological associations faster if they first hear the sound, and then see the corresponding letter/word, since crossmodal shifts from audition to vision were not sluggish.

In sum, the efficacy of low-level function programs needs to be more carefully documented, while phonics interventions appear to be the most efficient treatments to improve reading skills, although they seem to have more effects on reading accuracy and only a little on reading fluency. As the reading process becomes automatic, it demands less conscious effort, and the reader develops what is called automaticity. The development of reading fluency with the reduction of the effort for word identification is crucial for the comprehension of text (Norton & Wolf, 2012).

Starting from the hypothesis that fluency constitutes a critical parameter of skilled reading and time-constrained reading (that is, being forced to read at a rate faster than one's habitual reading rate) can significantly improve reading accuracy and comprehension (the "acceleration phenomenon"), Breznitz et al. (2013) proposed a reading acceleration training. The reading acceleration training (Horowitz-Kraus & Breznitz, 2013) is a program that presents texts in an accelerated mode, after determining the individual's typical reading rate. For each sentence, the letters disappeared one at a time, according to the participant's mean reading rate (ms/letter). As the reading skills improve, the erasure speed is adjusted to meet the new demands. The method gradually pushes the individual to improved reading speed, and it has been shown to have a positive effect during reading in children (Breznitz & Berman, 1997; Horowitz-Kraus et al., 2014). The computerized reading acceleration training protocol that introduced time constraints has also been proposed to adults with dyslexia to improve their reading fluency skills and reading comprehension. The acceleration manipulation significantly improved the ability to recognize words automatically (lexical representations), resulting in better reading fluency, as measured in seconds per word (Horowitz-Kraus, 2016), and the benefit in adults with dyslexia was retained 6 months post-training (Breznitz et al., 2013). Moreover, accelerating reading could reduce distractibility, circumvent working memory limitations, and increase readers' reliance on stimulus-driven word decoding (Horowitz-Kraus, 2016; Horowitz-Kraus & Breznitz, 2013).

A recent systematic review of the literature underlines the ameliorative effect on reading rate and fluency in children and adults with dyslexia after an Action Video Games (AVG) training (Peters et al., 2019), described as a fun, motivational, and engaging intervention for dyslexia (Peters et al., 2021). AVG are distinguished from other types of video games for specific characteristics like speed, high sensory-motor load, and presentation of multiple, peripheral, rapidly moving, and spatial-temporally unpredictable stimuli. By activating both spatial and temporal attention at the same time, AVG enable individuals to enlarge the size of their useful field of view and to improve the fast discrimination of a rapid sequence of visual stimuli as well as the perception of visual global motion in noise. AVG training produced learning that, by rapidly orienting the attentional spotlight, transfers beyond attentional components and has a positive effect on reading fluency. The spotlight of visual attention in individuals with dyslexia is sluggish and weaker in comparison to chronological age and reading level controls, and it is considered a crucial deficit in dyslexia (Roach et al., 2007; Bosse et al., 2007; Franceschini et al., 2013; Moores et al., 2015). The attentional deficit could reduce the success of traditional dyslexia treatments, because learning ability is hampered by spatial and temporal attention dysfunction. Thus, treatment of attentional deficits could be crucial in dyslexia remediation. This hypothesis was tested (Franceschini et al., 2013) by evaluating reading, phonological, and attentional skills in two matched groups of children with dyslexia before and after they played action or non-action video games for nine sessions of 80 min per day. Results documented that 12 hours of playing AVG improved children's visual attention and reading speed (as measured as time, in seconds, necessary to read the specific item, depending of the task), without any cost in terms of accuracy (as measured as the ratio between the correct response and the total number of items), more than 1 year of spontaneous reading. Moreover, Franceschini et al. (2017) have demonstrated that even in a language with a deep orthography as English, playing action video games has a positive effect on reading. In particular, regardless of orthography, children with dyslexia ameliorated their reading speed as well as visual, auditory, and cross-modal attentional shifting, with cascading effects on audio-visual processing and phonological working memory, without a direct targeting of phonological, orthographic, or grapheme-to-phoneme decoding. Recently, Peters et al. (2021) stated that short AVG training significantly improves reading accuracy, rate, comprehension, and rapid naming. Evidence for the efficacy of AVG in improving reading abilities has also been found in adult populations. Particularly, by comparing two groups of young adults who were either AVG players or non-players, Antzaka et al. (2017) documented that the effect of AVG on reading extended to thirty-six French adult expert readers. Moreover, a study investigating the combined effects of AVG and neuromodulation on young adults with dyslexia (Bertoni et al., 2024) demonstrated that the posterior parietal cortex stimulation during training improved temporal attention, reading of word texts, and pseudoword decoding. Moreover, the intervention resulted in an increased P300 amplitude, indicative of improved attentional control and the ability to resist distraction. The authors interpreted the results as an indication that the visual attention span (a component of visual attention defined as the number of distinct visual elements) could be a core component mediating this effect. The interpretation derived from the evidence is that AVG players performed a visual attention span task and a reading task better than the other group, and that performance on these tasks was correlated.

In conclusion, the exploration of various reading remediation strategies for adults with dyslexia highlights the ongoing potential for neuroplasticity throughout life, challenging earlier beliefs that cognitive improvements are predominantly confined to childhood. The efficacy of phonics training remains well-supported, enhancing reading accuracy and spelling, while recent advancements suggest that combining interventions, such as AVG with neuromodulation, can further improve reading fluency and attentional control. Additionally, novel approaches like rhythmic auditory training and acceleration techniques offer promising results in enhancing reading speed and comprehension. Despite these advancements, the challenge of generalizing interventions across different languages and individual needs persists. Future research should focus on refining these interventions, assessing their long-term effectiveness, and exploring how to best integrate various methods to support comprehensive literacy development in adults with dyslexia.

10.3 Neural Changes Following Remediation

Studies in children with dyslexia documented that remedial treatment improves not only reading abilities but also modifies activation in critical brain areas (Aylward et al., 2003; Richards et al., 2000; Shaywitz et al., 2004; Simos et al., 2002; Temple et al., 2003).

Before examining brain changes following remediation in dyslexia, it is helpful to first refer to Table 10.2, which provides an overview of the main neuroimaging techniques used to investigate reading-related brain mechanisms. Among these, functional magnetic resonance imaging (fMRI) has been instrumental in revealing the distributed neural systems that support reading: an anterior system, primarily located in the inferior frontal gyrus, and two essential posterior systems: one in the parieto-temporal region (dorsal stream) and another in the occipito-temporal region (ventral stream) (Philipose et al., 2007; Price, 2000; Shaywitz, 2003; Turkeltaub et al., 2002).

Figure 10.1 summarizes the main regions of interest (ROIs) within these networks, highlighting both their role in typical reading and the alterations observed in individuals with dyslexia. All of these regions have been found to have a role in the reading process (Graves et al., 2010; Turkeltaub et al., 2002), and some studies have investigated their specific contribution.

The anterior system seems particularly involved in the output of phonological and articulatory as well as semantic aspects of word reading (Jobard et al., 2003; Price, 2000). The first posterior dorsal system is considered crucial in

TABLE 10.2 Brain Imaging Techniques

Technique	Description
Magnetic Resonance Imaging (MRI)	MRI provides detailed, high-quality, and high-resolution brain images. The MRI machine is a giant magnet, drum-shaped with an opening on one end. Individuals lie on a movable bed that slowly enters the drum's opening. Through this process, a computer generates scans of the brain's tissues and replicates the brain's structure in amazing detail. Several "slices" of the brain are imaged: side, frontal, and horizontal views of the brain.
Positron Emission Tomography (PET)	PET uses trace amounts of short-lived radioactive material to map functional processes in the brain. Areas of high radioactivity are associated with brain activity. PET offers quantitative analyses, allowing relative changes over time to be monitored as a disease process evolves or in response to a specific stimulus.
Single-photon emission computed tomography (SPECT)	SPECT is a type of nuclear imaging test that shows how blood flows to tissues and the brain. Tests have shown that it might be more sensitive to brain injury than MRI scanning because it can detect reduced blood flow to injured sites.
Functional Magnetic Resonance Imaging (fMRI)	fMRI is one of the most important functional brain scanning techniques. It detects the changes in blood oxygenation and flow that occur in response to neural activity. fMRI can be used to produce activation maps showing which parts of the brain are involved in a particular cognitive process.
Diffusion Tensor Imaging (DTI)	DTI is a pivotal technique for assessing brain microstructure and connectivity. It measures the directional diffusion of water molecules in tissue, which is particularly constrained along white matter fiber tracts in the brain. By analyzing this anisotropic diffusion, DTI generates detailed maps of white matter pathways, revealing structural connectivity patterns critical for understanding brain function and integrity.
Electroencephalogram (EEG)	EEG is the measurement of the electrical activity of the brain by recording from electrodes placed on the scalp. EEGs are frequently used in experimentation because the process is non-invasive. The EEG is capable of detecting changes in electrical activity in the brain on a millisecond level. It is one of the few techniques available that has such high temporal resolution.
Magneto-encephalogram (MEG)	MEG is an imaging technique used to measure the magnetic fields produced by electrical activity in the brain. These measurements are commonly used in both research and clinical settings, including assisting surgeons in localizing a pathology, assisting researchers in determining the function of various parts of the brain, neurofeedback, and others.
Near infrared spectroscopy (NIRS)	NIRS is an optical technique for measuring blood oxygenation in the brain. How much the light is attenuated depends on blood oxygenation, and thus NIRS can provide an indirect measure of brain activity.

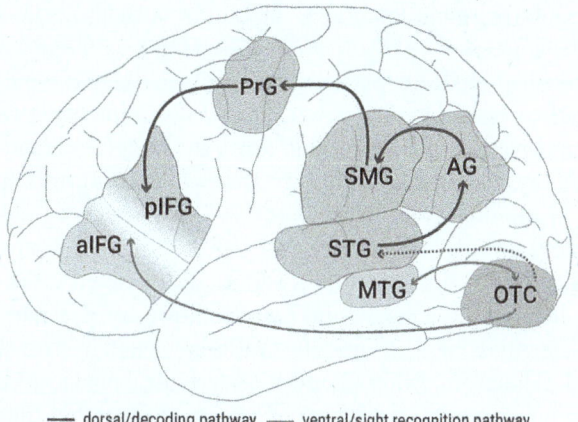

— dorsal/decoding pathway   — ventral/sight recognition pathway

FIGURE 10.1 A neurobiological dual-stream model of reading. Adapted from Turker and Hartwigsen (2022).

mapping the visual percept of print onto the sounds (phonology) of spoken language (Shaywitz, 2003), while the second posterior ventral system is particularly involved in skilled, fluent reading (i.e., rapid and automatic reading) (Cohen et al., 2000; Vinckier et al., 2007). In dyslexia, alterations in the two crucial posterior systems have been consistently found. Particularly, there is functional neuroimaging evidence of hypoactivation of the left parieto-temporal and occipito-temporal regions in both children and adults with dyslexia when they perform reading-related tasks (Hoeft et al., 2006, 2007; Richlan et al., 2009, 2011; Pugh et al., 2000; Shaywitz et al., 2002, 2007).

Successful reading is mediated by a growth of activation (Hoeft et al., 2011) in these posterior regions of the left hemisphere, found typically hypoactive in adults with dyslexia ("normalization") and in regions of the right hemisphere not usually involved in typical reading ("compensation").

Although effective remedial treatments determine the development of cognitive functions, the brain's aptitude to restructure itself and the neural plasticity are crucial for the remediation, the neurobiological correlates of reading improvement in adults with dyslexia have not been widely investigated (Ben-Soussan et al., 2014; Eden et al., 2004; Horowitz-Kraus, 2016; Pecyna & Pokorski, 2013). Neural plasticity refers to the ability of neurons to change in structure and function in response to an external stimulus. Neuroplasticity occurs as neurons respond to the activities of adjacent neurons that are spontaneously active or are activated by events in the external environment. Neural plasticity largely results from changes in the strengths of synaptic connections between neurons and the formation of new connections. Neural plasticity is essential for the normal development of brain circuits, creating the differences in those circuits that make us individuals. Neural plasticity mediates the acquisition of knowledge and skill, and brain repair after injury (Buonomano & Johnson, 2009).

Studies about treatment outcomes in adults with dyslexia are relatively small, and the functional reorganization following treatment is little known. The neurobiological basis for plasticity in adults is likely to be different from that in children, as reading and its associated skills in the pediatric population are dynamic and continuously changing throughout development (Eden et al., 2004). Specifically, the frontal lobes are the last to mature (Chugani, 1998; Fuster, 2002; Huttenlocher & Dabholkar, 1997) and are recruited by adults to a different extent than by children (Schlaggar et al., 2002; Simos et al., 2001; Turkeltaub et al., 2003) during reading and reading-related tasks.

Moreover, in adults, the behavioral manifestations of dyslexia are relatively stable, and plasticity is likely to manifest differently in a system that is mature and stabilized. Therefore, brain changes underlying behavioral plasticity can confidently be interpreted as treatment effects in adults rather than the interaction effect between the development of cognitive and sensorimotor systems and the time span of the treatment, which most likely happens in children. The neural correlates of reading remediation and effective intervention strategies for adults with dyslexia were derived both from findings in acquired reading disorders and in developmental dyslexia. Regarding acquired reading disorders, brain changes were found in a patient with stroke on the left frontotemporal cortex (Small et al., 1998), who, after a phonologically based reading intervention (training the decomposition of words into parts in order to make grapheme to phoneme conversion), increased the left lingual gyrus activity. A remedial training to teach word decoding and to identify individual sounds and blends in words (Adair et al., 2000) was proposed for an alexic patient with the right hemisphere inactive during nonword reading. After treatment, nonword reading increased activity in the posterior right perisylvian cortices homologous to the dominant hemisphere areas engaged by reading. Brain activity also increased in Broca's area of both hemispheres. More recently, Cohen et al. (2016) described a single-case longitudinal study of an individual with pure alexia due to a small left fusiform lesion, accompanied by a loss of *visual word form area* responsivity and by the degeneration of the associated white matter pathways. The patient was followed up for two years, and results showed a progressive improvement in reading that was not associated with the re-emergence of a new area selective to words, but with increasing responses in the spared occipital cortex posterior to the lesion and in the contralateral right occipital cortex. Moreover, those regions showed a nonspecific increase in activations over time and a functional correlation with distant language areas. Similarly, Kim and Lemke (2016) described a single-case longitudinal study with acquired aphasia after a left hemisphere stroke, presenting a spoken language profile consistent with anomic aphasia. After 12 weeks of oral reading treatment, the patient's eye movement patterns changed, indicating a shift towards a more efficient reading strategy. Specifically, before treatment, the patient tended to fixate closer to the beginning of words, while after treatment, his initial fixation position shifted towards the optimal viewing position, resulting in more efficient reading. However, contrary to expectations, the number of fixations, regressions, and fixation durations increased after treatment, indicating a higher level of cognitive processing during reading. Despite this increase, the patient's comprehension improved, suggesting that the increased eye movement parameters may be related to improved comprehension strategies rather than reading efficiency.

In sum, findings on brain changes after acquired reading disorders seemed to involve brain regions targeted by the specific training and an increase of activation in regions adjacent to those injured, but also in homologous contralateral regions.

Regarding developmental dyslexia, a first study aimed at examining the physiological consequences of reading intervention on adults was conducted by Eden et al. (2004). Authors employed a controlled design in which a group of adults with dyslexia received 112 hours of structured multisensory phonological intervention, and a control group of adults with dyslexia did not receive any treatment. While prior to the intervention, the two groups did not differ on measures of single-word, nonword, and text reading, after treatment, the abilities that were directly targeted by the instructional method (phonological processing through auditory and visual modalities) improved significantly only in the treated group. Significant improvements were also observed on nonword reading efficiency, text reading accuracy, but not on reading speed and comprehension. Following the instructional method, the adults with dyslexia showed improvement on skills directly targeted by the intervention (i.e., phonemic awareness and visual imagery) and on reading skills reliant on phonological awareness. The behavioral changes were also accompanied by neural changes. Indeed, high intervention-related brain activities were observed in the left hemisphere inferior parietal lobule, intraparietal sulcus, and fusiform gyrus during the phonological manipulation. In the right hemisphere, numerous foci of significant increases were observed, with more pronounced changes in the posterior superior temporal cortex, angular gyrus, superior parietal cortex, and inferior frontal cortex. These latter two regions are homotopic to areas seen in normal readers in the left hemisphere. In sum, neural correlates of phonologically based instruction indicate increased activity of the left parietal cortex (as observed for typical readers), as well as compensatory mechanisms in the right hemisphere perisylvian regions, most notably parietal cortex.

The progress made in understanding the neurophysiology of reading intervention in adults has been described in a recent systematic review of the literature (Braid & Richlan, 2022). Several studies have found increased brain activity in the left hemisphere reading areas after reading training in individuals with reading difficulties (Heim et al., 2015; Horowitz-Kraus et al., 2014). This suggests that with targeted training, the typical reading network functions can improve in people with dyslexia. Moreover, in some studies, the differences in brain activity between individuals with dyslexia and typical readers were less noticeable after training (Meyler et al., 2008; Richards et al., 2006). In other studies, an increased brain activity of the right hemisphere and sub-cortical regions was described, suggesting the activation of some compensatory process engaging regions outside the typical reading network in order to make up for the reading deficits (Meyler et al., 2008; Nugiel et al., 2019; Partanen et al., 2019).

Consistently across studies, the most notable improvements were seen in the right inferior frontal gyrus (IFG) (Horowitz-Kraus et al., 2014; Meyler et al., 2008; Partanen et al., 2019). The right IFG is active during reading even before training, and individuals who showed more activity there initially tended to show greater improvement after training (Hoeft et al., 2011). The right IFG seems to be involved in articulatory recoding, working memory, and attention during reading (Shaywitz et al., 2002; Hancock et al., 2017).

This result in adults with developmental dyslexia substantiated what was found in lesional studies, demonstrating that behavioral plasticity is realized by enhancing the activity of the left lateralized linguistic areas and of the right hemisphere regions. However, the right hemisphere engagement, found by authors (Eden et al., 2004) even prior to the intervention (perhaps reflecting a degree of compensation), dramatically increases after the training. This vast increase in adults with dyslexia could be related to training-dependent processes in the context of restricted availability of left-hemisphere regions, in much the same way as reported in stroke patients (Rijntjes & Weiller, 2002), and was larger than that observed in pediatric studies. Indeed, remediation studies on children with dyslexia did not consistently report such right hemisphere changes during phonological training (Aylward et al., 2003) or even showed a decrease in right hemisphere utilization following intervention (Simos et al., 2002).

The degree of plasticity exhibited by the mature brain might be greater than originally believed (Kaas, 2002; Nudo et al., 1996), but the formation of new intracortical connections is very limited (Kaas, 2002) and an unlikely cause of adult plasticity. The functional shifts to the right hemisphere observed in adults with developmental dyslexia in not unlike those following left hemisphere brain lesions acquired early in life, for example, inducing language representation in the homotopic areas of the undamaged right hemisphere (Staudt et al., 2002).

Brain changes after cognitive training in adults with developmental dyslexia were not only documented by neuroimaging studies. In order to improve reading performance, the Quadrato Motor Training, which targeted cerebellar functioning, was proposed to adults with developmental dyslexia (Ben-Soussan et al., 2014). Indeed, competent reading skills are sustained by implicit learning abilities based on cerebellar involvement. Evidence showed that children and adults with dyslexia are impaired on cerebellar implicit learning paradigms

(Fawcett et al., 2001; Fawcett & Nicolson, 1999; Ivry & Justus, 2001; Menghini et al., 2006; Sperling et al., 2004; Stoodley & Stein, 2011; Vicari et al., 2003). The Quadrato Motor Training is a structured sensorimotor training program that involves the sequencing of motor responses based on verbal commands. Using magnetoencephalography, the authors measured changes in alpha power and coherence following the training in twenty-two adult Hebrew readers (twelve with developmental dyslexia and ten controls). Reading performance was assessed pre- and post-training using a comprehensive battery of behavioral tests. Results demonstrated improved performance on a speeded reading task (a list of forty-five written words of increasing difficulty was presented, and participants were asked to accurately read as many words as possible from the list in 1 min) following 1 month of intensive training in both the adults with dyslexia and the control group. Participants with dyslexia, but not controls, showed a significant increase in cerebellar oscillatory alpha power following training. In addition, inter-hemispheric alpha coherence was higher in adults with dyslexia than in controls. These findings suggested that the combination of motor and language training embedded in the Quadrato Motor Training increased cerebellar oscillatory activity in adults with dyslexia and improved and supported the hypothesis that the cerebellum plays a role in skilled reading. Another study (Horowitz-Kraus, 2016) found electroencephalographic changes after treatment in adults with developmental dyslexia. Specifically, two event-related potential components were investigated, that is, the error-related and correct-response negativity, which changed after treatment in adults with dyslexia. Usually, the error-related negativity component is evoked when there is a mismatch between the neural representation of the correct and the actual response (Bernstein et al., 1995). In contrast, correct-response negativity reflects imprecise perception or incomplete processing of a stimulus, which causes uncertainty regarding the desired response (Scheffers & Coles, 2000). These two components are evoked when there is a mismatch between the neural representation of the correct and the actual response. The study (Horowitz-Kraus, 2016) verified whether a reading training (a reading acceleration program) improved the ability to recognize words automatically (lexical representations) in adults with developmental dyslexia. Since it was documented that individuals with developmental dyslexia have a less active error-detection mechanism during reading than typical readers, the study also hypothesized a beneficial effect on error detection during reading. Results indicated that after training, reading scores improved, as well as error-related negativity amplitudes that were smaller in individuals with developmental dyslexia than in typical readers before training. Moreover, pre-training and post-training differences between error-related and correct-response negativity components were larger in individuals with developmental dyslexia than in typical readers. The effect of the treatment in participants with dyslexia may attest to the plasticity of the brain, and the increased activation of the error-detection mechanism may indicate a more efficient processing between the correct and the actual responses.

In summary, both fMRI and electroencephalographic changes have been observed in adults with developmental dyslexia and have been mostly linked to the specific training performed. Cognitive remediation elicited brain changes by normalizing cerebral activity in the typical reading regions and by compensatory mechanisms in the contralateral homologues.

In order to develop more targeted and effective reading interventions, future studies should define more specific training with distinctive characteristics. The inclusion of multiple control groups that undergo a variety of interventions is needed to identify the most effective training technique. Long-term outcome studies with longitudinal evaluations of cognitive and brain measures should better identify changes in adults with developmental dyslexia after remedial treatment.

10.4 Brain-induced Plasticity by Neuromodulation

Given the critical role of specific brain regions in reading, the brain alterations found in adults with dyslexia, and the evidence of plasticity after a remediation program (Eden et al., 2004; Temple et al., 2003), directly inducing brain changes could open a new perspective in remedial reading disorders. The use of neuromodulation, including EEG-based Neurofeedback (NF) and non-invasive brain stimulation (NIBS) as transcranial magnetic stimulation (TMS) or transcranial electrical stimulation (tES), provides the opportunity to go beyond traditional cognitive treatments. Specifically, neuromodulation techniques (see Table 10.3 for more details) have been proposed as a promising tool to enhance cognitive functions in individuals with learning disabilities (Cancer et al., 2021; Eroğlu et al., 2022; Frye et al., 2008; Krause & Cohen Kadosh, 2013; Turker & Hartwigsen, 2022; Vicario & Nitsche, 2013a, 2013b). NIBS is a group of tools used to alter neural membrane polarization, inducing currents to and within the brain for therapeutic or research purposes (Krishnan et al., 2015). Given NIBS' capacity to modulate neural network activity, it may have a meaningful role in the diagnosis, monitoring, and treatment of a wide range of neurodevelopmental disorders. Compared to NIBS, NF has fewer exclusion criteria (Marzbani et al., 2016) and is frequently utilized in clinical settings for neurodevelopmental disorders across all age groups (e.g., ADHD patients; Holtmann et al., 2014).

If a limited number of studies are published on cognitive remediation and on brain modification after training in adults with developmental dyslexia, even fewer studies are conducted on the efficacy of neuromodulation (Turker & Hartwigsen, 2022).

One prominent NF protocol is Lubar's (Lubar, 1991), originally designed for ADHD patients, which has also been applied to individuals with dyslexia,

TABLE 10.3 Non-invasive Brain Stimulation (NIBS) Techniques

Transcranial Magnetic Stimulation (TMS)

TMS is a non-invasive method to stimulate neurons in the brain and induce immediate or long-term changes in activity. It is a cost-effective NIBS method used in a laboratory. It uses a rapidly changing electric current within a conducting coil to generate a strong, but relatively focal, magnetic field. The coil is connected to a pulse generator, or stimulator, that delivers electric current to the coil. When applied to the scalp, the magnetic field induces electrical activity in the underlying brain tissue, temporarily interfering with local cortical information processing. The stimulation is delivered to the brain by passing a strong, brief electrical current through an insulated wire coil placed on the skull. Depending on the frequency, duration of the stimulation, and the strength of the magnetic field, TMS can activate or suppress activity in cortical regions.

Transcranial Electrical Stimulation (tES)

tES induces a subthreshold modulation of neuronal membrane potentials, altering excitability and neurotransmitter activity. The peculiarity of the tool is that it alters spontaneous neural activity. tES consists in the application of two or more electrodes to an individual's scalp to induce an electrical current through the cortex. While a large amount of the current is conducted between electrodes through soft tissue and skull, a portion of the current penetrates the scalp and reaches the brain, where it can modify neuronal excitability. tES includes various techniques, including transcranial direct current stimulation (tDCS), alternating current stimulation (tACS), and random noise stimulation (tRNS). Although these techniques are similar in that they are applied through electrodes placed on the scalp, electrical patterns and, therefore, behavioral and neuronal outcomes differ.

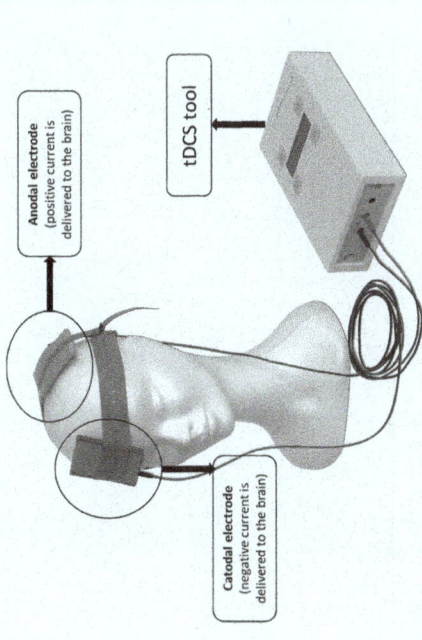

(*Continued*)

TABLE 10.3 (Continued)

EEG-based Neurofeedback (NF)	NF allows individuals to learn how to self-regulate their brain activity. By providing real-time information about brain functioning through an EEG pattern, NF enables individuals to observe and modify their brainwave, which is then displayed to the individual in the form of visual or auditory feedback, to achieve desired outcomes. One of the key principles underlying NF is operant conditioning, where individuals are rewarded for producing specific brainwave patterns associated with desired states of mind, such as relaxation or focus. Through repeated sessions of neurofeedback training, individuals can learn to modulate their brain activity and improve cognitive function, emotional regulation, and overall well-being.

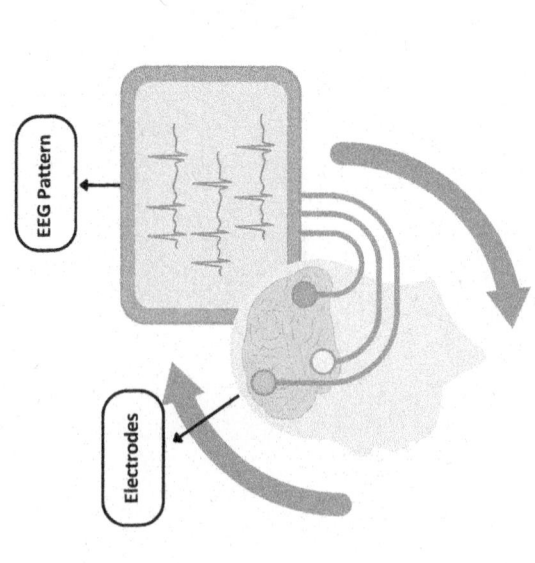

TMS vs tES

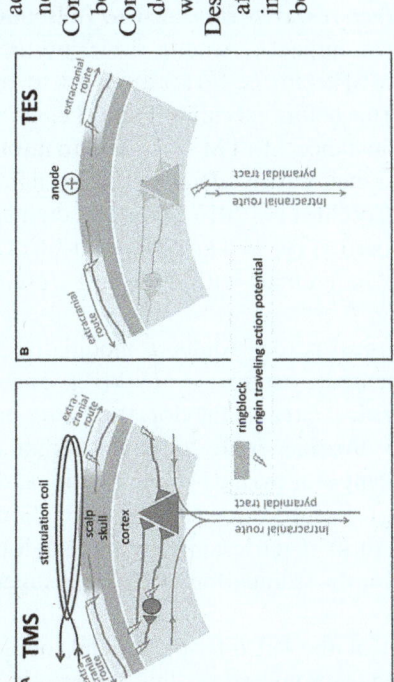

Differences between tES and TMS include presumed mechanisms of action, with TMS acting as a neuro-stimulator and tES as a neuromodulator.

Compared to tES, TMS has better spatial and temporal resolution and has better-established protocols.

Compared to TMS, tES has the advantage of being easier to use in double-blind or sham-controlled studies and easier to apply concurrently with behavioral tasks.

Despite their differences, both TMS and tES could induce long-term after-effects on cortical excitability that may translate into behavioral impacts that can last for months. These long-term after-effects are believed to engage mechanisms of neural plasticity.

due to the high comorbidity between the two conditions. The protocol aims to increase β frequencies while decreasing θ frequencies, enhancing attentional skills and visuo-motor integration. Research indicates that this approach can positively influence reading abilities and improve auditory vigilance and phonological awareness.

Other studies have similarly adopted the β/θ ratio. For example, Nazari et al. (2012) demonstrated significant enhancements in phonological awareness and reading skills, alongside changes in brainwave coherence, and designed personalized treatments, identifying hypo-coherence between specific brain regions. Sadeghi and Nazari (2015) observed behavioral improvements in visuo-spatial attention, and Raesi et al. (2017) reported improvements in accuracy, comprehension, and spelling after NF training. More recently, Eroğlu et al. (2020) utilized multiscale entropy analysis and individualized NF training based on participants' EEG activity, leading to increased brainwave complexity in participants with dyslexia. Moreover, in a recent study protocol by Cancer et al. (2021), it has been proposed that the evaluation of a single-session bilateral NF protocol targeting hemispheric imbalances in the temporo-parietal (TP) areas to improve reading in adults with dyslexia. The protocol aimed to increase the β/θ ratio in the left TP areas while decreasing the β/θ ratio in the contralateral area during linguistic tasks, with a focus on reinforcing attentional skills and visuo-motor integration (Au et al., 2014). Overall, these studies highlight the potential of NF training to address various cognitive and linguistic deficits associated with dyslexia; however, further research is needed to fully understand their effectiveness and long-term impacts. Among TMS protocols, high-frequency repetitive TMS (hf-rTMS) trains (≥ 5 Hz) are used to transiently enhance the excitability of the cortex before executing a task (Peinemann et al., 2004; Rothkegel et al., 2010). For instance, hf-rTMS was used to improve linguistic abilities in adults, producing ameliorative effects in picture naming (Cappa et al., 2002; Cotelli et al., 2008; Cotelli et al., 2010, 2006) and digit span (Duzel et al., 1996). It has been proposed (Frye et al., 2008) that hf-rTMS could also enhance reading abilities in individuals with dyslexia by exciting underactive neural pathways for reading.

In our previous study on Italian typical reader adults, a modulator 5Hz hf-rTMS effect on reading was documented(Costanzo et al., 2012). The coil was applied, bilaterally, over the two critical sites of the dorsal reading pathway (Cohen et al., 2000; Shaywitz, 2003; Vinckier et al., 2007), the left inferior parietal lobule and the right superior temporal gyrus, before specific reading tasks (word, nonword, and text reading). Results documented a reduction of nonword reading errors after the stimulation of the left inferior parietal lobule and an increase in text reading errors after the stimulation of the right superior temporal gyrus.

Our results support the involvement of the left inferior parietal lobule in grapheme/phoneme transduction needed for nonword reading. Moreover, it is possible that the negative outcome after stimulation of the right superior temporal gyrus comes from the interhemispheric competitive effect, with the right superior temporal gyrus having an inhibitory influence on the left homologous area, generally involved in whole word and text reading (Vinckier et al., 2007).

A similar stimulation protocol was applied in a group of Italian adults with dyslexia (Costanzo et al., 2013) to improve their reading abilities. For this purpose, 5Hz hf-rTMS was applied over the same critical sites of our previous study (Costanzo et al., 2012) underactive in individuals with dyslexia during reading and reading-related tasks (Pugh et al., 2000; Shaywitz et al., 2002). Results showed that 5Hz hf-rTMS over the left inferior parietal lobule improved nonword reading accuracy (number of errors) and over the left superior temporal gyrus increased word reading speed total time in seconds) and text reading accuracy. Moreover, nonword reading accuracy also improved after the right inferior parietal lobule stimulation. A recent study conducted by Turker et al. (2023), based on previous results, investigated the effects of TMS in typical adult readers on the left temporo-parietal cortex (TPC), a region that plays a key role in phonological decoding and that seems to be inhibited in dyslexia (Habib, 2021). Indeed, the authors found that the effects of TPC inhibition on reading performance displayed significant variability among participants and promoted short-term plasticity that could be a compensatory mechanism to prevent performance disruption (Turker et al., 2023).

These findings indicate that in adults with dyslexia, the two sites of the left dorsal reading pathway have a differential role in word, nonword, and text reading. The result of a right inferior parietal lobule involvement suggests there is an additional compensatory recruitment of the right hemisphere regions in adults with dyslexia. In conclusion, for the first time, it was proven that distinctive facilitation of a neural pathway known to be underactive in dyslexia may transitorily improve reading abilities in adults with dyslexia. Such an ameliorative effect opens new perspectives for the development of NIBS treatment protocols in both adults and children with developmental dyslexia.

As concerns electrical stimulation, transcranial direct current stimulation (tDCS), transcranial alternating current stimulation (tACS), and transcranial random noise stimulation (tRNS) belong to a group of tools that are used to alter neural membrane polarization, inducing currents to and within the brain for therapeutic or research purposes (Bertoni et al., 2024; Krishnan et al., 2015; Marchesotti et al., 2020; Reed & Cohen Kadosh, 2018). Of importance, previous studies conducted in both adults and children demonstrated the tolerability of these techniques (Antal et al., 2017; Bikson et al., 2016; Bikson et al., 2023). tDCS is a polarity-dependent technique that consists of the application of a weak direct electrical current (1–2 mA) to the scalp, facilitating the flow of current from the electrodes (i.e., anode and cathode) to the scalp. Similarly, tACS applies electrical stimulation to the scalp, but in the form of alternating current, while tRNS applies electrical current at a random frequency and amplitude within a specific range. All these techniques are portable, comfortable, cost-effective, and can be used repeatedly with potential long-term efficacy, making them suitable for a wide range of applications and disorders.

tDCS, tACS, and tRNS have been used in typical reading adults to improve reading efficiency (Bertoni et al., 2024; Marchesotti et al., 2020; Rufener & Zaehle, 2021; Thomson et al., 2015; Turkeltaub et al., 2012). Specifically, Turkeltaub et al. (2012) studied the effect on reading in adults, enhancing left lateralization of the posterior temporal cortex by tDCS. They hypothesized that reading efficiency (derived from the Test of Word Reading Efficiency – TOWRE – in which participants read aloud a list of real words or nonwords as quickly as possible) and reading-related skills (i.e., access to lexical, semantic, or phonological representation) might increase, and that individuals with low reading skills might receive higher benefit in reading from NIBS. Twenty-five right-handed native English speakers were recruited for the study, and after 20-minute stimulation sessions (1.5 mA real tDCS and sham), participants underwent several reading tasks. The results indicated that only the word reading efficiency improved after 1.5 mA real tDCS and that the beneficial effect was higher in participants with low reading skills than in more fluent readers. The study documented that enhancing left lateralization of the posterior temporal cortex using tDCS short-term positive effect in reading (in word reading efficiency), especially in participants with low reading skills. Thus, tDCS could be considered a useful tool, particularly for individuals with reading difficulties, and the first promising neuromodulatory remediation for dyslexia.

A following study by Thomson and collaborators (2015) was conducted in a group of thirty-nine typical adult readers. This double-blind crossover study was aimed at determining the impact of 20 min 2 mA tDCS stimulation (anodal vs cathodal) over homologous brain regions (left vs right temporo-parietal junction) on reading and phonological abilities. The results revealed a significant effect of hemisphere stimulation on reading efficiency (from TOWRE-2; Torgesen et al., 2011). The largest hemispheric change was seen for word efficiency, with a performance decrement seen for the left hemisphere stimulation. However, a positive effect on reading speed was found following the right hemisphere anodal stimulation. Nevertheless, concerning phonological abilities, no significant effect of hemisphere or polarity effects was obtained. Relating these findings, the results obtained by Turkeltaub et al. (2012) appeared discrepant given the known dominance of the left hemisphere in language processing. Authors speculated that NIBS techniques are demonstrating the complex interplay between hemispheres and that the more widespread excitatory effect of anodal tDCS could result in unnatural competition from surrounding areas, thus reducing efficiency at the main processing site for a given skill. They also conjectured that when an individual's left hemisphere linguistic system is already functioning at an optimal level, there is less scope for left anodal tDCS to result in further improvement. In contrast, the activity of the right hemisphere may have more potential for enhancement, and there are precedents for such an explanation in other processing domains (Boggio et al., 2006).

The first study using tDCS in reading deficits was conducted in an adult with mild pure alexia due to chronic brain injury (Lacey et al., 2015). In this case report, 20 min 2 mA real high definition anodal tDCS was delivered over the left posterior temporal cortex for 5 days, and sham tDCS was delivered 10 days later for 5 days, both in combination with a reading training. Results revealed that tDCS may accelerate reading training effects in alexia therapy, such that fewer sessions are needed to train the same amount of material. The study documented that recovery of specific areas of the left hemisphere was crucial to reading recovery, and the left lateralization of posterior temporal activity was associated with improved reading performance.

A tDCS treatment protocol was also applied to adults with developmental dyslexia by Heth and Lavidor (2015). The study was designed within the framework of the magnocellular deficit theory and aimed at better understanding the contribution of the dorsal system to word reading. According to the Magnocellular-Dorsal (M-D) deficit, an impaired growing process of a group of neurons (magnocells) could lead to several difficulties in visual elaboration in individuals with dyslexia (see Boden & Giaschi, 2007). The magnocellular system is sensitive to low spatial and high temporal frequencies. It involves light/dark contrast detection and steady binocular fixation for the development of proper orthographic skills. First studies by Galaburda and Livingstone (1993) and Livingstone et al. (1991) reported anatomically abnormal magnocells in the lateral geniculate nucleus, a thalamic structure that receives information from the retina and projects to primary visual cortex (V1). Electrophysiological (Jednoróg et al., 2011) and fMRI (Demb et al., 1997) studies have also corroborated these findings by highlighting abnormal neural responses to magnocellular stimuli (as motion detection, perception of contrast sensitivity).

Twenty-three Hebrew adults with dyslexia were recruited (males and females, 18 years and older) and were randomly assigned to two groups (real tDCS and sham tDCS). Different tasks (including oral text reading, RAN, and symbol search) were administered before, immediately after, and 1 week after the end of the 20-minute 1.5 mA anodal tDCS over the left visual-extrastriate area MT/V5. Before and immediately after stimulation, reading speed did not significantly differ between real and sham tDCS groups. However, there was a significant difference in reading speed between the two groups 1 week after stimulation. No effect on reading errors was found. However, a recent study by Cummine et al. (2020) found weak-to-no evidence for an added effect of anodal stimulation on reading performance/speed for either skilled or impaired readers. The authors applied anodal tDCS to the left supramarginal gyrus (SMG) with the aim of improving reading performance in adult adults with dyslexia, including text reading, word reading, pseudoword reading, and rapid automatized naming. However, no significant improvement in reading performance following anodal tDCS of the left SMG/TPJ was reported, as well as following phoneme segmentation training. This suggests that either the left SMG does not play a critical role in reading in adults with dyslexia, or methodological limitations, such as training selection, contributed to the null findings. It is particularly surprising that phoneme segmentation training had no positive effects on performance, as improvements would typically be expected in this domain even among adults with dyslexia after adequate training (Turker & Hartwigsen, 2022).

Nevertheless, these results support the potential of NIBS in promoting reading abilities in dyslexia, even in the adult population. More encouraging results come from a study using tDCS treatment in children and adolescents with dyslexia (Battisti et al., 2022; Costanzo et al., 2016a, 2016b; Rahimi et al., 2022). Children and adolescents with dyslexia who received 18 sessions of 20 minutes of 1 mA anodal tDCS over left temporo-parietal regions (Costanzo et al., 2016b) and a cognitive phonological training ameliorated their performances in some reading tasks compared to participants who underwent the sham tDCS. The effects persisted even 1 month after the end of the treatment. A few years later, Rios et al. (2018) conducted an open-label, offline, tDCS study implementing changes to previous protocols for dyslexic children. They applied stimulation over the left anodal/right cathodal temporal cortex and supraorbital region, extended sessions to 30 minutes, and increased current intensity to 2mA. Results showed significant improvements in reading accuracy for text and nonword post-treatment. Two studies conducted between 2019 and 2020 investigated the effects of tDCS on reading measures. Costanzo et al. (2019), building on a previous trial, found that 26 participants in the active tDCS group showed improvements in low-frequency word reading accuracy and non-word reading speed, with effects lasting up to 6 months. Lazzaro et al. (2021a) explored clinical reading measures and individual variables, reporting enhanced word reading fluency after 20 minutes of active tDCS at 1mA compared to sham, with outcomes influenced by baseline reading performance, age, and IQ.

More recently, Lazzaro et al. further studied a tDCS-induced modulation of reading performance while assessing other processes relevant to reading, such as motion perception and visuospatial working memory (Lazzaro et al., 2021b). Left anodal/right cathodal tDCS of the left TPC (as in previous studies) improved text reading accuracy, word recognition, and motion perception. However, word or pseudoword reading was not significantly modulated as previously reported from studies of the same group. At the same time, stimulation changed the focus of attention. Moreover, improvement in text reading performance was explained by a change in visuospatial working memory following TPC stimulation. In a more recent clinical study (Battisti et al., 2022), children and adolescents with dyslexia received tDCS to enhance left neural excitability while decreasing right neural excitability of the TPC (LA/RC condition). Results showed an improvement in nonword reading, as reported in previous literature (Turker & Hartwigsen, 2022).

These results indicate that tDCS-induced improvements may be explained by modulation of basic reading processes, but may also reflect improvements in general domain support functions such as working memory and attention. Further research is needed to confirm this preliminary finding, but it highlights the complex interaction between regions and the functions to which they contribute (Turker & Hartwigsen, 2022).

Despite its central role in semantic and phonological processes, only one study to date has specifically investigated the influence of the left IFG in adults with dyslexia (Rodrigues de Almeida et al., 2019). In this study, researchers explored how different phonological workload conditions interacted with tDCS. In the experimental protocol, participants were involved in a total of six sessions, with two sessions dedicated to each of the three tDCS conditions: anodal, cathodal, and sham. Each experimental session involved performing specific tasks, such as categorical perception, lexical decision, and word naming. Stimuli were presented during the fMRI sessions. This approach allowed for systematic testing of each stimulation condition and comparison of the results obtained under different tDCS conditions.

Both anodal and cathodal tDCS were applied to the left IFG during activities such as word reading, lexical decision-making, and speech comprehension (categorical perception). Given the essential role of the left IFG in pseudoword processing, the authors expected to see improvements in pseudoword reading following stimulation. However, surprisingly, anodal tDCS improved speech comprehension but had no effect on speech production or word reading. A subsequent fMRI session was included to correlate behavioral changes with potential modulations in brain activity within the reading network, but no significant effects of tDCS on brain activation patterns in the left IFG or the TPC were found. Consequently, the reasons for these unexpected results remain unclear (Rodrigues de Almeida et al., 2019).

A detailed analysis of the results from tDCS studies, particularly those examining the left TPC, reveals a consistent pattern, especially in children. Stimulating the left TPC not only speeds up and improves accuracy in pseudoword reading for children and adolescents with dyslexia but may also positively influence the reading of low-frequency words and texts. However, since neurostimulation primarily affects the decoding process, it is unlikely to have a direct impact on text reading, especially in adolescents who, despite their difficulties, tend to rely on visual word reading. Therefore, further investigation is needed to understand how this "decoding" center may influence text comprehension. Regarding adults with dyslexia, the effect of tDCS on TPC seemed to improve both word-reading speed and text comprehension accuracy. Although these results should be interpreted with caution due to the limited number of studies, they clearly suggest that reading is mediated by large-scale brain networks rather than by localized brain modules. In summary, evidence indicates that non-invasive brain stimulation can enhance reading performance through complex, distributed mechanisms rather than simply acting on specific brain areas (Turker & Hartwigsen, 2022 review).

Other tES protocols have been applied to improve reading using tACS or tRNS, based on neurophysiological hypotheses regarding the alteration of oscillations in dyslexia. In particular, it has been suggested that compromised auditory sampling and a particular lack of hemispheric specialization for gamma oscillations have been observed in adults with dyslexia (Lehongre et al., 2011; Morillon et al., 2012) and could influence the perception of acoustic cues and sensitivity to linguistic stimuli. Modulation of the auditory system may therefore lead to enhanced accuracy and reduced variability in categorical phoneme perception, potentially impacting phonological processing and thereby reading.

The study conducted by Rufener and colleagues examined the effectiveness of 40 Hz tACS and tRNS on the left auditory cortex to improve phonemic categorization in adolescents and adults with dyslexia. During three stimulation sessions while performing a phonemic categorization task, it was found that tACS significantly enhanced accuracy in categorizing voice onset time in adolescents, while tRNS showed positive effects in adult participants. Using EEG to assess the amplitude of auditory response (P50-N1), tACS was observed to increase this amplitude compared to placebo, indicating a relevant neurophysiological effect. In contrast, tRNS showed less pronounced effects both behaviorally and neurophysiologically in adults. These results suggest that tACS and tRNS may modulate auditory responses differently in individuals with dyslexia, with potential implications for optimizing stimulation techniques in neuromodulatory treatments (Rufener et al., 2019).

Furthermore, considering that tDCS does not target specific brain rhythms, the recent study conducted by Marchesotti et al. (2020) explores the potential of tACS as an intervention for adults with developmental dyslexia. By applying tACS, the authors aimed to modulate neural oscillations in the cortex, including auditory gamma peak frequencies. The study found a positive relationship between gamma oscillations and phonological awareness, suggesting a causal link between low-gamma activity in the left auditory cortex and deficits in phonological processes. Interestingly, tACS delivered at 30 Hz has been shown to be effective in enhancing phoneme processing and auditory temporal resolution. Similarly, Rufener and Zaehle (2021) suggest 40 Hz gamma-tACS over the auditory cortex as an effective clinical tool for modulating phoneme processing. These findings are significant for basic aspects of speech-processing research, as the relationship between low-gamma neural activity and phonemic encoding had previously only been theorized or inferred through correlational studies. Finally, aiming to advance the optimization of tES protocols for the treatment of dyslexia, a very recent ongoing study is comparing the effects of tDCS and tRNS on temporo-parietal regions in children and adolescents with dyslexia (Battisti et al., 2024).

Despite several studies being conducted on the use of NIBS for reading disorders, demonstrating positive effects on reading abilities in dyslexia, further evidence is needed to better define experimental parameters. In particular, it is crucial to clarify electrode configurations, the optimal stimulation protocol, the duration, and the long-term effectiveness of NIBS to open new treatment perspectives for reading disorders (Santos et al., 2021).

10.5 Perspective and Clinical Practice

Although the definition of dyslexia is widely accepted among specialists (APA, 2022), the effectiveness of treatments remains debated, particularly for adults, creating an uncertain landscape regarding interventions. For adults, a comprehensive support system is essential to address not only reading difficulties but also the cognitive challenges associated with dyslexia, as well as the secondary psychological effects of living with a developmental disorder. Without adequate support, dyslexia can lead to lower-than-expected educational outcomes, an increase in psychiatric disorders, and higher unemployment rates, thereby raising the risk of social marginalization (Aro et al., 2019; Eloranta et al., 2019; Livingston et al., 2018).

There is a pressing need for scientifically validated methods to support individuals with dyslexia, particularly adults, as evidence-based interventions remain limited (Costantini et al., 2020; Doyle & McDowall, 2019; Gerber, 2012; Hock, 2012). Current interventions are primarily focused on children and address various aspects of reading skills. Snowling et al. (2020) emphasize that phonological interventions, which include phonemic awareness training and letter knowledge combined with structured reading practice, are especially effective for children with dyslexia. However, age affects the efficacy of interventions: phonological approaches show greater effectiveness in early elementary school, while comprehension-focused or mixed strategies become more beneficial later on (Galuschka et al., 2020). Nonetheless, phonology-based training programs have also demonstrated positive effects in adults (Eden et al., 2004).

Several studies on reading comprehension interventions have shown effectiveness in both children and adults with dyslexia, particularly when explicit and strategy-focused methods are used. However, effect sizes vary from mild to moderate (0.20–0.70), and the ability to apply learned strategies in new contexts remains inconsistent (Shaywitz et al., 2008). It has also been stressed that the importance of developing treatment plans that address the comorbidities often associated with dyslexia, as these can influence how individuals respond to interventions (Costantini et al., 2020; Snowling et al., 2020).

Recovery programs for adults with dyslexia, focusing on computer-based accelerated reading programs (e.g., Fast ForWord), cross-modal attention (e.g., action video games), or sensorimotor responses guided by verbal commands (e.g., Motor Square Training), have shown potential for improving reading skills. However, promising intervention practices for adults with dyslexia have included sessions lasting several hours (De Lima et al., 2020), and research on psychosocial interventions for adults with dyslexia remains limited (Costantini et al., 2020).

Given the positive results of NIBS in enhancing reading efficiency in adults, a future avenue for rehabilitation may be NIBS training to boost brain plasticity. NIBS has emerged as a critical tool in managing dyslexia in children and adults, as reviewed by Turker and Hartwigsen (2022). Interventions targeting the left and right TPC have shown positive effects on the reading abilities of dyslexic adults (Turker & Hartwigsen, 2022). To maximize the effects of neuromodulation, it may be beneficial to combine brain stimulation with targeted training programs, further enhancing the behavioral performance of individuals with dyslexia (Costanzo et al., 2016a, 2019; Younger & Booth, 2018).

Overall, brain stimulation offers promising potential for the treatment of dyslexia in adults. tES techniques are portable, painless, inexpensive, safe, and suitable for home-based treatment and are already self-administered at home for some diseases, such as chronic pain. Home-based tDCS treatment may thus represent a very near future perspective for remediation practice in adults with dyslexia. However, it is crucial to consider individual variability in brain plasticity to develop more effective and personalized therapeutic interventions (Cancer & Antonietti, 2018; Turker & Hartwigsen, 2022; Westwood et al., 2017).

10.6 Conclusion

The concept of brain plasticity has surpassed the old idea that the adult brain is "hard-wired" after critical developmental periods in childhood. While it is true that the brain is significantly more plastic during early years, and this capacity declines with age, recent research suggests that plasticity continues throughout life. Following this understanding, various reading remediation protocols effective in children have been proposed for adults with dyslexia, showing positive effects on reading. However, there remains a lack of evidence from randomized controlled trials supporting the efficacy of certain treatments in improving different components of reading. Specifically, improvements in higher-level comprehension, the ultimate goal of reading, have not been conclusively demonstrated. Phonics training, the most common treatment for reading deficits, primarily improves nonword reading accuracy and has moderate effects on word reading accuracy, reading fluency, spelling, letter-sound knowledge, and phonological output. Other methods, such as acceleration manipulation training, visual/sensorimotor processing training (like Quadrato Motor Training), and AVG training, have been shown to improve reading fluency in adults with developmental dyslexia.

These reading improvements are associated with neural changes in typically hypoactive regions of the left hemisphere in adults with dyslexia and in regions of the right hemisphere not usually involved in typical reading. Recently, studies using NIBS have documented positive effects on reading by directly targeting brain regions involved in the reading process. This suggests that NIBS protocols could represent a promising rehabilitative tool for both children and adults with dyslexia.

In future studies, researchers should combine NIBS protocols with neuroimaging to map stimulation-induced changes at a larger network level to increase the current understanding of the neural correlates associated with behavioral modulation. Such studies will provide a more comprehensive picture of how the reading network in adult dyslexic readers works and responds to neurostimulation. Since the effects of NIBS protocols are often less focal than expected and the functional relevance of remote effects has been demonstrated in previous work, a network perspective will help to better understand the functional relevance and interaction of different key areas for reading (e.g., Hartwigsen et al., 2017). Moreover, such combinations will also provide insight into potential compensatory changes in response to disruptive NIBS protocols at a larger network level. Finally, future controlled and randomized studies are necessary to better define effective remedial protocols for adults with dyslexia, with particular attention to developing mechanisms to improve reading comprehension and to reduce the impact of associated deficits and comorbidities.

Note

1 The Cochrane Library is a collection of databases in medicine and other healthcare specialties provided by Cochrane and other organizations. At its core is the collection of Cochrane Reviews, a database of systematic reviews and meta-analyses, which summarize and interpret the results of medical researches. The Cochrane Library aims to make the results of well-conducted controlled trials readily available and is a key resource in evidence-based medicine.

References

Adair, J. C., Nadeau, S. E., Conway, T. W., Gonzalez-Rothi, L. J., Heilman, P. C., Green, I. A., & Heilman, K. M. (2000). Alterations in the functional anatomy of reading induced by rehabilitation of an alexic patient. *Neuropsychiatry, Neuropsychology, and Behavioral Neurology*, *13*, 303–311.

American Psychiatric Association. (2022). *Diagnostic and statistical manual of mental disorders* (5th ed., text rev.). American Psychiatric Publishing.

Antal, A., Alekseichuk, I., Bikson, M., Brockmöller, J., Brunoni, A. R., Chen, R., Cohen, L. G., Dowthwaite, G., Ellrich, J., Flöel, A., Fregni, F., George, M. S., Hamilton, R., Haueisen, J., Herrmann, C. S., Hummel, F. C., Lefaucheur, J. P., Liebetanz, D., Loo, C. K., ... Paulus, W. (2017). Low intensity transcranial electric stimulation: Safety, ethical, legal regulatory and application guidelines. *Clinical Neurophysiology: Official Journal of the International Federation of Clinical Neurophysiology, 128*(9), 1774–1809.

Antzaka, A., Lallier, M., Meyer, S., Diard, J., Carreiras, M., & Valdois, S. (2017). Enhancing reading performance through action video games: The role of visual attention span. *Scientific Reports, 7*, 14563.

Aro, T., Eklund, K., Eloranta, A. K., Närhi, V., Korhonen, E., & Ahonen, T. (2019). Associations between childhood learning disabilities and adult-age mental health problems, lack of education, and unemployment. *Journal of Learning Disabilities, 52*(1), 71–83.

Au, A., Ho, G. S., Choi, E. W., Leung, P., Waye, M. M., Kang, K., & Au, K. Y. (2014). Does it help to train attention in dyslexic children: Pilot case studies with a ten-session neurofeedback program. *International Journal on Disability and Human Development, 13*(1), 45–54.

Aylward, E. H., Richards, T. L., Berninger, V. W., Nagy, W. E., Field, K. M., Grimme, A. C., Richards, A. L., Thomson, J. B., & Cramer, S. C. (2003). Instructional treatment associated with changes in brain activation in children with dyslexia. *Neurology, 61*, 212–219.

Battisti, A., Lazzaro, G., Costanzo, F., Varuzza, C., Rossi, S., Vicari, S., & Menghini, D. (2022). Effects of a short and intensive transcranial direct current stimulation treatment in children and adolescents with developmental dyslexia: A crossover clinical trial. *Frontiers in Psychology, 13*, 986242.

Battisti, A., Lazzaro, G., Varuzza, C., Vicari, S., & Menghini, D. (2024). Effects of online tDCS and hf-tRNS on reading performance in children and adolescents with developmental dyslexia: A study protocol for a cross sectional, within-subject, randomized, double-blind, and sham-controlled trial. *Frontiers in Neurology, 15*, 1338430.

Ben-Soussan, T. D., Avirame, K., Glicksohn, J., Goldstein, A., Harpaz, Y., & Ben-Shachar, M. (2014). Changes in cerebellar activity and inter-hemispheric coherence accompany improved reading performance following Quadrato motor training. *Frontiers in Systems Neuroscience, 8*, 81.

Bernstein, P. S., Scheffers, M. K., & Coles, M. G. (1995). "Where did I go wrong?" a psychophysiological analysis of error detection. *Journal of Experimental Psychology Human Perception & Performance, 21*, 1312–1322.

Bertoni, S., Franceschini, S., Mancarella, M., Puccio, G., Ronconi, L., Marsicano, G., & Facoetti, A. (2024). Action video games and posterior parietal cortex neuromodulation enhance both attention and reading in adults with developmental dyslexia. *Cerebral Cortex, 34*(4), bhae152.

Bikson, M., Ganho-Ávila, A., Datta, A., Gillick, B., Joensson, M. G., Kim, S., Kim, J., Kirton, A., Lee, K., Marjenin, T., Onarheim, B., Rehn, E. M., Sack, A. T., & Unal, G. (2023). Limited output transcranial electrical stimulation 2023 (LOTES-2023): Updates on engineering principles, regulatory statutes, and industry standards for wellness, over-the-counter, or prescription devices with low risk. *Brain Stimulation, 16*(3), 840–853.

Bikson, M., Grossman, P., Thomas, C., Zannou, A. L., Jiang, J., Adnan, T., Mourdoukoutas, A. P., Kronberg, G., Truong, D., Boggio, P., Brunoni, A. R., Charvet, L., Fregni, F., Fritsch, B., Gillick, B., Hamilton, R. H., Hampstead, B. M., Jankord, R., Kirton, A., ... Woods, A. J. (2016). Safety of Transcranial direct current stimulation: Evidence based update 2016. *Brain Stimulation, 9*(5), 641–661.

Bishop-Liebler, P., Welch, G., Huss, M., Thomson, J. M., & Goswami, U. (2014). Auditory temporal processing skills in musicians with dyslexia. *Dyslexia*, 20, 261–279.

Boden, C., & Giaschi, D. (2007). M-stream deficits and reading-related visual processes in developmental dyslexia. *Psychological Bullettin*, 133, 346–366.

Boggio, P. S., Castro, L. O., Savagim, E. A., Braite, R., Cruz, V. C., Rocha, R. R., Rigonatti, S. P., Silva, M. T., & Fregni, F. (2006). Enhancement of non-dominant hand motor function by anodal transcranial direct current stimulation. *Neuroscience Letters*, 404, 232–236.

Bosse, M. L., Tainturier, M. J., & Valdois, S. (2007). Developmental dyslexia: The visual attention span deficit hypothesis. *Cognition*, 104, 198–230.

Braid, J., & Richlan, F. (2022). The functional neuroanatomy of reading intervention. *Frontiers in Neuroscience*, 16, 921931.

Brem, S., Bach, S., Kucian, K., Guttorm, T. K., Martin, E., Lyytinen, H., et al. (2010). Brain sensitivity to print emerges when children learn letter-speech sound correspondences. *Proceedings of the National Academy of Sciences USA*, 107, 7939–7944.

Breznitz, Z., & Berman, L. (1997). The underlying factors of word recognition in regular and dyslexic readers. *Reading and Writing*, 9(4), 331–348. https://doi.org/10.1023/A:1024696101081

Breznitz, Z., Shaul, S., Horowitz-Kraus, T., Sela, I., Nevat, M., & Karni, A. (2013). Enhanced reading by training with imposed time constraint in typical and dyslexic adults. *Nature Communications*, 4, 1486.

Buonomano, D. V., & Johnson, H. A. (2009). Cortical plasticity and learning: Mechanisms and models. In L. R. Squire (Ed.), *Encyclopedia of neuroscience*. London: Academic Press.

Cancer, A., & Antonietti, A. (2018). tDCS modulatory effect on reading processes: A review of studies on typical readers and individuals with dyslexia. *Frontiers in Behavioral Neuroscience*, 12, 162.

Cancer, A., Stievano, G., Pace, G., Colombo, A., Brembati, F., Donini, R., & Antonietti, A. (2023). Remedial interventions for developmental dyslexia: Comparing the rhythmic reading training to the "Abilmente" approach. *Psychology of Music*, 51(3), 938–951.

Cancer, A., Vanutelli, M. E., Lucchiari, C., & Antonietti, A. (2021). Using neurofeedback to restore inter-hemispheric imbalance: A study protocol for adults with dyslexia. *Frontiers in Psychology*, 12, 768061.

Cappa, S. F., Sandrini, M., Rossini, P. M., Sosta, K., & Miniussi, C. (2002). The role of the left frontal lobe in action naming: rTMS evidence. *Neurology*, 59, 720–723.

Cheema, K., Fleming, C., Craig, J., Hodgetts, W. E., & Cummine, J. (2023). Reading and spelling profiles of adult poor readers: Phonological, orthographic and morphological considerations. *Dyslexia*, 29(2), 58–77.

Chugani, H. T. (1998). A critical period of brain development: Studies of cerebral glucose utilization with PET. *Preventive Medicine*, 27, 184–188.

Cogo-Moreira, H., Andriolo, R. B., Yazigi, L., Ploubidis, G. B., Brandão de Ávila, C. R., & Mari, J. J. (2012). Music education for improving reading skills in children and adolescents with dyslexia. *Cochrane Database Systematic Review*, 8, CD009133.

Cogo-Moreira, H., Brandão de Ávila, C. R., Ploubidis, G. B., & Mari, J. (2013). Effectiveness of music education for the improvement of reading skills and academic achievement in young poor readers: A pragmatic cluster-randomized, controlled clinical trial. *PLoS One*, 8(3), e59984.

Cohen, L., Dehaene, S., McCormick, S., Durant, S., & Zanker, J. M. (2016). Brain mechanisms of recovery from pure alexia: A single case study with multiple longitudinal scans. *Neuropsychologia*, 91, 36–49.

Cohen, L., Dehaene, S., Naccache, L., Lehericy, S., Dehaene-Lambertz, G., Henaff, M. A., & Michel, F. (2000). The visual word form area: Spatial and temporal characterization of an initial stage of reading in normal subjects and posterior split- brain patients. *Brain*, *123*, 291–307.

Costantini, A., Ceschi, A., & Sartori, R. (2020). Psychosocial interventions for the enhancement of psychological resources among dyslexic adults: A systematic review. *Sustainability*, *12*(19), 7994.

Costanzo, F., Menghini, D., Caltagirone, C., Oliveri, M., & Vicari, S. (2012). High frequency rTMS over the left parietal lobule increases non-word reading accuracy. *Neuropsychologia*, *50*(11), 2645–2651.

Costanzo, F., Menghini, D., Caltagirone, C., Oliveri, M., & Vicari, S. (2013). How to improve reading skills in dyslexics: The effect of high frequency rTMS. *Neuropsychologia*, *51*, 2953–2959.

Costanzo, F., Rossi, S., Varuzza, C., Varvara, P., Vicari, S., & Menghini, D. (2019). Long-lasting improvement following tDCS treatment combined with a training for reading in children and adolescents with dyslexia. *Neuropsychologia*, *130*, 38–43.

Costanzo, F., Varuzza, C., Rossi, S., Sdoia, S., Varvara, P., Oliveri, M., Giacomo, K., Vicari, S., & Menghini, D. (2016a). Evidence for reading improvement following tDCS treatment in children and adolescents with dyslexia. *Restorative Neurology and Neuroscience*, *34*, 215–226.

Costanzo, F., Varuzza, C., Rossi, S., Sdoia, S., Varvara, P., Oliveri, M., Koch, G., Vicari, S., & Menghini, D. (2016b). Reading changes in children and adolescents with dyslexia after transcranial direct current stimulation. *Neuroreport*, *27*, 295–300.

Cotelli, M., Calabria, M., Manenti, R., Rosini, S., Zanetti, O., Cappa, S. F., & Miniussi, C. (2010). Improved language performance in Alzheimer disease following brain stimulation. *Journal of Neurology, Neurosurgery, and Psychiatry*, *82*(7), 794–797.

Cotelli, M., Manenti, R., Cappa, S. F., Geroldi, C., Zanetti, O., Rossini, P. M., & Miniussi, C. (2006). Effect of transcranial magnetic stimulation on action naming in patients with Alzheimer disease. *Archives of Neurology*, *63*, 1602–1604.

Cotelli, M., Manenti, R., Cappa, S. F., Zanetti, O., & Miniussi, C. (2008). Transcranial magnetic stimulation improves naming in Alzheimer disease patients at different stages of cognitive decline. *European Journal of Neurology*, *15*, 1286–1292.

Cummine, J., Villarena, M., Onysyk, T., & Devlin, J. T. (2020). A study of null effects for the use of Transcranial direct current stimulation (tDCS) in adults with and without reading impairment. *Neurobiology of Language*, *1*(4), 434–451.

Dayan, E., & Cohen, L. G. (2011). Neuroplasticity subserving motor skill learning. *Neuron*, *72*(3), 443–454.

De Lima, R. F., Salgado-Azoni, C. A., Dell'Agli, B. A. V., Baptista, M. N., & Ciasca, S. M. (2020). Behavior problems and depressive symptoms in developmental dyslexia: Risk assessment in Brazilian students. *Clinical Neuropsychiatry*, *17*(3), 141.

Demb, J. B., Boynton, G. M., & Heeger, D. J. (1997). Brain activity in visual cortex predicts individual differences in reading performance. *Proceedings of the National Academy of Sciences*, *94*, 13363–13366.

Doyle, N. E., & McDowall, A. (2019). Context matters: A review to formulate a conceptual framework for coaching as a disability accommodation. *PLoS One*, *14*(8), e0199408.

Draganski, B., Gaser, C., Busch, V., Schuierer, G., Bogdahn, U., & May, A. (2004). Neuroplasticity: Changes in grey matter induced by training. *Nature*, *427*, 311–312.

Draganski, B., Gaser, C., Kempermann, G., Kuhn, H. G., Winkler, J., Buchel, C., & May, A. (2006). Temporal and spatial dynamics of brain structure changes during extensive learning. *Journal of Neuroscience*, *26*, 6314–6317.

Duzel, E., Hufnagel, A., Helmstaedter, C., & Elger, C. (1996). Verbal working memory components can be selectively influenced by transcranial magnetic stimulation in patients with left temporal lobe epilepsy. *Neuropsychologia, 34*, 775–783.

Eden, G. F., Jones, K. M., Cappell, K., Gareau, L., Wood, F. B., Zeffiro, T. A., & Flowers, D. L. (2004). Neural changes following remediation in adult developmental dyslexia. *Neuron, 44*(3), 411–422.

Eloranta, A. K., Närhi, V., & Ahonen, T. (2019). The development of reading and spelling skills, and self-concept in children with and without dyslexia. *Annals of Dyslexia, 69*(1), 60–79.

Eroğlu, G., Gürkan, M., Teber, S., Ertürk, K., Kırmızı, M., Ekici, B., et al. (2020). Changes in EEG complexity with neurofeedback and multi-sensory learning in children with dyslexia: A multiscale entropy analysis. *Applied Neuropsychology: Child, 9*, 1–12. https://doi.org/10.1080/21622965.2020.1772794

Eroğlu, G., Teber, S., Ertürk, K., Kırmızı, M., Ekici, B., Arman, F., & Çetin, M. (2022). A mobile app that uses neurofeedback and multi-sensory learning methods improves reading abilities in dyslexia: A pilot study. *Applied Neuropsychology: Child, 11*(3), 518–528.

Fattinger, S., de Beukelaar, T. T., Ruddy, K. L., Volk, C., Heyse, N. C., Herbst, J. A., & Huber, R. (2017). Deep sleep maintains learning efficiency of the human brain. *Nature Communications, 8*(1), 15405.

Fawcett, A., Nicolson, R., & Maclagan, F. (2001). Cerebellar tests differentiate between groups of poor readers with and without IQ discrepancy. *Journal of Learning Disabilities, 34*, 119–135.

Fawcett, A. J., & Nicolson, R. I. (1999). Performance of dyslexic children on cerebellar and cognitive tests. *Journal of Motor Behavior, 31*, 68–78.

Fitch, R. H., Miller, S., & Tallal, P. (1997). Neurobiology of speech perception. *Annual Review of Neuroscience, 20*, 331–353.

Fletcher, J., & Grigorenko, E. (2017). Neuropsychology of learning disabilities: The past and the future. *Journal of the International Neuropsychological Society, 23*, 930–940.

Franceschini, S., Gori, S., Ruffino, M., Viola, S., Molteni, M., & Facoetti, A. (2013). Action video games make dyslexic children read better. *Current Biology, 23*, 462–466.

Franceschini, S., Trevisan, P., Ronconi, L., Bertoni, S., Colmar, S., Double, K., Facoetti, A., & Gori, S. (2017). Action video games improve reading abilities and visual-to-auditory attentional shifting in English-speaking children with dyslexia. *Scientific Reports, 7*, 5863.

Frye, R. E., Rotenberg, A., Ousley, M., & Pascual-Leone, A. (2008). Transcranial magnetic stimulation in child neurology: Current and future directions. *Journal of Child Neurology, 23*, 79–96.

Fuster, M. (2002). Frontal lobe and cognitive development. *Journal of Neurocytology, 31*, 373–385.

Gabrieli, J. D. E., Norton, E. S., & Krafnick, A. J. (2009). Neural systems of reading and dyslexia: Insights from functional neuroimaging. *Current Directions in Psychological Science, 18*(6), 360–366. https://doi.org/10.1111/j.1467-8721.2009.01668.x

Galaburda, A., & Livingstone, M. (1993). Evidence for a magnocellular defect in developmental dyslexia. *Annals of the New York Academy of Sciences, 682*, 70–82.

Galuschka, K., Görgen, R., Kalmar, J., Haberstroh, S., Schmalz, X., & Schulte-Körne, G. (2020). Effectiveness of spelling interventions for learners with dyslexia: A meta-analysis and systematic review. *Educational Psychologist, 55*(1), 1–20.

Galuschka, K., Ise, E., Krick, K., & Schulte-Körne, G. (2014). Effectiveness of treatment approaches for children and adolescents with reading disabilities: A meta-analysis of randomized controlled trials. *PLoS One, 9*, e89900.

Gerber, P. J. (2012). The impact of learning disabilities on adulthood: A review of the evidence-based literature for research and practice in adult education. *Journal of Learning Disabilities, 45*(1), 31–46. https://doi.org/10.1177/0022219411426858

Goswami, U., Thomson, J., Richardson, U., Stainthorp, R., Hughes, D., Rosen, S., & Scott, S. K. (2000). Amplitude envelope onsets and developmental dyslexia: A new hypothesis. *Proceedings of the National Academy of Sciences of the United States of America, 99*(16), 10911–10916. https://doi.org/10.1073/pnas.122368599

Graves, W. W., Desai, R., Humphries, C., Seidenberg, M. S., & Binder, J. R. (2010). Neural systems for reading aloud: A multiparametric approach. *Cerebral Cortex, 20*(8), 1799–1815.

Habib, M. (2000). The neurological basis of developmental dyslexia: An overview and working hypothesis. *Brain, 123*(12), 2373–2399.

Habib, M. (2021). The neurological basis of developmental dyslexia and related disorders: A reappraisal of the temporal hypothesis, twenty years on. *Brain Sciences, 11*(6), 708.

Habib, M., Lardy, C., Desiles, T., Commeiras, C., Chobert, J., & Besson, M. (2016). Music and dyslexia: A new musical training method to improve reading and related disorders. *Frontiers in Psychology, 7*, 26.

Hancock, R., Richlan, F., & Hoeft, F. (2017). Possible roles for fronto-striatal circuits in reading disorder. *Neuroscience & Biobehavioral Reviews, 72*, 243–260.

Harrar, V., Tammam, J., Perez-Bellido, A., Pitt, A., Stein, J., & Spence, C. (2014). Multisensory integration and attention in developmental dyslexia. *Current Biology, 24*, 531–535.

Hartwigsen, G., Bzdok, D., Klein, M., Wawrzyniak, M., Stockert, A., Wrede, K., & Saur, D. (2017). Rapid short-term reorganization in the language network. *eLife, 6*, e25964.

He, Y., Chen, Z. J., & Evans, A. C. (2007). Small-world anatomical networks in the human brain revealed by cortical thickness from MRI. *Cerebral Cortex, 17*(10), 2407–2419.

Heim, S., Pape-Neumann, J., van Ermingen-Marbach, M., Brinkhaus, M., & Grande, M. (2015). Shared vs. specific brain activation changes in dyslexia after training of phonology, attention, or reading. *Brain Structure and Function, 220*, 2191–2207.

Heth, I., & Lavidor, M. (2015). Improved reading measures in adults with dyslexia following transcranial direct current stimulation treatment. *Neuropsychologia, 70*, 107–113.

Hock, M. F. (2012). Effective literacy instruction for adults with specific learning disabilities: Implications for adult educators. *Journal of Learning Disabilities, 45*(1), 64–78.

Hoeft, F., Hernandez, A., McMillon, G., Taylor-Hill, H., Martindale, J. L., Meyler, A., Keller, T. A., Siok, W. T., Deutsch, G. K., Just, M. A., Whitfield-Gabrieli, S., & Gabrieli, J. D. (2006). Neural basis of dyslexia: A comparison between dyslexic and non dyslexic children equated for reading ability. *Journal of Neuroscience, 26*, 10700–10708.

Hoeft, F., McCandliss, B. D., Black, J. M., Gantman, A., Zakerani, N., Hulme, C., Lyytinen, H., Whitfield-Gabrieli, S., Glover, G. H., Reiss, A. L., & Gabrieli, J. D. (2011). Neural systems predicting long-term outcome in dyslexia. *Proceedings of the National Academy of Sciences USA, 108*, 361–366.

Hoeft, F., Meyler, A., Hernandez, A., Juel, C., Taylor-Hill, H., Martindale, J. L., McMillon, G., Kolchugina, G., Black, J. M., Faizi, A., Deutsch, G. K., Siok, W. T., Reiss, A. L., Whitfield-Gabrieli, S., & Gabrieli, J. D. (2007). Functional and morphometric brain dissociation between dyslexia and reading ability. *Proceedings of the National Academy of Sciences of the United States of America, 104*, 4234–4239.

Holtmann, M., Sonuga-Barke, E., Cortese, S., & Brandeis, D. (2014). Neurofeedback for ADHD: A review of current evidence. *Child and Adolescent Psychiatric Clinics, 23*(4), 789–806.

Horowitz-Kraus, T. (2016). Improvement of the error-detection mechanism in adults with dyslexia following Reading acceleration training. *Dyslexia*, *22*, 173–189.

Horowitz-Kraus, T., & Breznitz, Z. (2013). Compensated dyslexics have a more efficient error detection system than non-compensated dyslexics. *Journal of Child Neurology*, *2896*, 1266–1276.

Horowitz-Kraus, T., Cicchino, N., Amiel, M., Holland, S. K., & Breznitz, Z. (2014). Reading improvement in English- and Hebrew-speaking children with reading difficulties after reading acceleration training. *Annals of Dyslexia*, *64*(3), 183–201.

Huss, M., Verney, J. P., Fosker, T., Mead, N., & Goswami, U. (2011). Music, rhythm, rise time perception and developmental dyslexia: Perception of musical meter predicts reading and phonology. *Cortex*, *47*(6), 674–689.

Huttenlocher, R., & Dabholkar, A. S. (1997). Regional differences in synaptogenesis in human cerebral cortex. *Journal of Comparative Neurology*, *387*, 167–178.

Ivry, R. B., & Justus, T. C. (2001). A neural instantiation of the motor theory of speech perception. *Trends in Neurosciences*, *24*, 513–515.

Jednoróg, K., Marchewka, A., Tacikowski, P., Heim, S., & Grabowska, A. (2011). Electrophysiological evidence for the magnocellular-dorsal pathway deficit in dyslexia. *Developmental Science*, *14*, 873–880.

Jensen, J., Lindgren, M., Andersson, K., Ingvar, D. H., & Levander, S. (2000). Cognitive intervention in unemployed individuals with reading and writing disabilities. *Applied Neuropsychology*, *7*(4), 223–236.

Jobard, G., Crivello, F., & Tzourio-Mazoyer, N. (2003). Evaluation of the dual route theory of reading: A metanalysis of 35 neuroimaging studies. *NeuroImage*, *20*(2), 693–712.

Kaas, J. H. (2002). Sensory loss and cortical reorganization in mature primates. *Progress in Brain Research*, *138*, 167–176.

Ki-Ju, K. (2022). Phonics instruction and reading acquisition in Korean learners: Cross-linguistic evidence for phonological processing. *Reading and Writing*, *35*(3), 645–667.

Kim, E. S., & Lemke, S. F. (2016). Behavioural and eye-movement outcomes in response to text-based reading treatment for acquired alexia. *Neuropsychological Rehabilitation*, *26*(1), 60–86.

Kitz, W. R., & Nash, R. T. (1992). Testing the effectiveness of the project success summer program for adult dyslexics. *Annals of Dyslexia*, *42*, 1–24.

Krause, B., & Cohen Kadosh, R. (2013). Can transcranial electrical stimulation improve learning difficulties in atypical brain development? A future possibility for cognitive training. *Developmental Cognitive Neuroscience*, *6*, 176–194.

Krishnan, C., Santos, L., Peterson, M. D., & Ehinger, M. (2015). Safety of noninvasive brain stimulation in children and adolescents. *Brain Stimulation*, *8*, 76–87.

Kyle, F. E., Kujala, J., Richardson, U., Lyytinen, H., & Goswami, U. (2013). Assessing the effectiveness of two theoretically motivated computer assisted reading interventions in the United Kingdom: GG rime and GG phoneme. *Reading Research Quarterly*, *48*, 61–76.

Lacey, E. H., Jiang, X., Friedman, R. B., Snider, S. F., Parra, L. C., Huang, Y., & Turkeltaub, P. E. (2015). Transcranial direct current stimulation for pure alexia: Effects on brain and behavior. *Brain Stimulation*, *8*, 305–307.

Landerl, K., Ramus, F., Moll, K., Lyytinen, H., Leppänen, P. H., Lohvansuu, K., O'Donovan, M., Williams, J., Bartling, J., Bruder, J., Kunze, S., Neuhoff, N., Tóth, D., Honbolygó, F., Csépe, V., Bogliotti, C., Iannuzzi, S., Chaix, Y., Démonet, J. F., ... Schulte-Körne, G. (2013). Predictors of developmental dyslexia in European orthographies with varying complexity. *Journal of Child Psychology and Psychiatry*, *54*, 686–694.

Lazzaro, G., Bertoni, S., Menghini, D., Costanzo, F., Franceschini, S., Varuzza, C., Ronconi, L., Battisti, A., Gori, S., Facoetti, A., & Vicari, S. (2021b). Beyond Reading modulation: Temporo-parietal tDCS alters Visuo-spatial attention and motion perception in dyslexia. *Brain Sciences, 11*(2), 263.

Lazzaro, G., Costanzo, F., Varuzza, C., Rossi, S., De Matteis, M. E., Vicari, S., & Menghini, D. (2021a). Individual differences modulate the effects of tDCS on reading in children and adolescents with dyslexia. *Scientific Studies of Reading, 25*(6), 470–485.

Lehongre, K., Ramus, F., Villiermet, N., Schwartz, D., & Giraud, A. L. (2011). Altered low-gamma sampling in auditory cortex accounts for the three main facets of dyslexia. *Neuron, 72*(6), 1080–1090.

Livingston, E. M., Siegel, L. S., & Ribary, U. (2018). Developmental dyslexia: Emotional impact and consequences. *Australian Journal of Learning Difficulties, 23*(2), 107–135.

Livingstone, M. S., Rosen, G. D., Drislane, F. W., & Galaburda, A. M. (1991). Physiological and anatomical evidence for a magnocellular defect in developmental dyslexia. *Proceedings of the National Academy of Sciences, 88*, 7943–7947.

Lubar, J. F. (1991). Discourse on the development of EEG diagnostics and biofeedback for attention-deficit/hyperactivity disorders. *Biofeedback and Self-Regulation, 16*, 201–225.

Marchesotti, S., Nicolle, J., Merlet, I., Arnal, L. H., Donoghue, J. P., & Giraud, A. L. (2020). Selective enhancement of low-gamma activity by tACS improves phonemic processing and reading accuracy in dyslexia. *PLoS Biology, 18*(9), e3000833.

Marzbani, H., Marateb, H. R., & Mansourian, M. (2016). Neurofeedback: A comprehensive review on system design, methodology and clinical applications. *Basic and Clinical Neuroscience, 7*(2), 143.

McArthur, T., Lam-McArthur, J., & Fontaine, L. (Eds.) (2018). In *Oxford companion to the English language*. Oxford University Press.

Menghini, D., Hagberg, G. E., Caltagirone, C., Petrosini, L., & Vicari, S. (2006). Implicit learning deficits in dyslexic adults: An fMRI study. *NeuroImage, 33*, 1218–1226.

Merzenich, M. M., & Jenkins, W. M. (1998). Cortical plasticity, learning, and learning dysfunction. In B. Julesz & I. Kavocs (Eds.), *Maturational windows in adult cortical plasticity* (pp. 247–272). New York: Addison-Wesley.

Meyler, A., Keller, T. A., Cherkassky, V. L., Gabrieli, J. D., & Just, M. A. (2008). Modifying the brain activation of poor readers during sentence comprehension with extended remedial instruction: A longitudinal study of neuroplasticity. *Neuropsychologia, 46*(10), 2580–2592.

Moores, E., Cassim, R., & Talcott, J. B. (2015). Adults with dyslexia exhibit large effects of crowding and detrimental effects of distractors in a visual tilt discrimination task. *PLoS One, 10*(9), e0137328. https://doi.org/10.1371/journal.pone.0137328

Morillon, B., Liégeois-Chauvel, C., Arnal, L. H., Bénar, C. G., & Giraud, A. L. (2012). Asymmetric function of theta and gamma activity in syllable processing: An intra-cortical study. *Frontiers in Psychology, 3*, 248.

Morishita, H., Miwa, J. M., Heintz, N., & Hensch, T. K. (2010). Lynx1, a cholinergic brake, limits plasticity in adult visual cortex. *Science, 330*(6008), 1238–1240.

Nazari, M. A., Mosanezhad, E., Hashemi, T., & Jahan, A. (2012). The effectiveness of neurofeedback training on EEG coherence and neuropsychological functions in children with reading disability. *Clinical EEG and Neuroscience, 43*(4), 315–322.

Norton, E. S., & Wolf, M. (2012). Rapid automatized naming (RAN) and reading fluency: Implications for understanding and treatment of reading disabilities. *Annual Review of Psychology, 63*, 427–452.

Nudo, R. J., Wise, B. M., SiFuentes, F., & Milliken, G. W. (1996). Neural substrates for the effects of rehabilitative training on motor recovery after ischemic infarct. *Science, 272*, 1791–1794.

Nugiel, T., Roe, M. A., Taylor, W. P., Cirino, P. T., Vaughn, S. R., Fletcher, J. M., & Church, J. A. (2019). Brain activity in struggling readers before intervention relates to future reading gains. *Cortex*, *111*, 286–302.

Nukari, J. M., Poutiainen, E. T., Arkkila, E. P., Haapanen, M. L., Lipsanen, J. O., & Laasonen, M. R. (2020). Both individual and group-based neuropsychological interventions of dyslexia improve processing speed in young adults: A randomized controlled study. *Journal of Learning Disabilities*, *53*(3), 213–227.

Partanen, M., Siegel, L. S., & Giaschi, D. E. (2019). Effect of reading intervention and task difficulty on orthographic and phonological reading systems in the brain. *Neuropsychologia*, *130*, 13–25.

Pecini, C., Spoglianti, S., Bonetti, S., Di Lieto, M. C., Guaran, F., Martinelli, A., & Chilosi, A. M. (2019). Training RAN or reading? A telerehabilitation study on developmental dyslexia. *Dyslexia*, *25*(3), 318–331.

Pecyna, M. B., & Pokorski, M. (2013). Near-infrared hemoencephalography for monitoring blood oxygenation in prefrontal cortical areas in diagnosis and therapy of developmental dyslexia. *Advances in Experimental Medicine and Biology*, *788*, 175–180.

Peinemann, A., Reimer, B., Löer, C., Quartarone, A., Münchau, A., Conrad, B., & Siebner, H. R. (2004). Long-lasting increase in corticospinal excitability after 1800 pulses of subthreshold 5Hz repetitive TMS to the primary motor cortex. *Clinical Neurophysiology*, *115*(7), 1519–1526.

Peters, J. L., Crewther, S. G., Murphy, M. J., & Bavin, E. L. (2021). Action video game training improves text reading accuracy, rate and comprehension in children with dyslexia: A randomized controlled trial. *Scientific Reports*, *11*(1), 18584.

Peters, J. L., De Losa, L., Bavin, E. L., & Crewther, S. G. (2019). Efficacy of dynamic visuo-attentional interventions for reading in dyslexic and neurotypical children: A systematic review. *Neuroscience & Biobehavioral Reviews*, *100*, 58–76.

Philipose, L. E., Gottesman, R. F., Newhart, M., Kleinman, J. T., Herskovits, E. H., Pawlak, M. A., Marsh, E. B., Davis, C., Heidler-Gary, J., & Hillis, A. E. (2007). Neural regions essential for reading and spelling of words and pseudowords. *Annals of Neurology*, *62*, 481–492.

Price, C. J. (2000). The anatomy of language: Contributions from functional neuroimaging. *Journal of Anatomy*, *197*, 335–359.

Pugh, K. R., Mencl, W. E., Jenner, A. R., Katz, L., Frost, S. J., Lee, J. R., Shaywitz, S. E., & Shaywitz, B. A. (2000). Functional neuroimaging studies of reading and reading disability (developmental dyslexia). *Mental Retardation and Developmental Disabilities Research Reviews*, *6*, 207–213.

Raesi, S., Pourmohammad, M., & Nili Ahmadabadi, M. (2017). Visual attention and reading ability: A study of children with developmental dyslexia. *Reading and Writing*, *30*(6), 1273–1292.

Rahimi, V., Mohammadkhani, G., Rad, J. A., Mousavi, S. Z., & Khalili, M. E. (2022). Modulation of auditory temporal processing, speech in noise perception, auditory-verbal memory, and reading efficiency by anodal tDCS in children with dyslexia. *Neuropsychologia*, *177*, 108427.

Ramus, F., Rosen, S., Dakin, S. C., Day, B. L., Castellote, J. M., White, S., & Frith, U. (2003). Theories of developmental dyslexia: Insights from a multiple case study of dyslexic adults. *Brain*, *126*(4), 841–865. https://doi.org/10.1093/brain/awg076

Reed, T., & Cohen Kadosh, R. (2018). Transcranial electrical stimulation (tES) mechanisms and its effects on cortical excitability and connectivity. *Journal of Inherited Metabolic Disease*, *41*, 1123–1130.

Richards, T. L., Aylward, E. H., Field, K. M., Grimme, A. C., Raskind, W., Richards, A. L., & Berninger, V. W. (2006). Converging evidence for triple word form theory in children with dyslexia. *Developmental Neuropsychology*, *30*(1), 547–589.

Richards, T. L., Corina, D., Serafini, S., Steury, K., Echelard, D. R., Dager, S. R., Marro, K., Abbott, R. D., Maravilla, K. R., & Berninger, V. W. (2000). Effects of a phonologically driven treatment for dyslexia on lactate levels measured by proton MR spectroscopic imaging. *American Journal of Neuroradiology, 21*, 916–922.

Richlan, F., Kronbichler, M., & Wimmer, H. (2009). Functional abnormalities in the dyslexic brain: A quantitative meta-analysis of neuroimaging studies. *Human Brain Mapping, 30*(10), 3299–3308.

Richlan, F., Kronbichler, M., & Wimmer, H. (2011). Meta-analyzing brain dysfunctions in dyslexic children and adults. *NeuroImage, 56*(3), 1735–1742.

Rijntjes, M., & Weiller, C. (2002). Recovery of motor and language abilities after stroke: The contribution of functional imaging. *Progress in Neurobiology, 66*, 109–122.

Rios, D. M., Correia Rios, M., Bandeira, I. D., Queiros Campbell, F., de Carvalho Vaz, D., & Lucena, R. (2018). Impact of Transcranial direct current stimulation on Reading skills of children and adolescents with dyslexia. *Child Neurology Open, 5*, 2329048X18798255.

Roach, N. W., Edwards, V. T., & Hogben, J. H. (2007). The tale is in the tail: An alternative hypothesis for psychophysical performance variability in dyslexia. *Perception, 36*(6), 955–974. https://doi.org/10.1068/p5467

Rodrigues de Almeida, L., Pope, P. A., & Hansen, P. C. (2019). Task load modulates tDCS effects on language performance. *Journal of Neuroscience Research, 97*(11), 1430–1454.

Rothkegel, H., Sommer, M., & Paulus, W. (2010). Breaks during 5Hz rTMS are essential for facilitatory after effects. *Clinical Neurophysiology, 121*(3), 426–430.

Rufener, K. S., Krauel, K., Meyer, M., Heinze, H. J., & Zaehle, T. (2019). Transcranial electrical stimulation improves phoneme processing in developmental dyslexia. *Brain Stimulation, 12*(4), 930–937.

Rufener, K. S., & Zaehle, T. (2021). Dysfunctional auditory gamma oscillations in developmental dyslexia: A potential target for a tACS-based intervention. *Progress in Brain Research, 264*, 211–232.

Sadeghi, N., & Nazari, M. A. (2015). Effect of neurofeedback on visual-spatial attention in male children with reading disabilities: An event-related potential study. *Neuroscience & Medicine, 6*(02), 71.

Saine, N. L., Lerkkanen, M.-K., Ahonen, T., Tolvanen, A., & Lyytinen, H. (2010). Predicting word-level reading fluency outcomes in three contrastive groups: Remedial and computer-assisted remedial reading intervention, and mainstream instruction. *Learning and Individual Differences, 20*, 402–414.

Saine, N. L., Lerkkanen, M.-K., Ahonen, T., Tolvanen, A., & Lyytinen, H. (2011). A computer-assisted remedial reading intervention for school beginners at-risk for reading disability. *Child Development, 82*, 1013–1028.

Santos, F. H., Mosbacher, J. A., Menghini, D., Rubia, K., Grabner, R. H., & Kadosh, R. C. (2021). Effects of transcranial stimulation in developmental neurocognitive disorders: A critical appraisal. *Progress in Brain Research, 264*, 1–40.

Scheffers, M. K., & Coles, M. G. (2000). Performance monitoring in a confusing world: Error-related brain activity, judgments of response accuracy, and types of errors. *Journal of Experimental Psychology Human Perception & Performance, 26*, 141–151.

Schlaggar, B. L., Brown, T. T., Lugar, H. M., Visscher, K. M., Miezin, F. M., & Petersen, S. E. (2002). Functional neuroanatomical differences between adults and school-age children in the processing of single-words. *Science, 296*, 1476–1479.

Seymour, P. H., Aro, M., & Erskine, J. M. (2003). Foundation literacy acquisition in European orthographies. *British Journal of Psychology, 94*, 143–174.

Shaywitz, B. A., Morris, R., & Shaywitz, S. E. (2008). The education of dyslexic children from childhood to young adulthood. *Annual Review of Psychology, 59*, 451–475. https://doi.org/10.1146/annurev.psych.59.103006.093633

Shaywitz, B. A., Shaywitz, S. E., Blachman, B. A., Pugh, K. R., Fulbright, R. K., Skudlarski, P., Mencl, W. E., Constable, R. T., Holahan, J. M., Marchione, K. E., Fletcher, J. M., Lyon, G. R., & Gore, J. C. (2004). Development of left occipitotemporal systems for skilled reading in children after a phonologically-based intervention. *Biological Psychiatry*, 55, 926–933.

Shaywitz, B. A., Shaywitz, S. E., Pugh, K. R., Mencl, W. E., Fulbright, R. K., Skudlarski, P., & Gore, J. C. (2002). Disruption of posterior brain systems for reading in children with developmental dyslexia. *Biological Psychiatry*, 52(2), 101–110.

Shaywitz, B. A., Skudlarski, P., Holahan, J. M., Marchione, K. E., Constable, R. T., Fulbright, R. K., Zelterman, D., Lacadie, C., & Shaywitz, S. E. (2007). Age-related changes in reading systems of dyslexic children. *Annals of Neurology*, 61, 363–370.

Shaywitz, S. E. (2003). *Overcoming dyslexia: A new and complete science-based program for reading problems at any level*. New York: Knopf.

Shaywitz, S. E., & Shaywitz, B. A. (2008). Paying attention to reading: The neurobiology of reading and dyslexia. *Development and Psychopathology*, 20, 1329–1349.

Simos, P. G., Breier, J. I., Fletcher, J. M., Foorman, B. R., Mouzaki, A., & Papanicolaou, A. C. (2001). Age-related changes in regional brain activation during phonological decoding and printed word recognition. *Developmental Neuropsychology*, 19, 191–210.

Simos, P. G., Fletcher, J. M., Bergman, E., Breier, J. I., Foorman, B. R., Castillo, E. M., Davis, R. N., Fitzgerald, M., & Papanicolaou, A. C. (2002). Dyslexia-specific brain activation profile becomes normal following successful remedial training. *Neurology*, 58, 1203–1213.

Small, S. L., Kendall Flores, D., & Noll, D. C. (1998). Different neural circuits subserve reading before and after therapy for acquired dyslexia. *Brain and Language*, 62, 298–308.

Snowling, M. J., Gallagher, A., & Frith, U. (2000). Family risk of dyslexia: The relationship between phonological awareness, language, and literacy skills in early reading development. *Journal of Child Psychology and Psychiatry*, 44(7), 923–940. https://doi.org/10.1111/1469-7610.00509

Snowling, M. J., Hayiou-Thomas, M. E., Nash, H. M., & Hulme, C. (2020). Dyslexia and developmental language disorder: Comorbid disorders with distinct effects on reading comprehension. *Journal of Child Psychology and Psychiatry*, 61(6), 672–680.

Sperling, A., Lu, Z.-L., Manis, F. (2004). Slower implicit categorical learning in adult poor readers. *Annals of Dyslexia*, 54, 281–303.

Staudt, M., Lidzba, K., Grodd, W., Wildgruber, D., Erb, M., & Krageloh-Mann, I. (2002). Right-hemispheric organization of language following early left-sided brain lesions: Functional MRI topography. *NeuroImage*, 16, 954–967.

Stoodley, C. J., & Stein, J. F. (2011). The cerebellum and dyslexia. *Cortex*, 47, 101–116.

Strong, G. K., Torgerson, C. J., Torgerson, D., & Hulme, C. (2010). A systematic meta-analytic review of evidence for the effectiveness of the 'fast ForWord' language intervention program. *Journal of Child Psychology and Psychiatry*, 52(3), 224–235. https://doi.org/10.1111/j.1469-7610.2010.02329.x

Szelag, E., & Skolimowska, J. (2012). Cognitive function in elderly can be ameliorated by training in temporal information processing. *Restorative Neurology and Neuroscience*, 30(5), 419–434.

Tallal, P. (1980). Auditory temporal perception, phonics, and reading disabilities in children. *Brain and Language*, 9, 182–198.

Temple, E., Deutsch, G. K., Poldrack, R. A., Miller, S. L., Tallal, P., Merzenich, M. M., & Gabrieli, J. D. (2003). Neural deficits in children with dyslexia ameliorated by behavioural remediation: Evidence from functional MRI. *Proceedings of the National Academy of Sciences USA*, 100, 2860–2865.

Thomson, J. M., Doruk, D., Mascio, B., Fregni, F., & Cerruti, C. (2015). Transcranial direct current stimulation modulates efficiency of reading processes. *Frontiers in Human Neuroscience, 9*, 114.

Tierney, A., & Kraus, N. (2013). The ability to move to a beat is linked to the consistency of neural responses to sound. *Journal of Neuroscience, 33*(38), 14981–14988.

Torgesen, J., Wagner, R., & Rashotte, C. (2011). *Test of word Reading efficiency – 2 (TOWRE-2)* (2nd ed.). Austin, TX: Pro-Ed.

Turkeltaub, E., Gareau, L., Flowers, D. L., Zeffiro, T. A., & Eden, G. F. (2003). Development of neural mechanisms for reading. *Nature Neuroscience, 6*, 767–773.

Turkeltaub, P. E., Benson, J., Hamilton, R. H., Datta, A., Bikson, M., & Coslett, H. B. (2012). Left lateralizing transcranial direct current stimulation improves reading efficiency. *Brain Stimulation, 5*, 201–207.

Turkeltaub, P. E., Eden, G. F., Jones, K. M., & Zeffiro, T. A. (2002). Meta-analysis of the functional neuroanatomy of single-word reading: Method and validation. *NeuroImage, 16*, 765–780.

Turker, S., & Hartwigsen, G. (2022). The use of noninvasive brain stimulation techniques to improve reading difficulties in dyslexia: A systematic review. *Human Brain Mapping, 43*(3), 1157–1173.

Turker, S., Kuhnke, P., Schmid, F. R., Cheung, V. K. M., Weise, K., Knoke, M., & Hartwigsen, G. (2023). Adaptive short-term plasticity in the typical reading network. *NeuroImage, 281*, 120373.

Vicari, S., Marotta, L., Menghini, D., Molinari, M., & Petrosini, L. (2003). Implicit learning deficit in children with developmental dyslexia. *Neuropsychologia, 41*, 108–114.

Vicario, C. M., & Nitsche, M. A. (2013a). Non-invasive brain stimulation for the treatment of brain diseases in childhood and adolescence: State of the art, current limits and future challenges. *Frontiers in Systems Neuroscience, 7*, 94.

Vicario, C. M., & Nitsche, M. A. (2013b). Transcranial direct current stimulation: A remediation tool for the treatment of childhood congenital dyslexia? *Frontiers in Systems Neuroscience, 7*, 139.

Vinckier, F., Dehaene, S., Jobert, A., Dubus, J. P., Sigman, M., & Cohen, L. (2007). Hierarchical coding of letter strings in the ventral stream: Dissecting the inner organization of the visual word-form system. *Neuron, 55*(1), 143–156.

Vonthron, F., Yuen, A., Pellerin, H., Cohen, D., & Grossard, C. (2024). A serious game to train rhythmic abilities in children with dyslexia: Feasibility and usability study. *JMIR Serious Games, 12*, e42733.

Weiss, A. H., Granot, R. Y., & Ahissar, M. (2014). The enigma of dyslexic musicians. *Neuropsychologia, 54*, 28–40.

Westwood, S. J., Olson, A., Miall, R. C., Nappo, R., & Romani, C. (2017). Limits to tDCS effects in language: Failures to modulate word production in healthy participants with frontal or temporal tDCS. *Cortex, 86*, 64–82.

Younger, J. W., & Booth, J. R. (2018). Parietotemporal stimulation affects acquisition of novel grapheme-phoneme mappings in adult readers. *Frontiers in Human Neuroscience, 12*, 109.

Ziegler, J. C., Perry, C., Ma-Wyatt, A., Ladner, D., & Schulte-Körne, G. (2003). Developmental dyslexia in different languages: Language-specific or universal? *Journal of Experimental Child Psychology, 86*, 169–193.

11
THE DEFINITION OF DYSLEXIA, STILL DEBATED AFTER ALL THESE YEARS

Franck Ramus

11.1 Introduction

In 2014, Joe Elliott and Elena Grigorenko took the dyslexia world by storm by launching "the Dyslexia Debate", proposing to do away with the term "dyslexia", and to simply treat all poor readers as one indistinct lump (Elliott & Grigorenko, 2014). Shocked, like many investigators in the field, I promptly reacted to defend the view that, despite many points well taken, not all poor readers were alike, and that it was a grave mistake to refuse to distinguish between them (Ramus, 2014).

Ten years later, Elliott and Grigorenko are back at it, with a fully updated literature review on dyslexia (Elliott & Grigorenko, 2024; henceforth, E&G). Again, the literature review is thorough and up-to-date, so I found little to dispute there. Most interestingly, while most of their argument remains unchanged, they have significantly modified their conclusion. Having become aware of the many interests that the word "dyslexia" serves, they no longer recommend its abandonment. Rather, they agree with continuing its use, under the condition that it should be strictly equated with reading disability or poor reading, without distinguishing between varieties of poor readers.

Simultaneously, several groups of researchers have felt a similar need to revisit the definition of dyslexia in the light of updated scientific knowledge. The International Dyslexia Association (IDA) has published a special issue of Annals of Dyslexia (Odegard et al., 2024), including several papers invited to reflect on a potential update of the IDA's original definition (Lyon et al., 2003). A group of researchers from the UK has also conducted a Delphi consensus procedure in order to establish a list of consensus statements on the definition of dyslexia (Carroll et al., 2025) and on practices for dyslexia (Holden et al.,

2025). Meanwhile, my views on dyslexia and on diagnostic categories have evolved as well, to such an extent that we might well end up meeting in the middle ground.

11.2 Different Views of Disease

For the first 15 years of my research on dyslexia, I had a clear idea of what dyslexia was: a distinct clinical entity with specific characteristics, making it stand apart qualitatively from "garden variety" or expected poor reading, from other clinical entities, and from normal functioning. Dyslexia was a natural kind, and the goal of research was to delineate its contours by "carving nature at its joints". I think that this feeling is shared by most researchers and clinicians who have seen many individuals with dyslexia, and who know dyslexia when they see it. Of course, I was aware that reading and other abilities were continuously distributed and that diagnostic criteria required somewhat arbitrary thresholds. Nevertheless, I considered that this naturally followed from measurement error and the multitude of factors other than dyslexia that influence reading ability, and that this therefore did not contradict the notion of a qualitatively distinct natural kind. I was also aware that researchers' and clinicians' impression of knowing what dyslexia is was somewhat circular: our intuition about what did and what did not characterise dyslexia relied to a large extent on what we had been taught that dyslexia was. Was there any real dyslexia entity, or was there only an arbitrary cognitive profile that we had learnt to recognise? Yet, together with most practitioners and researchers, I stuck to what could be termed a realist or a "lesion" view of disorders (Kendell, 1975).

By studying medical classifications more broadly, I have come to realise that the problem is not specific to dyslexia, nor is it specific to psychological, psychiatric, or neurological disorders. There is no such thing as an objectively defined disease. No disorder is a natural kind that we can just see by looking where the medical joints. This is quite obvious at the level of symptoms, which are all continuously distributed, whether a score in a reading test or a measure of blood pressure. Even more radical symptoms, such as bone fractures, infarcts, or cancers, come in graded versions with pathology smoothly fading into normality. This is also true at the etiological level, where some diseases are defined: even for chromosomal abnormalities that seem to give rise to obvious natural kinds (think of Down or Turner syndrome), there is in fact a whole continuum of partial trisomies or monosomies that engender a whole continuum of effects. Even at the level of the single gene, there can be a multitude of different mutations that very gradually modify the function or the level of expression of the protein. Discontinuity is nowhere to be seen.

This is not to say that all distributions are normal, or even unimodal. For various reasons, some mutations are more likely (or viable) than others, some causes are more frequent than others, some symptoms tend to cluster together, leading some distribution modes to be noticeable and therefore some categories to seem more natural than others. But this is the exception more than the rule. In most cases, distributions have only one mode and no obvious discontinuity separating normality from pathology. Those of us who have had the chance to see distributions of reading or cognitive scores from large, representative populations have failed to see any "hump" that might reveal a distinct population with reading disability (e.g., Di Folco et al., 2022).

Thus, a purely realist view of diseases is ill-founded. Diagnostic categories are what we define them to be. This doesn't imply that they are entirely arbitrary. Rather, their definition must be justified by their expected usefulness: to identify the individuals most in need of help and to provide them with the most appropriate treatment. Thus, definitions of diseases must incorporate a normative judgement considering the conditions that are sufficiently harmful to justify treatment, hence the classic conceptualisation of disease as "harmful dysfunction" (Wakefield, 1992, 2007), which is widely applied both in the World Health Organization's International Classification of Diseases and in the American Psychiatric Association's Diagnostic and Statistical Manual.

In ICD-11's definition of *Developmental learning disorder with impairment in reading*, the "significant and persistent difficulties in learning academic skills related to reading" criterion defines the nature of the dysfunction, while the "significant impairment in the individual's academic or occupational functioning" criterion defines what is considered harmful (World Health Organization, 2022). Similarly, in DSM-5's definition of *Specific learning disorder with impairment in reading*, "Difficulties learning and using reading skills" defines the nature of the dysfunction, while "cause significant interference with academic or occupational performance, or with activities of daily living" defines the harmfulness. In both cases, additional criteria provide more precise definitions of the dysfunction, of the severity threshold, and of potential exclusions.

It is interesting to note that both the ICD-11 and the DSM-5 definitions are purely statistical, based on applying thresholds on distributions of skills. This is obvious for the dysfunction criteria, but even the harmfulness criterion can be seen as applying a threshold on a distribution of academic or occupational functioning. These definitions thus stand out in a sea of definitions of dyslexia that largely seem to be based on a realist view of disorders and that include whatever people think reflects "what dyslexia really is": a certain type of cognitive deficit (Rose, 2009; Snowling & Hulme, 2024), a presumed neurobiological or genetic basis (Wolf et al., 2024), or any other putative essential trait of dyslexia.

Indeed, neither the ICD nor the DSM provides a definition of dyslexia per se. Their avoidance of the term is not fortuitous. It is probably motivated by the fact that they aim to include all varieties of reading disability, whether they affect word reading accuracy, reading fluency, reading comprehension, or any combination thereof. This contrasts with the traditional notion of dyslexia as affecting specifically word reading accuracy and/or fluency. Reading comprehension can, of course, be affected by reading accuracy and fluency difficulties, but it is not systematically so. Furthermore, there is evidence for a different, specific type of reading comprehension difficulties ("poor comprehenders") that arise later, independently from reading accuracy and fluency difficulties, and that seem to more directly reflect oral language comprehension difficulties (Nation et al., 2010).

Interestingly, as we have previously analysed (Di Folco et al., 2022), the two classifications differ mainly in two crucial criteria: 1) the ICD-11 maintains a reading-IQ discrepancy criterion ("performance in reading is markedly below what would be expected for chronological age and level of intellectual functioning"), while the DSM-5 dropped it. 2) The DSM-5 requires that the symptoms have persisted "despite the provision of interventions that target those difficulties", while the ICD-11 makes no such requirement. This latter criterion is synonymous with "poor response to intervention", and effectively ensures that transitory reading delays that may be due to suboptimal teaching are not diagnosed as a specific learning disorder.

The controversial reading-IQ discrepancy criterion, although statistical, can be seen as a remnant of a realist view, whereby dyslexia is not merely the tail of the distribution of reading ability, but is something more special, a specific cognitive deficit relative to other cognitive abilities. This criterion was disputed mostly on the grounds that it was unreliable (Stanovich, 2005) and that it did not seem to usefully distinguish children who might benefit from different interventions (Stuebing et al., 2011). In that sense, by doing away with this criterion, the DSM has adopted a more thoroughly anti-realist stance than the ICD, focusing strictly on the usefulness of diagnostic criteria rather than on ideas about what the disorder "really is".

This trend seems further reinforced by the second difference between ICD-11 and DSM-5. Indeed, by ensuring that diagnosis is targeted at children who have resisted first-intention educational interventions and who therefore really need more complex or intensive interventions, the DSM-5 definition theoretically ensures that the diagnosis of specific learning disorder is made maximally useful. It may therefore be an optimal solution to the conundrum of dyslexia definitions, as advocated by Miciak and Fletcher (Miciak & Fletcher, 2020) and Vaughn et al. (2024).

Surprisingly, although E&G enthusiastically comment on the advantages of this approach to the definition of dyslexia (which they label Dyslexia 3), they eventually dismiss it on the grounds that 1) this approach requires multi-tiered systems of support (MTSS) or response-to-intervention (RTI) frameworks to operate[1]; 2) even where such systems exist, they may not be implemented consistently, in particular with respect to the criteria for adequate or insufficient response to intervention, and 3) that it will meet resistance from many stakeholders and the dyslexia industry (p. 286).

11.3 E&G's Recommendations

In their conclusion, E&G reluctantly accept the continued use of the term "dyslexia", subject to 11 conditions. I list them below, together with my comments:

i Dyslexia should be used solely to reference a severe and persistent difficulty in accurate and fluent word reading in the individual's first language.

   Everybody agrees on "severe and persistent". Yet, taken alone, these criteria are consistent with diagnosing a child who has not received evidence-based teaching and first-intention educational remediation. Consistent with E&G's worry that the dyslexia label should not be used too liberally, I think it would make more sense to add DSM-5's insufficient response to intervention criterion, in order to promote good teaching practices and pedagogical interventions, and to avoid the transitory labelling of children who will outgrow simple reading delays. In my view, the term dyslexia could be reserved for pupils who reach Tier 3 within MTSS, or even (more conservatively) for those who don't respond sufficiently well to Tier 3. Such a criterion is that MTSS is designed with a minimal pace between tiers. If it takes 3 years to reach Tier 3, that's probably too late.

ii The use of dyslexia as a term synonymous with a medical diagnosis, with symptoms and an underlying cause, should be discontinued.

   E&G does not make it clear what is wrong with the notion of symptoms and underlying cause. This is a sound way to describe disorders that manifest behaviourally, but whose symptoms can be understood as the consequence of a complex network of causes at distinct levels (cognitive, neural, genetic).

   E&G's second recommendation resonates with the "this is not a disease" discourse, popular with some (but not all) individuals with learning disorders, autism spectrum disorders, and psychiatric disorders. This view considers that the words disease, disorder, or dysfunction carry a value judgement that is not legitimate. The alternative view is to consider that calling something a disease is a deliberate choice, made to draw attention to and help a certain category of population. And the best criterion to do so is the notion of "harmful dysfunction". As I have shown above, ICDs and APAs' definitions do implement the double criterion of harmful dysfunction to reading disability. In that sense, dyslexia can legitimately be defined as a disorder, without this implying any value judgement, of course.

   The idea that dyslexia should not be a medical diagnosis is also sometimes argued on the grounds that evidence-based interventions are not medical but rather pedagogical. But this is not in itself the sole valid criterion to decide to call something a disorder. Not all diseases call for medical treatment (e.g., diet for phenylketonuria, glasses for myopia, behavior therapy for Down syndrome). Furthermore, even for dyslexia, this may only be true for first-intention interventions (stage 2 of MTSS). While Tier 3 interventions remain of the same nature, there are still pupils who fail to progress in Tier 3 interventions. For those pupils, extensive neuropsychological and language testing is appropriate, and other types of intervention should be considered, including speech and language therapy, orthoptics, psychomotor remediation, etc. In other words, beyond Tier 3 (the stage where use of the word dyslexia may be useful), paramedical/medical interventions may be relevant.

So, to the extent that Tier 3 dyslexia is a "harmful dysfunction", there is every reason for dyslexia to remain in the ICD and in the DSM as a disorder.

iii It should no longer be considered appropriate to divide struggling readers into diagnosable dyslexic and non-dyslexic categories.

It depends on what one means by "struggling readers". If one considers all struggling readers who may qualify for Tier 2 interventions, some are temporarily struggling readers, while others will show persistent difficulties (Tier 3). I think that E&G agree that only the latter should qualify for a diagnosis of dyslexia. Now, once children meet the criteria for sufficiently persistent difficulty and resistance to intervention, I agree that there is no reason to divide them into diagnosable dyslexic and non-dyslexic categories, in particular based on an IQ discrepancy criterion. However, there may be reasons to divide them into distinct subtypes of dyslexia, depending on the linguistic, visual, or visuo-attentional nature of their difficulty (Potier Watkins et al., 2023; Saksida et al., 2016).

iv It should be recognised that some reading difficulties are primarily a consequence of intellectual disability and severe sensory impairment (i.e., hearing or vision). Such difficulties are likely to require modified approaches to the teaching of reading.

Yes. This is similar to Statement #40 in the Delphi consensus study (Carroll et al., 2025). And as our understanding of the different subtypes of dyslexia progresses, other types of reading difficulties should be recognised as well, depending on the nature of the underlying cognitive deficits.

v The assessment of reading difficulties should focus primarily on relevant literacy skills and how these can best be enhanced.

At stage 2, yes. At stage 3 and beyond, more specific assessments of the underlying cognitive skills are likely to be useful.

vi Given the probabilistic, multifactorial nature of reading difficulty, the use of the term dyslexia should carry no assumptions as to etiology in respect of any individual reader.

Absolutely. Given the chaotic, many-to-many relationships between factors at the genetic, neural, and cognitive levels, it is unlikely that the observation of any set of symptoms will allow one to draw meaningful conclusions about other levels of description, beyond weak probabilistic associations.

vii Co-occurring comorbidities should be acknowledged, where appropriate, but these should not be seen to be indicative of an underlying dyslexic condition.

Absolutely. No comorbidity or associated characteristic is in itself a criterion for or an indication of dyslexia.

viii The expanded understanding of the dyslexia construct, spreading far beyond reading disability, should be discontinued.

Absolutely. Dyslexia should not be made synonymous with any "neuro-diverse condition". For the term to be meaningful, it must remain strictly a severe and persistent reading difficulty.

ix Where required by national or regional education systems, formal labelling of difficulty in academic areas should employ broad classificatory terms such as learning disability or specific learning disability. This should specify the particular areas of difficulty encountered by the individual (accurate and fluent word reading, reading comprehension, spelling, math, etc.).

This is consistent with the current medical classifications in DSM-5 and ICD-11.

x Professional training of educators should focus upon the prevention of, recognition of, and intervention for literacy difficulties (including problems of word recognition/decoding).

Yes. And on how to implement MTSS, since this is the only rational approach to the identification of dyslexic readers and to the provision of suitable, proportionate help.

xi The notion that those hitherto diagnosed as dyslexic require a different instructional approach to that appropriate for other struggling readers should be actively dispelled.

This is certainly true at Tier 2. However, at Tier 3 and beyond, the instructional approach needs to be increasingly individualised and tailored to the specific needs of each child. Furthermore, as a child's cognitive deficits are becoming well identified and as the limits of remediation become apparent, compensation strategies and adaptations allowing the child to circumvent their difficulties and have full access to education should be implemented. In other words, the instructional approach appropriate for Tier 3 dyslexic readers may partly differ from that appropriate for Tier 2 struggling readers.

11.4 Conclusions

There is much to like in E&G's 2024 version of the Dyslexia Debate. For one thing, the word "dyslexia" has regained its right to existence. For another, it keeps rejecting any realist notion of "what dyslexia is" to focus on "what the most useful definition of dyslexia is", a stance with which I am now much more aligned. Furthermore, it focuses on difficulties in word reading, as opposed to other forms of reading difficulty. This is consistent with the current academic understanding of dyslexia, but at odds with international classifications that also include difficulties in reading comprehension.

However, E&G has not changed its preferred way of defining the relevant category of individuals. Dyslexia is simply equated with a particularly broad notion of "reading disability", in which no additional inclusion or exclusion criterion can be applied beyond "a severe and persistent difficulty in accurate and fluent word reading". While they mention several good reasons to avoid making the definition too specific, in particular the risk of excluding some reading-disabled individuals from interventions from which they would benefit, this definition remains too broad in several ways. First, rather than excluding uncorrected sensory impairments from the definition of dyslexia, they indicate that they "are likely to require modified approaches to the teaching of reading" (point iv). One wonders what kind of modified teaching would be more appropriate than visual correction or hearing aids, and why not spare these children an inadequate dyslexia label? Second, E&G's preferred definition, while requiring that the difficulty be persistent, does not spell out the conditions under which persistence is to be appreciated. In particular, it does not require the provision of evidence-based reading instruction (MTSS's Tier 1), nor does it require the provision of a more intensive reading intervention (Tier 2). Thus, it risks including cases of educational disadvantage and cases of temporary difficulty due to a lack of appropriate educational intervention. Finally, E&G's definition also lacks an impact criterion, ensuring that only those individuals whose disorder has a significant impact on their academic or occupational functioning are diagnosed.

The notion of harmful dysfunction proposed by Wakefield (1992) remains to this day the most conceptually consistent definition of a disorder. It requires a double assessment: one for the nature of the dysfunction (here, in reading), and one for the harm caused (in academic or occupational functioning). The unambiguous identification of the dysfunction requires the application of a number of exclusion criteria, in particular concerning sensory disorders and inadequate educational instruction. The harm criterion requires an assessment of educational impact (in children). The RTI-MTSS approach provides the most sound and evidence-based framework to assess educational impact: it materialises as an insufficient response to targeted educational intervention. Depending on how the MTSS is organised (e.g., what specific criteria for inclusion in Tier 2 and Tier 3) and on the nature of the interventions proposed in Tier 3 and beyond, a sound diagnosis of dyslexia might require an insufficient response to intervention either at Tier 2 or at Tier 3.

Having the diagnosis of dyslexia crucially rest on the notion of response to intervention is consistent both with DSM-5 and with proposals by Miciak and Fletcher (Miciak & Fletcher, 2020) and Vaughn et al. (2024). For the DSM-5 to be perfectly consistent with the advocated notion of dyslexia, it would only need to split the current "impairment in reading" specifier into two more specific ones: "impairment in word reading accuracy or fluency" (dyslexia) and "impairment in reading comprehension" (poor comprehension).

While recognising the "scientific merit" of the proposal and "the promise of RTI/MTSS", E&G oppose the rather weak rebuttal that "there are likely to be too many competing personal and professional perspectives, interests, and agendas for their conception of dyslexia to gain and retain widespread purchase". Although it would be silly to give up the most scientifically sound definition just by anticipation of opposition, it remains true that MTSS are the exception rather than the rule, particularly outside North America. One may therefore worry that having a definition of dyslexia rest on a framework that is locally unavailable may make a diagnosis of dyslexia inaccessible to most of the children concerned. Yet, the immense merit of adopting such a definition would be to incite educational systems to adopt and widely deploy RTI/MTSS approaches, which is likely to benefit all poor readers in the long term. A flexible approach to the transition, with multiple definitions temporarily co-existing (as is currently the case in many countries with no official guidelines on dyslexia diagnosis), would simply be needed to ensure continuity of service for all reading-disabled children.

Acknowledgements

This work has received support under the programme "Investissements d'Avenir" launched by the French Government and implemented by ANR with the references ANR-17-EURE-0017 and ANR-10-IDEX-0001-02.

Note

1 Multi-tiered systems of support can be operationalised in different ways, but the most common approach consists in Tier 1: evidence-based teaching approaches for all pupils; Tier 2: for those pupils who fail to learn appropriately despite Tier 1, a specific educational intervention, in small groups with similar needs; Tier 3: for those pupils who fail to learn appropriately despite Tier 2, further intervention, typically more intensive, individualised, and potentially based on a more detailed assessment of cognitive skills and individual needs.

References

Carroll, J. M., Holden, C., Kirby, P., Thompson, P. A., Snowling, M. J., & the Dyslexia Delphi Panel. (2025). Toward a consensus on dyslexia: Findings from a Delphi study. *Journal of Child Psychology and Psychiatry*, *66*(7), 1065–1076. https://doi.org/10.1111/jcpp.14123

Di Folco, C., Guez, A., Peyre, H., & Ramus, F. (2022). Epidemiology of reading disability: A comparison of DSM-5 and ICD-11 criteria. *Scientific Studies of Reading*, *26*(4), 337–355. https://doi.org/10.1080/10888438.2021.1998067

Elliott, J. G., & Grigorenko, E. L. (2014). *The dyslexia debate*. Cambridge University Press.

Elliott, J. G., & Grigorenko, E. L. (2024). *The dyslexia debate revisited*. Cambridge University Press.

Holden, C., Kirby, P., Snowling, M. J., Thompson, P. A., & Carroll, J. M. (2025). Towards a consensus for dyslexia practice: Findings of a Delphi study on assessment and identification. *Dyslexia (Chichester, England)*, *31*(1), e1800. https://doi.org/10.1002/dys.1800

Kendell, R. E. (1975). *The concept of disease and its implications for psychiatry*. University of Edinburgh Edinburgh.

Lyon, G. R., Shaywitz, S. E., & Shaywitz, B. A. (2003). A definition of dyslexia. *Annals of Dyslexia*, *53*, 1–14.

Miciak, J., & Fletcher, J. M. (2020). The critical role of instructional response for identifying dyslexia and other learning disabilities. *Journal of Learning Disabilities*, *53*(5), 343–353. https://doi.org/10.1177/0022219420906801

Nation, K., Cocksey, J., Taylor, J. S., & Bishop, D. V. (2010). A longitudinal investigation of early reading and language skills in children with poor reading comprehension. *Journal of Child Psychology and Psychiatry*, *51*, 1031–1039.

Odegard, T. N., Farris, E. A., & Middleton, A. E. (2024). Dyslexia in the 21st century: Revisiting the consensus definition. *Annals of Dyslexia*, *74*(3), 273–281. https://doi.org/10.1007/s11881-024-00316-9

Potier Watkins, C., Dehaene, S., & Friedmann, N. (2023). Characterizing different types of developmental dyslexias in French: The Malabi screener. *Cognitive Neuropsychology*, *40*(7–8), 319–350. https://doi.org/10.1080/02643294.2024.2327665

Ramus, F. (2014). Should there really be a "dyslexia debate"? *Brain*, *137*, 3371–3374. https://doi.org/10.1093/brain/awu295

Rose, J. (2009). *Identifying and teaching children and young people with dyslexia and literacy difficulties*. Department for Education and Skills.

Saksida, A., Iannuzzi, S., Bogliotti, C., Chaix, Y., Démonet, J. F., Bricout, L., Billard, C., N'Guyen-Morel, M. A., Le Heuzey, M.-F., Soares-Boucaud, I., George, F., Ziegler, J. C., & Ramus, F. (2016). Phonological skills, visual attention span, and visual stress in developmental dyslexia: Insights from a population of French children. *Developmental Psychology*, *52*(10), 1503–1516.

Snowling, M., & Hulme, C. (2024). Do we really need a new definition of dyslexia? A commentary *Annals of Dyslexia*, *74*(3), 355–362. https://doi.org/10.1007/s11881-024-00305-y

Stanovich, K. E. (2005). The future of a mistake: Will discrepancy measurement continue to make the learning disabilities field a pseudoscience? *Learning Disability Quarterly*, *28*, 103–106. https://doi.org/10.2307/1593604

Stuebing, K. E., Barth, A. E., Molfese, P. J., Weiss, B., & Fletcher, J. M. (2011). IQ is not strongly related to response to reading instruction: A meta-analytic interpretation. *Exceptional Children*, *76*, 31–51.

Vaughn, S., Miciak, J., Clemens, N., & Fletcher, J. M. (2024). The critical role of instructional response in defining and identifying students with dyslexia: A case for updating existing definitions. *Annals of Dyslexia*, *74*(3), 325–336. https://doi.org/10.1007/s11881-024-00303-0

Wakefield, J. C. (1992). The concept of mental disorder. *American Psychologist*, *47*(3), 373–388. https://doi.org/10.1037/0003-066X.47.3.373

Wakefield, J. C. (2007). The concept of mental disorder: Diagnostic implications of the harmful dysfunction analysis. *World Psychiatry: Official Journal of the World Psychiatric Association (WPA)*, *6*(3), 149–156.

Wolf, M., Gotlieb, R. J. M., Kim, S. A., Pedroza, V., Rhinehart, L. V., Tempini, M. L. G., & Sears, S. (2024). Towards a dynamic, comprehensive conceptualization of dyslexia. *Annals of Dyslexia, 74*(3), 303–324. https://doi.org/10.1007/s11881-023-00297-1

World Health Organization. (2022). *International classification of diseases eleventh revision (ICD-11)*. World Health Organization. https://icdcdn.who.int/icd11referenceguide/en/html/index.html

12
COMPENSATORY MECHANISMS IN UNIVERSITY STUDENTS WITH DYSLEXIA

Pascale Colé, Lynne G. Duncan and Eddy Cavalli

12.1 Introduction

Research predominantly highlights the cognitive and neural deficits underlying the persistence of reading difficulties among university students with dyslexia (see Chapters 1–7 and 9 of this book). However, focusing solely on these deficits does not fully explain how these individuals manage to read. In recent years, research has started to turn its attention to the compensatory strategies that may help account for how dyslexic students cope with the intense exposure to written material required for higher education and the attainment of post-secondary degrees. Indeed, university students with dyslexia represent an ideal population for investigating the compensatory mechanisms associated with dyslexia.

It is estimated that 22–25% of children with dyslexia manage to overcome their initial reading difficulties (Lefly & Pennington, 1991). An investigation by Cavalli et al. (2018) of a large sample of 83 university students with dyslexia found that 18% ($N=15$) performed within the normative range on the Alouette standardized test of reading aloud a meaningless text (see Figure 12.1).

The test used by Cavalli et al. (2018), which is considered a measure of reading fluency-a core component of reading comprehension abilities (Wallot, O'Brien, Haussmann, Kloos, & Lyby, 2014)-shows that only a small percentage of these students have achieved this compensation. Thus, even within a population of adults with dyslexia regarded as high-functioning (Law, Veispak, Vanderauwera, & Ghesquière, 2018), relatively few appear to have compensated for their reading difficulties. These findings raise questions about the behavioural manifestations of compensation in dyslexia, as reading is considered a complex cognitive activity that engages a broad set of functions, skills, and

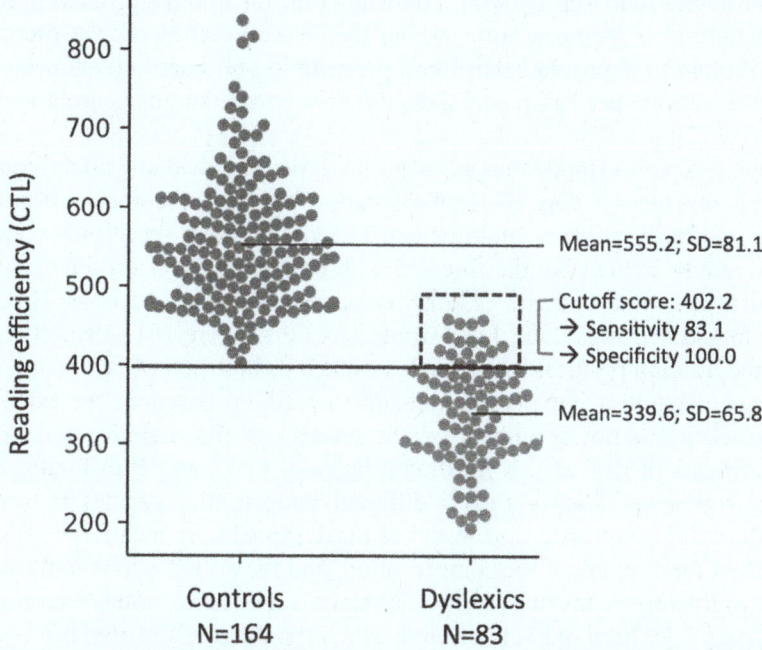

FIGURE 12.1 Distribution of efficiency scores (CTL index) obtained by a group of control adult readers ($N = 164$) and a group of adults with dyslexia ($N = 83$) on the Alouette reading test. The CTL index takes account of both accuracy and reading time, and the test has a sensitivity of 83% and a specificity of 100%. The red horizontal line represents the optimal value for the screening threshold (see Cavalli et al., 2018). The red dashed rectangle represents the 15 dyslexic participants who achieved a performance within the control sample's normal range. Adapted from Cavalli et al. (2018).

processing mechanisms (see the introductory chapter, Cutting & Scarborough, 2012). Further, the nature of compensations, whether behavioural or neurocognitive, has been the subject of limited research and the very concept of compensation requires further clarification.

12.2 The Concept of Compensation

As Livingston and Happé (2017) note, there is currently no agreed definition of compensation that describes its behavioural, cognitive, and neural characteristics. In light of this observation and based on a review of research on dyslexia, the authors propose that "compensation signifies some discrepancy between the perceived ability of an individual, exhibited in their behaviour (i.e., degree of observable symptoms), and actual ability, exhibited in underlying cognitive and/or neural function" (p. 731). Following this, the authors propose a working definition of compensation, which they conceptualize as "the processes contributing to improved behavioural presentation of a neurodevelopemental disorder, despite persisting core deficit(s) at cognitive and/or neurobiological levels" (p. 731).

Livingston and Happé thus suggest that dyslexic individuals can be considered *compensated* if they exhibit behavioural markers of compensation (initially, and brain markers could be considered later) that specifically concern their reading abilities but they must also show persistence of certain cognitive impairments that underlie reading deficits (as studies, such as Hatcher, Snowling, & Griffiths, 2002; Law, Wouters, & Ghesquière, 2015, demonstrate). A compensation profile is therefore determined by both compensation markers and neurocognitive impairments related to reading. However, the extent of compensation is not dependent on the severity of the cognitive and neural impairments of dyslexia, as illustrated by cases C, D, and E in Figure 12.2, where "the same" severity leads to different compensation profiles. In this figure, the weights represent the severity of the dyslexic impairments, the balloons represent the strength of the compensation, and the dotted arrows indicate the behavioural improvement in dyslexic symptoms. The horizontal line represents the diagnostic threshold value, below which the diagnosis of dyslexia is confirmed and above which the behavioural criteria for dyslexia are not met.

Only case D can be considered a successful case of compensation but can it be considered "total" (i.e., the individual no longer suffers from reading

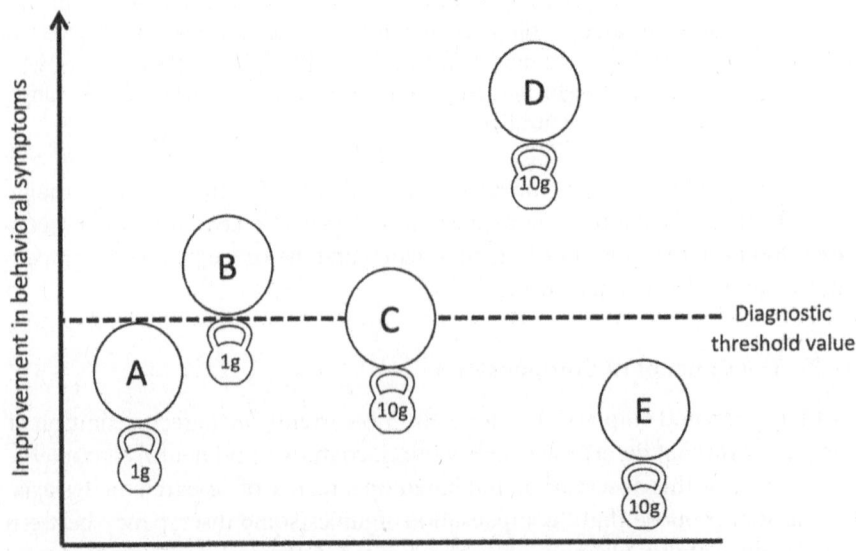

FIGURE 12.2 Compensation according to Livingston and Happé (2017).

difficulties)? As we will see in Section 12.4, for the proposals of Livingston and Happé to be fully operational, they must take into account the evaluation of different components of reading (decoding, word recognition, reading fluency, and reading comprehension) in order to distinguish between compensation profiles, as reading compensation cannot be seen as an "all or nothing" phenomenon. Furthermore, which indicator(s) of reading skills would be relevant? Should we use, for example, the level of reading comprehension required to acquire academic knowledge (which is the ultimate goal of reading), or the "core" marker of dyslexia, namely word recognition skills (Sprenger-Charolles & Colé, 2013)?

To address what the components of a compensation system might be, the multifactorial approach to dyslexia (Pennington, 2006) provides an interesting theoretical framework (which will be discussed in Section 12.5) for considering an interactive multi-level system to characterize this compensation system. According to Haft, Myers, and Hoeft (2016), the concept of compensation can be understood as a set of cognitive, neurobiological, and socio-emotional skills underlying the processes implemented by the cognitive system to compensate for the deficits causing dyslexia. These skills are considered as protective factors that have the potential to help mitigate (to varying degrees) some of the detrimental effects of the deficits at the root of dyslexia. Figure 12.2 illustrates the idea that compensatory processes, even if minimally effective, are consistently implemented by the cognitive system in an attempt to provide an appropriate response to the task at hand (reading a word, sentence, text, and comprehension). Finally, it is not possible to consider a diagnosis of dyslexia without identifying both the deficits and the compensations, as this will enable the most appropriate intervention and support.

12.3   Compensatory Strategies in Dyslexia

Livingston and Happé (2017) identify three general compensatory mechanisms in developmental dyslexia that help to reduce the behavioural symptoms and enable a level of reading sufficient for pursuing higher education. The first mechanism is where the phonological deficit at the cognitive level (which many researchers consider to be the root cause of dyslexia, see Chapter 2 and Sprenger-Charolles & Colé, 2013) can be fully corrected, leading to reading abilities within the normal range. The second is that phonological processing is not deficient but rather "delayed," meaning that it takes more time for a dyslexic individual to reach near-typical reading efficiency. However, the literature offers little support for these first two hypotheses. The results presented in Chapter 2 show that one indicator of a phonological processing deficit, namely phonological awareness, remains impaired in adults with dyslexia. For example, Bruck (1992, 1993) demonstrated poor phonological awareness in adults with dyslexia compared to typically reading individuals of the same chronological age and to reading-age-matched controls. Miller-Shaul (2005) further noted that this deficit tends to worsen compared to chronological age controls, especially in relation to the time taken to complete these tasks (see also Cavalli et al., 2016).

In fact, almost all studies report deficits in phonological awareness among adults with dyslexia and the meta-analysis by Swanson and Hsieh (2009) shows that tasks measuring phonological processing produce some of the largest effect sizes in comparisons with controls (Cohen's d = 1.60; see also the more recent meta-analysis by Reis, Araújo, Morais, and Faísca (2020) for tasks involving complex phoneme manipulation). Additionally, Cavalli et al. (2016) showed in a multiple-case study that 100% of a dyslexic student group performed significantly worse than the control group on a phoneme deletion task when speed was examined, and 90% showed lower accuracy.

Deficits are also observed in other forms of phonological processing, such as phonological short-term memory and the decoding procedure in reading (see, e.g., Castet, Descamps, Denis-Noël, & Colé, 2019; Szenkovits & Ramus, 2005). Supporting these behavioural findings, it is observed that the cortical areas dedicated to phonological processing are generally under-activated in individuals with dyslexia (see Chapter 7 of this book), and a reduction in grey matter is recorded in the left superior temporal sulcus (Eckert, Berninger, Vaden Jr., Gebregziabher, & Tsu, 2016; Richlan, Kronbichler, & Wimmer, 2013), a region considered central to phonological processing (but see Boets et al., 2013 on this point).

The third compensatory mechanism involves the possibility that dyslexic individuals may develop neurocognitive reading pathways that are independent of the deficient phonological route. We will revisit this point in Section 12.6.2 (see also Chapter 3 of this book, which provides valuable insights into this topic).

Although it seems reasonable to assume that the population of adults with dyslexia who are able to pursue university studies might contain a significant proportion of compensated dyslexics, a review of the research dedicated to this group does not provide entirely clear evidence. This is because the majority of these studies focus on identifying deficits, with compensation not being a central issue (except, e.g., Patael et al., 2018; Parrila, Georgiou, & Corkett, 2007; see also Figure 0.3 in the introductory chapter). In addition, these studies are mostly group-based (except for, e.g., Cavalli et al., 2016; Ramus et al., 2003) and the use of averages to characterize dyslexic and typically-reading students may obscure behavioural profiles of compensation within the dyslexic group. Cavalli et al. (2018) conducted a study with a large sample of dyslexic students and found that 18% of them achieved reading performance within the normal range. These individuals should, in theory, experience minimal difficulty with reading. One might then consider that their persistent problems could arise from other areas, such as spelling (a skill that is often still impaired in this population, Callens, Tops, & Brysbaert, 2012, and in the meta-analysis by Swanson & Hsieh, 2009, where the effect size for spelling difficulties was 1.77), or other areas related to reading (such as a visual disorder, e.g., see Castet et al., 2019), which could interfere with reading and general learning situations. Ramus et al. (2003) report from a sample of 16 dyslexic students that although all showed a phonological deficit (100%), only 5 of them exhibited this as a single deficit (31.2%). The remaining 11 students also exhibited associated deficits, such as auditory, visual, or motor impairments (68.7% of individuals showed associated deficits). This raises questions about how to conceptualise developmental dyslexia, particularly with respect to comorbidity with other disorders (a topic we will address in detail in Section 12.5).

An additional analysis in the study by Cavalli et al. (2018), conducted exclusively on the 15 dyslexic participants who achieved a reading score on the Alouette test above the screening threshold (i.e., within the normal range for control readers), enabled identification of individual deficit profiles related to phonological processing. Table 12.1 below reports the number of adults with dyslexia presenting deficits through the use of an efficiency measure (accuracy/time ratio) for tasks evaluating phonological skills (i.e., pseudoword reading, phonemic awareness, phonological short-term memory).

One might consider these individuals to be compensated dyslexics, since, according to Livingston and Happé's (2017) definition, their reading performance is normal (at least as measured by the test used), but the cognitive impairments underlying dyslexia appear to persist (such as the phonological deficit). However, the reading test used (the Alouette test) involves reading aloud a text that, although meaningless, may still provide occasional cues that help with reading. This may explain why, in the absence of context, 73% of these same individuals show deficient performance in pseudoword reading efficiency. In fact, Bruck (1990) showed that dyslexic university students often rely heavily or systematically on context to anticipate words, even when sentences provide minimal predictive value for the words to be read.

TABLE 12.1 Number (and percentage) of the 15 dyslexic participants whose Alouette reading score was within the typical reader range (CTL score > 402.2) in the Cavalli et al. (2018) study, who showed a deficit in pseudoword reading, phonemic awareness or phonological short-term memory (STM).

Task	N (%)
Pseudoword	11/15 (73)
Phonological awareness	7/15 (47)
Phonological STM	9/15 (60)

12.4 Behavioural Indicators of Compensation in Dyslexia: Data from University Students with Dyslexia

Adults with dyslexia who are able to pursue higher education offer valuable insights into the behavioural manifestations of dyslexia compensation. The evidence further suggests that all components of reading should be assessed, including reading fluency, basic reading processes (decoding and reading isolated words), reading comprehension, and spelling. Group studies have reported that while university-level dyslexic students continue to experience significant difficulties in decoding (pseudoword reading) and word recognition (isolated word reading), they may exhibit reading comprehension performance comparable to that of typically reading controls (Brèthes et al., 2022; Hatcher et al., 2002; Hebert, Zhang, & Parrila, 2018; Miller-Shaul, 2005), particularly when time pressure is removed (Deacon, Cook, & Parrila, 2012; Parrila et al., 2007). A meta-analysis conducted by Reis et al. (2020) reports that approximately one-third of adult participants diagnosed with dyslexia in the reviewed studies achieve reading comprehension performance within the normative range, suggesting that this ability may be less consistently impaired in adulthood. In contrast, most of these studies reported consistent deficits in phonemic awareness. However, these studies reported group averages that may mask significant individual differences in reading abilities, and, in addition, used tests and reading comprehension indicators with varying linguistic levels, such as sentences, paragraphs, and short or long texts, which engage word recognition skills to differing extents (Keenan, Betjemann, & Olson, 2008).

One of the first studies to examine the reading abilities of compensated and non-compensated dyslexics was conducted by Lefly and Pennington (1991). These authors compared two groups of adults with dyslexia matched for chronological age (mean of 45 years), total years of education (mean between 14 and 16 years), socio-economic status, and IQ. A control group of typical readers was also included in the study. Both dyslexic groups had significantly lower scores on the Adult Reading History Questionnaire (ARHQ; a screening assessment for reading difficulties during schooling; see, e.g., Bjornsdottir et al., 2014) and on a reading quotient (which compares observed reading and spelling performance with expected performance based on age and education level) relative to the control group. The compensated dyslexic group achieved identical performance to the control group on the Peabody Individual Achievement Test (PIAT) measures of word recognition and reading comprehension (silent reading of sentences with multiple-choice responses). However, they differed on oral reading fluency (Gray Oral Reading Test), Wide Range Achievement Test (WRAT) spelling, and the reading quotient. The non-compensated dyslexics differed from the control group on all measures. Compensated and non-compensated dyslexics differed on all measures except for reading comprehension. Law et al. (2015) also observed that compensated adult dyslexics performed better than non-compensated dyslexics on word recognition (WRAT-III) but, in contrast to Lefly and Pennington (1991), also found that the compensated dyslexics showed better reading comprehension as well (Woodcock-Johnson III (WJ-III); silent passage reading plus cloze procedure). Interestingly, these dyslexic groups did not differ from each other in a composite phonological measure comprising phonological awareness, digit span, nonword recall, and Rapid Automatised Naming (RAN). The dyslexic group as a whole differed from controls in each of the phonological subtests, suggesting the persistence of a primary phonological deficit across both compensated and non-compensated dyslexics (see also Pennington, Van Orden, Smith, Green, & Haith, 1990, for a similar conclusion).

Parrila et al. (2007) reported that 21 out of the 28 dyslexic students (75%) they evaluated demonstrated similar reading comprehension performance to control readers, using an untimed comprehension measure based on the comprehension questions answered according to what the participant was able to read in the Nelson-Denny Reading Test text. When timing is considered, using the reading fluency rate (which calculates the oral reading speed during the first minute), only eight participants (28%) exhibited performance similar to the control group. However, with the exception of two participants, all dyslexic adults in the study showed persistent difficulties in two or more areas of word reading, decoding, and spelling. Regarding phonological awareness, 15 out of 28 (53%) continued to demonstrate difficulties, but since the test involved words, interviews revealed that the participants had used orthographic strategies to complete the task (see Martin, Frauenfelder, & Colé, 2013, for a similar conclusion). Finally, 15 of the 28 dyslexic participants (53%) also showed difficulties in a RAN task, suggesting a persistent issue with the activation of phonological representations. Therefore, the majority of the dyslexic students in the study appeared to be compensated to the point where they can read for learning (provided they can read at their own pace), but continue to experience significant difficulties in the foundational skills of reading (decoding, word recognition). It seems that higher-level reading processes are easier to compensate for because they rely on a range of different abilities (vocabulary, general knowledge, and semantic processing). Supporting this hypothesis, Ransby and Lee Swanson (2003) found that the variance in reading comprehension performance is only minimally explained by phonological abilities, whereas general knowledge and vocabulary have a strong explanatory power, both for adults with dyslexia and control readers. Additionally, as Keenan et al. (2008) showed, the ability to comprehend texts is poorly explained by word-reading ability (around 7% of the variance), but much more variance is explained by oral comprehension abilities (around 30%). The opposite is observed for sentences that provide limited semantic context. More recently, Hebert et al. (2018) observed that although university-level dyslexic students exhibited reading comprehension performance similar to that of the control group (percentage of correct answers without time constraints), when word reading speed and text reading speed are controlled, they remained slower in responding to questions (vocabulary, literal and inferential questions) and required more time to activate knowledge related to the text. The authors concluded that these students needed more time to understand a text, not only due to their slower word and text reading speed but also for other reasons, such as underdeveloped metacognitive strategies, slower retrieval of necessary information for comprehension, lack of confidence in their responses, etc. (see also Simmons & Singleton, 2000).

Finally, the study by Deacon et al. (2012) highlights the importance of the timing of diagnosis on the reading profiles of dyslexic students. The researchers compared two groups of adults with dyslexia: one group that had received a dyslexia diagnosis following a comprehensive assessment, and another group composed of students who scored within the potential dyslexia range on the ARHQ but had not received an official dyslexia diagnosis (although 14/31 of them had received accommodations such as tutoring and additional time in exams). Their performance on word and pseudoword reading tasks, text fluency, and text comprehension (with and without time constraints), as well as on a phonemic awareness task with pseudowords, was compared to that of a control group. In the latter task, both dyslexic groups performed worse than the control group but did not differ from each other. Interestingly, the scores of the adults with dyslexia showed a delay of about four school years, suggesting persistent difficulties in the phonological processing involved in this task. For the reading tasks, the control group outperformed both dyslexic groups, regardless of the measure used. The two dyslexic groups had nearly identical performance, except that the diagnosed group performed within normal range for reading comprehension without time pressure, while the other group showed this result in the text fluency task. According to the authors, these profiles reflect different adaptive strategies: the diagnosed group is likely to have learned to use effective compensatory comprehension strategies, which the other group may not have developed, as they placed emphasis instead on achieving a more typical reading rate.

The precise identification of the behavioural components of reading compensation in adults with dyslexica remains a relatively under-researched issue. However, the cited studies strongly suggest that complete compensation for reading difficulties across all components of reading is more of an exception than the rule (only 2 out of 28, according to Parrila et al., 2007, or 7% of the sample), even for adults with dyslexia who engage in intensive daily reading. On the other hand, when reading comprehension is prioritized as the criterion, the study by Parrila et al. shows that 75% of the examined sample (21/28) could be considered to exhibit compensation. The most frequent sign of compensation appears to be in reading comprehension tasks without time pressure. It also seems that the profile of deficits in the foundational processes of reading (word reading, decoding) is specific to each individual, suggesting that compensation profiles and degrees of compensation may also vary. Finally, the nearly universal observation of phonological disorders, particularly as measured by phonemic awareness tasks, may be interpreted as evidence that the cognitive difficulties underlying dyslexia cannot be fully compensated.

More recently, the cognitive profile approach adopted by Faísca, Reis, and Araújo (2023) is particularly interesting in addressing the question of cognitive indicators of dyslexia compensation. This study, conducted with Portuguese university students diagnosed with dyslexia during childhood, along with their matched skilled adult control readers, assessed their reading and cognitive abilities. A cluster analysis of the data from participants with dyslexia revealed two distinct profiles. Cluster 1 consisted of participants with clear phonological deficits and associated reading difficulties (64.5% of dyslexic participants), while Cluster 2 demonstrated better performance on most core reading skills and higher general cognitive abilities (35.5%). This suggests that individuals in Cluster 2 have partially overcome their phonological limitations through continued exposure to reading and writing. Therefore, the analysis identified two groups of university students with dyslexia, showing clearly different levels of reading performance and related skills. Although neither group reached normative reading levels, the more efficient group (Cluster 2) performed similarly to typical control readers in phonological awareness (phoneme deletion and spoonerism), phonological short-term memory, alphanumeric RAN, verbal working memory, and vocabulary. Additionally, compared to control readers, Cluster 2 exhibited higher general cognitive abilities, including composite non-verbal IQ and performance on the picture completion subtest, as well as a better visuospatial memory span. This result suggests that general cognitive abilities can serve as protective factors, helping students to compensate for their reading difficulties.

12.5 Models of Compensation in Dyslexia: The Multifactorial Approach

To understand the compensatory system developed by individuals with dyslexia, it is necessary to have detailed models of both reading and the cognitive functions involved, as well as a comprehensive description of all of the causal (or etiological) factors underlying dyslexia.

Morton and Frith (1993, 2001) were among the first to propose a "causal" model of dyslexia involving three levels of description: cerebral, cognitive, and behavioural. An environmental component was also outlined, which may influence any of these three levels. According to this model, dyslexia is caused by a genetic disorder that triggers a series of neurobiological issues, which in turn lead to cognitive and behavioural disorders. Morton and Frith (1993) refer to the cognitive deficits leading to dyslexic disorders as "cognitive primitives" (irreducible), as there are no more elementary cognitive processes to explain them. The cognitive level is not seen as an intermediary causal level between the cerebral and behavioural levels because cognitive primitives are neurologically hardwired; they realize the functional instantiation of the underlying brain circuitry. Thus, for example, phonological processing is considered a cognitive primitive in dyslexia, representing the functional instantiation of the brain circuitry associated with this processing. Moreover, environmental factors can modulate cognitive difficulties, for example, the transparency of orthographic systems in reading (which we will discuss further in Section 12.6.5). In Frith and Morton's model, a single cognitive deficit (phonological processing) would be necessary and sufficient to cause (and thus explain) all the behavioural characteristics of dyslexia. The hypothesis of a phonological processing deficit as the cause of dyslexia remains dominant in many studies in the field. However, Pennington (2006) challenged the reality of a there being a single deficit in dyslexia, regardless of the nature of the deficit being proposed (e.g., phonological, visual, auditory). He pointed out several of the weaknesses in a single-deficit model. First, a single cognitive deficit cannot explain all the behavioural symptoms of dyslexia. For instance, not all dyslexic individuals exhibit a phonological deficit (Pennington et al., 2012; White et al., 2006). Conversely, not all individuals with a phonological deficit display dyslexia (Snowling, 2008). A constellation of deficits may therefore lead to dyslexic symptoms. Second, single-deficit models do not easily account for the comorbidity of dyslexia with other neurodevelopmental disorders such as dyscalculia, specific language impairments, speech disorders (oral development disorders, particularly in the intelligible production of speech), and attention-deficit hyperactivity disorder (ADHD). For example, Pennington (2006) reports that the comorbidity of dyslexia with speech disorders or ADHD is about 30%, suggesting these disorders do not occur independently. More specifically, according to Willcutt and Pennington (2000a), the comorbidity of dyslexia and ADHD ranges from 25% to 40% and molecular genetic methods suggest numerous shared genes between these two neurodevelopmental disorders (Gayán et al., 2005).

Finally and recently, Marchetti et al. (2023) demonstrated a significant co-occurrence of articulatory deficits in adults with dyslexia. Two groups of university students with dyslexia were recruited: one without associated disorders and the other with Developmental Coordination Disorder (DCD). A diadochokinesis (DDK) task, designed to evaluate articulatory performance, was administered to both groups. Specifically, the aim was to determine whether the fine and gross motor deficits observed in the DCD group were also associated with an articulatory/orofacial deficit. In this task, participants were instructed to produce the tri-syllabic pseudoword /pataka/ as quickly and accurately as possible for 30 seconds, at a pitch and volume they found comfortable. Interestingly, both dyslexic groups exhibited slower articulatory rates compared to the skilled reader control group, with the DCD dyslexic group showing additional difficulties in respiratory control (evidenced by a reduced proportion of speech and an increased pause duration). A phoneme awareness task (Initial Phoneme Deletion Task) involving pseudoword strings was also administered. While both dyslexic groups performed worse than the control group, their performances were comparable, suggesting that impaired phoneme representations in dyslexia may be partly explained by articulatory deficits that hinder access to these representations.

Moreover, a single deficit model explains the comorbidity of dyslexia and speech disorders through the severity hypothesis, which posits that both disorders are caused by the same underlying phonological deficit. According to this model, speech disorders are considered an earlier developmental manifestation of this deficit compared to dyslexia. In this framework, cases of comorbidity involve individuals with the most severe phonological deficits. If the deficit is less severe, speech disorders may not be clinically detected, although dyslexia might still be identified. To account for cases where individuals present with very early speech disorders but do not later develop dyslexia, the model must consider the possibility of a distinct subtype of speech disorder. Alternatively, it could be hypothesized that the phonological deficit in these cases resolves by the time children begin learning to read. However, longitudinal studies, such as those by Snowling, Bishop, and Stothard (2000) and Peterson and Pennington (2009), have reported that children who exhibited very early speech disorders (at age 4) demonstrated normal reading abilities at age 15 while continuing to exhibit phonological deficits. Thus, the phonological deficits observed in these children without dyslexia but which are similar to those with dyslexia are inconsistent with the hypothesis of a single cognitive deficit.

More generally, genetic studies of dyslexia suggest that its origin is not deterministic (caused by a single gene, which would make dyslexia a discrete "all-or-nothing" condition) but probabilistic (and therefore polygenic, with dyslexia resulting from deficits influenced by multiple genes and their interactions). Each gene contributes only modestly to the etiology of dyslexia (Bishop, 2015; Fisher & Francks, 2006; Pennington, 2006). Giraud and Ramus (2013) have proposed a model in which the phonological deficits associated with dyslexia are caused by genetic anomalies affecting the cortical microarchitecture of the temporal lobe.

Moreover, behavioural genetics studies (see DeFries, Fulker, & Olson, 2005, for an overview of the methodology) showed that in dyslexia, the relationship between traits (e.g., reading skills and inattention) is stronger in monozygotic twins (derived from the same egg and sharing the same genetic makeup) than in dizygotic twins (derived from two different eggs and sharing, on average, half their genetic heritage) (Willcutt et al., 2000). This finding supports a genetic overlap between dyslexia and ADHD. Willcutt et al. (2000) also reported that a deficit in processing speed is characteristic not only of dyslexia but also of ADHD, suggesting that processing speed may represent a shared cognitive risk factor (for more recent findings, see McGrath et al., 2011). Shared deficits have been reported in other comorbidities of dyslexia, such as the phonological deficit observed in Specific Language Impairment (Bishop, McDonald, Bird, & Hayiou-Thomas, 2009) and a processing speed deficit in dyscalculia (van der Sluis, de Jong, & van der Leij, 2004). These studies therefore suggest a cognitive and etiological overlap between dyslexia and other neurodevelopmental disorders, which argues against a single-deficit model as it cannot fully account for their co-occurrence at higher rates than would be expected by chance (Willcutt & Pennington, 2000a). Accordingly, Pennington (2006) proposed a multiple-deficit model, summarized in Figure 12.3.

The term *pleiotropy* is derived from the field of genetics and broadly refers to the phenomenon where a single biological cause can lead to multiple cognitive deficits (Pennington, 2006).

In this model, both genetic and environmental risk factors operate probabilistically, increasing the susceptibility to the emergence of a disorder (conversely, protective factors reduce this susceptibility). Etiological factors give rise to the behavioural symptoms observed in neurodevelopmental disorders by influencing the development of neural systems and the cognitive processes involved. There is no single etiological or cognitive factor sufficient to cause the disorder. Instead, multiple cognitive deficits (each stemming from multiple etiological factors) are necessary to produce a disorder at the behavioural level.

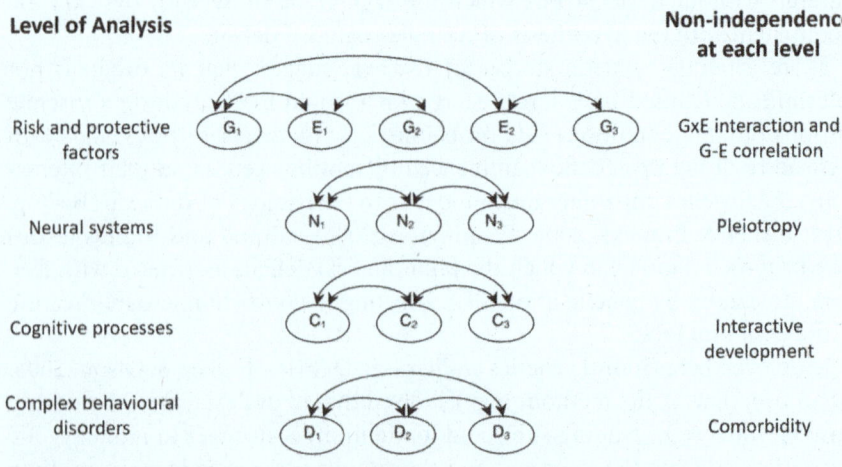

KEY: G=genetic risk or protective factor; E=environmental risk or protective factor; N=neural system; C=cognitive process; D=disorder

FIGURE 12.3 A multifactorial model of dyslexia. Adapted from Pennington (2006).

Some of the etiological and cognitive risk factors are shared across multiple disorders. Consequently, comorbidity in neurodevelopmental disorders is to be expected. One implication of this model is that the distribution of susceptibility to a disorder is often continuous and quantitative rather than discrete and categorical. As a result, the threshold for the disorder to manifest is somewhat arbitrary. This implies that observed comorbidity arises from both disorder-specific profiles of etiological and cognitive risk factors and the sharing of these risk factors across disorders.

In this model, there are four levels of analysis: etiological, neural, cognitive, and symptomatological (behavioural), where sets of symptoms define complex behavioural disorders. At each level, the bidirectional arrows indicate that the potential causes of the disorder are not independent. For instance, at the etiological level, interactions between genes and the environment can be considered. At the neural level, a single genetic or environmental risk factor will often affect more than one neural system (*pleiotropy, phenotypic determinism*). Even if the risk factor initially impacts only one neural system, this alteration may have downstream effects on the development of other neural systems. At the cognitive level, potential causes are correlated because cognition involves the interaction of multiple functions whose development is also interdependent. It is this overlap or interaction between functions that leads to the observed comorbidity at the symptom level. Consequently, whereas a single deficit model conceptualizes the relationship between these disorders in terms of double dissociation (e.g., between dyslexia and ADHD), the multiple-deficit model frames it in terms of partial overlap. At the symptom level, there is comorbidity (i.e., more frequent co-occurrence than would be expected by chance) of complex behavioural disorders. In this framework, feedback loops from behaviour to the brain, and even to etiology, are not represented due to the lack of available data on this question.

This model was tested by McGrath et al. (2011) with 614 children and adolescents aged 8–16 years who exhibited dyslexic and ADHD-related difficulties. Participants were recruited from the Colorado Learning Disabilities Research Center as part of a study on the etiology of these two disorders. Consistent with Pennington's (2006) model, each disorder (reading and attention) has both disorder-specific and shared predictors. For dyslexia, the predictors include performance on a phonemic awareness task (e.g., removing the initial or final phoneme from a word or pseudoword) and rapid naming speed (e.g., quickly naming images, letters, or numbers). Both predictors were found to predict performance on isolated word reading tasks. Inhibition abilities (e.g., pressing a button whenever a "1" is followed by a "9," with or without distractors in between) specifically predict ADHD symptoms in the domains of inattention and hyperactivity-impulsivity. Processing speed (e.g., quickly copying symbols associated with numbers based on a given code) predicts both disorders.

Recently, van Bergen, van der Leij, and de Jong (2014) proposed an extension of Pennington's (2006) model (see Figure 12.4; see also Chapter 9), incorporating underexplored factors in the explanation of dyslexia, namely familial and extra-familial influences. Since the work of DeFries and Fulker (1985), the familial transmission of dyslexia has been well established. However, most research has focused on the genetic component, referred to in the model as *passive genetic transmission*. In recent years, efforts have also been made to identify the influence of phenotypic transmission from parents (i.e., parents shaping the child's environment) on children's reading deficits. Parental (familial) influence is thought to result both from observable parental behavioural traits (phenotypic), referred to as *passive cultural transmission*, and from the interaction between the parental genotype and the environment, referred to as *passive gene-environment correlation transmission*. For example, the importance parents place on reading, which leads them to closely monitor their child's reading development, illustrates the influence of parental phenotypic traits. Regarding *passive gene-environment transmission*, parents with strong (genotypic) reading skills are more likely to spend significant time reading, thus modelling this behaviour for their children. They may also have higher levels of

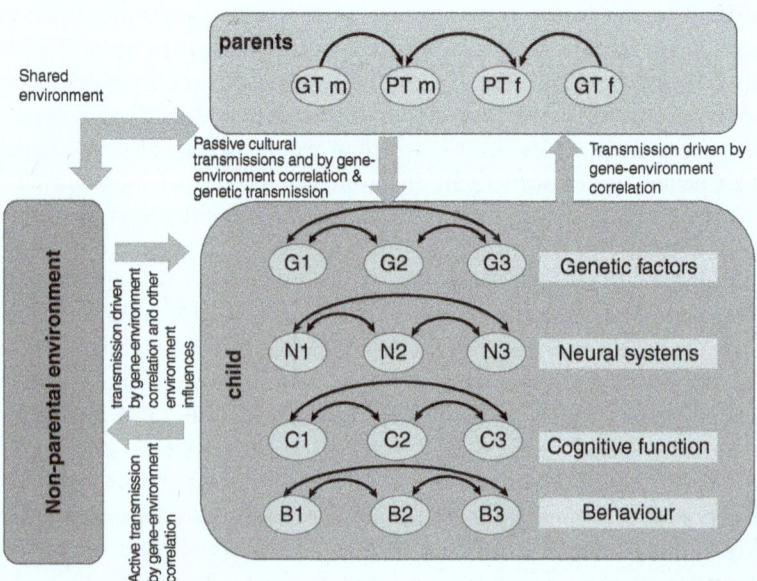

FIGURE 12.4 The dyslexia transmission model proposed by van Bergen et al. (2014), including both familial and extra-familial transmission. Adapted from van Bergen et al., 2014.

GT: genotype (m: mother and f: father), PT: phenotype, G: genetic factors, N: neural systems, C: cognitive function, B: behaviour.

education and enrol their children in better schools. The child is not merely passive in this process. Passive transmission is coupled with child-initiated or child-elicited transmission, referred to as *evocative gene-behaviour transmission*. Children who are genetically predisposed to become skilled readers are more likely to make frequent and early requests for reading activities, books, library visits, and story-time.

Alongside the family unit, environmental factors are also considered in the etiology of reading disorders in various ways. Thus, the extra-familial environment, whether shared or not by family members, can have either a positive or negative effect on the development and reinforcement of reading skills in both parents and children. This extra-familial environment can be shared, referring to all environmental factors that influence the reading phenotypes of both parents and children. For example, socio-economic conditions may limit access to printed or digital books, thereby impacting the reading abilities of both parents and children.

However, the child's environment is not solely shaped by the parents. As the child grows, they spend less and less time with their parents. Part of the environmental influence, therefore, is not shared with the parents. Gradually, the child themselves selects and actively creates their environment. This extra-parental environmental influence is thus considered *elicited* (elicited environmental influence and gene-environment correlation), with, for instance, teachers providing more challenging reading material to skilled readers. Additionally, the child exerts an active influence on their environment by selecting peers (e.g., friends) who enjoy reading (active gene-environment transmission).

Haft et al. (2016) add a socio-emotional level of analysis to this multifactorial framework of dyslexia, which refers to the psychosocial adjustment skills of individuals in relation to certain personality traits (e.g., the ability to engage in positive thinking). According to the authors, dyslexia could function as a risk factor for socio-emotional difficulties, either because these difficulties occur alongside dyslexia, potentially due to information processing difficulties and impulsivity (Parhiala et al., 2015), or because these socio-emotional problems manifest as a secondary emotional reaction triggered by the stress of repeated reading failures (Vaughn, Elbaum, & Boardman, 2001). Studies show that individuals with dyslexia are more likely than their typically developing peers to have low self-esteem and to develop anxiety or depression (Willcut & Pennington, 2000b). Thus, a vicious circle develops, in which negative emotions and social experiences interact with the individual's dyslexia, limiting cognitive abilities and reinforcing reading failure (see Haft et al., 2016 for a review on this point). Conversely, socio-emotional skills can act as protective factors for dyslexia (see Section 12.6.4). However, while the authors align with Pennington's (2006) framework, the status of this level of analysis is not clearly defined. It can be considered either as a component of the cognitive level of analysis itself or as a socio-emotional component of cognitive processes. The socio-emotional level fits into both Pennington's (2006) model and Van Bergen et al.'s (2014) model, but to understand its interactions with the other levels, its exact status must be clarified.

The value of the models reviewed lies in the fact that their level of description provides various possibilities for compensation (and not just deficits), for which the available data is limited. Nevertheless, they offer the important advantage of enabling us to interpret the data currently available.

12.6 A Synthesis of Potential Protective Factors in Dyslexia

12.6.1 Genetic Factors

There are a few studies on the interactions between genetic and environmental influences on the behavioural manifestations of dyslexia, and although it is unlikely that the mechanisms of compensation can be directly extracted from these studies, they remain valuable. Indeed, it is still difficult to identify the genes responsible for dyslexia, as some identified genes are not specific to the neural circuits involved in reading or even to the human brain (see Fischer et al., 2006 on this point). However, a few studies have explored the relationships between genetic mutations and reading deficits. For example, Zhang et al. (2012) sought to highlight a link between three variants of the DYX1C1 gene and reading and spelling skills in a sample of 284 Chinese children, followed over a period of 7–10 years. Every year, spelling and reading skills were assessed. The results of this study reveal a connection between the presence of an allele of the DYX1C1 gene and poor spelling skills, but not reading skills, suggesting that this allele may be an important risk factor for spelling abilities. Similarly, the study conducted by Bates et al. (2010) on adolescents (average age 17.5 years) suggests the presence of links between multiple variants of the DYX1C1 gene and a set of cognitive skills such as spelling of words and pseudowords, pseudoword reading, and digit span. Other genes have been proposed as candidate genes for susceptibility to dyslexia in at least two studies published in international journals, including the KIAA0319 gene (Francks et al., 2004), DCDC2 (Meng et al., 2005), MRPL19/GCFC2 (Anthoni et al., 2007), ROBO1 (Tran et al., 2014), and the FOXP2 gene (Sánchez-Morán et al., 2018), which has been identified as a candidate gene for the comorbidity between dyslexia and ADHD. However, it remains crucial to interpret these results with caution, as the likely interaction of multiple deficient genes complicates the issue. Finally, any intervention at this level in humans undeniably raises ethical concerns that must be considered.

However, Friend, DeFries, and Olson (2008), with a sample of 549 pairs of monozygotic and dizygotic twins (average age: 11.5 years), show that the parents' level of education (a proxy measure of socio-economic status) modulates the genetic influence of dyslexia. They observed a stronger genetic influence and a weaker environmental effect in children with parents who had a higher level of education (and thus a higher socio-economic status), compared to children with parents who had a lower level of education and socio-economic status. According to the authors, these data support an eco-biological model in which genetic heritability is stronger in an environment that stimulates the activation of genetic potential (in this case, the potential leading to reading, with the environment stimulating this activity as a factor of success). Recently, a large study involving 876 pairs of twins (300 monozygotic and 300 dizygotic) focused on the relationships between phonological skills and other more general cognitive abilities, such as verbal IQ and performance IQ (participants were tested at an average age of 16.2 years ±1.27 standard deviations), as well as the genetic or environmental source of this influence (Lazaroo et al., 2019). Overall, the results suggest a strong influence of genetic factors on all cognitive skills, including phonological abilities (i.e., the correlations between twins on different cognitive skills were stronger in monozygotic twins than in dizygotic twins). The results show that a general genetic factor (i.e., associated with crystallized learning and acquired knowledge) accounts for nearly 20% of the variance in phonological skills in reading, although the nature of this relationship is not explained. Shared environmental effects, on the other hand, do not explain the relationship between reading skills and academic performance. This study, although very informative, did not provide information on the reading level of the participants.

It would be interesting to identify among the twins those who present reading delays, reading disorders, and those who compensate for their reading difficulties, in order to relate these observations to genetic and environmental factors to determine whether these relationships are the result of pleiotropy (phenotypic determinism) or a causal effect of phonological decoding skills and/or academic abilities.

In this context, a recent study (Gialluisi et al., 2019), conducted as part of a Genome-Wide Association Study (GWAS), investigated genomic variants associated with cognitive performance in a large population, including 9 cohorts of children with dyslexia (N total = 2562) and control children (N total = 3468). The results suggest an association between a variant of the MIR924HG gene on chromosome 18q12.2 (a gene involved in the differentiation of cells into neurons) and performance on the rapid naming task of letters (RAN), with an effect size $\beta > 0.7$. This variant also shows, albeit with smaller effect sizes (β between 0.3 and 0.6), multivariate associations across the genome with other cognitive traits analyzed in the study, including rapid naming of letters, numbers, and objects, word and pseudoword reading, spelling, and phonological awareness. Thus, the study identified a genetic effect at the genome-wide level on RAN letter performance, suggesting a pleiotropic genetic relationship (shared effects between traits due to their reciprocal relationships) across the entire RAN domain (rapid naming of letters, numbers, and objects), and, to a lesser extent, with reading skills. Interestingly, the study also reports genome-wide results (i.e., polygenic risk score) supporting the hypothesis of a partly shared genetic etiology between dyslexia and ADHD, two disorders that are highly comorbid.

12.6.2 Neurobiological Factors in Compensation

The neurocognitive mechanisms involved in the compensation of individuals with dyslexia remain poorly studied and understood, especially with regard to dyslexic adults. Compensation has been proposed as a mechanism to overcome deficits in the neurocognitive networks associated with reading that individuals with dyslexia exhibit. Although this hypothesis is compelling, the neural mechanisms involved in compensation are currently unknown, partly due to the lack of a precise conceptualization of compensation in neuroscience, as discussed earlier in this chapter. Indeed, the most common conceptualization of compensation in the literature suggests is increased brain activity in clinical populations, without consideration of spatial aspects (i.e., the localization of this neural overactivity), the underlying cognitive processes or the fact that this overactivation may be related to an epiphenomenon, such as increased cognitive effort (Hoeft et al., 2007; Richlan et al., 2013). Currently, the most precise definition of compensation at the neuronal level involves a change in neuronal activity or connectivity in neural networks outside the typical networks for the cognitive processes of interest (here, reading), which facilitates and/or enhances behavioural performance in individuals with the clinical condition of interest (here, dyslexia) (Hillary, 2008; Livingston & Happé, 2017). These mechanisms inevitably develop with age and (reading) experience, reaching maximal effectiveness in adulthood. Indeed, as previously noted, studies conducted on university students with dyslexia provide promising leads for further understanding the architecture and functioning of compensation mechanisms in dyslexia.

Studies of compensation have highlighted that dyslexic individuals use a wide range of linguistic and non-linguistic strategies to improve their reading ability, and some of these strategies are also employed by typical readers. A key approach to understanding the neural phenomena involved in compensation is the Interactive Compensatory Model of Reading (Stanovich, 1980, 1984). According to this model, dyslexic individuals experience significant difficulties in low-level reading processes, particularly in word recognition, which leads to a greater reliance on higher-level processing that provides additional sources of information for more fluent reading. For example, greater reliance on contextual information, semantic knowledge, and morphological knowledge has been shown to contribute positively to reading success (see, e.g., Frith & Snowling, 1983; Elbro & Arnbak, 1996). At the neural level, these processing strategies have often been associated with activation of the left ventral reading pathway, particularly the activation of the left Inferior Frontal Gyrus (for a magnetoencephalography study on dyslexic adults and morphological knowledge, see, e.g., Cavalli et al., 2018).

Oral language skills have also been linked to compensatory mechanisms that allow individuals with dyslexia to overcome deficits in lower-level reading processes (e.g., decoding and word recognition). This approach aligns with the work stemming from the simple view of reading model (Gough & Tunmer, 1986; Wagner, Herrera, Spencer, & Quinn, 2015), which supports the idea that oral language skills (e.g., listening comprehension, vocabulary) directly interact with decoding skills and not just with reading comprehension skills (Colé et al., 2018; Tunmer & Chapman, 2012). Regarding this approach, to our knowledge, there is no neuroimaging literature addressing this question in dyslexic adults. However, for a detailed review of the literature on this topic within the context of dyslexia, readers are referred to Chapter 3 of this book, which focuses on oral language, morpho-semantic skills, and their neural correlates in dyslexic adults. While most studies presented in Chapter 3 address cognitive protective factors in dyslexia, and while these studies rarely evaluate both oral/semantic language skills and decoding/phonological skills together (but see Cavalli, Duncan, Elbro, El Ahmadi, & Colé, 2017), a recent study conducted using anatomical neuroimaging with dyslexic adolescents investigated the brain bases (gray matter brain volume; see Chapter 7 of this book for information about this measurement) that could be related to different cognitive profiles of reading (Patael et al., 2018). Specifically, the authors of this study focused on the brain bases of two types of reading profiles, which could be placed on a continuum between decoding skill and reading comprehension. Participants (with an average age of 13.4 years) either demonstrated equivalent levels of decoding and reading comprehension (i.e., control group) or a dissociation between these two skills (i.e., discrepant readers). Participants with low decoding skills but relatively good reading comprehension were described in this study as resilient adults with dyslexia; participants with low comprehension but relatively good decoding skills were described as having specific reading comprehension disorders. The results of this study revealed that the magnitude of the dissociation in the two dissociated reader groups was related to brain volume in the dorsolateral prefrontal cortex, a region heavily involved in executive control mechanisms and working memory. The volume of this brain region was larger in resilient adults with dyslexia than in the other reading groups. Interestingly, the results of a second experiment conducted with pre-reading children showed that the brain volume of the dorsolateral prefrontal cortex is a strong predictor of the magnitude of the dissociation visible three years later in these same readers. These findings suggest the involvement of the fronto-parietal network and the cognitive functions associated with this brain network (i.e., cognitive control and working memory) in compensatory mechanisms for the disorders exhibited by individuals with dyslexia.

Finally, other processes have been linked to the hyperactivation of certain brain regions, particularly those involved in articulatory processes, which may serve as compensatory mechanisms in dyslexic readers (Richlan et al., 2011; Pugh et al., 2000). Indeed, as outlined in Chapter 7 of this book, the brain regions involved in articulatory mechanisms and subvocalization largely overlap and primarily engage the sensorimotor regions of the left hemisphere, the fronto-parietal cortex, and the left fronto-striatal articulatory loop (Hancock, Richlan, & Hoeft, 2017). Accordingly, in line with this hypothesis, the hyperactivations identified in individuals with dyslexia primarily concern these brain regions (see the meta-analysis by Richlan et al., 2011), thus supporting the role of an articulatory network in the compensatory mechanisms in dyslexia. Finally, other brain regions, notably those in the right hemisphere, have also been identified and linked to compensatory mechanisms in dyslexia. A recent fMRI study by Cavalli et al. (2024) suggests that high-functioning adults with dyslexia exhibit impairments in processing orthographic information in the left Inferior Frontal Gyrus (IFG) and left Fusiform Gyrus (FG), and the more severely impaired adults with dyslexia (those who present weaker reading fluency scores) seem to rely on right-homologues of the FG to process orthographic information.

12.6.3 Cognitive Factors in Compensation

As described in previous chapters, the main symptoms of dyslexia observed in children and adolescents persist into adulthood (even among those classified as compensated or high-functioning). However, Miller-Shaul (2005) observes that certain characteristics of dyslexia can change significantly with age, as these adults with dyslexia have developed compensations (or adaptations) driven both by continuous exposure to written language and strong motivation to learn.

The study by Miller-Shaul (2005) is one of the few to compare performance on a broad set of tasks (phonological, orthographic, decoding, fluency, and reading comprehension) between a group of adult dyslexic readers (aged 20–27 years) and a group of dyslexic children (Grade 4), with each compared to their respective age-matched control group. Although this is not a longitudinal study (and thus these results should be interpreted with caution, as there are no other studies of this type to our knowledge), it provides interesting insights into the potential evolution of cognitive profiles of dyslexia across the lifespan. It was observed that while performance differences on phonological tasks (such as rhyme judgment tasks) worsen with age (effect sizes may be up to twice as large for adults as for children with dyslexia), this is not the case for abilities in recognizing word spelling (e.g., orthographic choice tasks), where adults with dyslexia may, in certain tasks, show effect sizes ranging from null to moderate, even when time is taken into account.

However, orthographic skills are often considered deficient and remain the subject of debate (Share & Geva, 1995; Stanovich, West, & Cunningham, 1991). Nevertheless, given their phonological difficulties, several researchers have proposed that the orthographic pathway might be favoured in dyslexia (Horowitz-Kraus & Breznitz, 2014). Shafrir and Siegel (1994) offer some support for this by demonstrating that adults with dyslexia, due to their persistent difficulties in decoding written words, tend to "scan" them, whereas their typically developing peers decode them. Despite this, as we have emphasized, complete compensation, including word recognition, is very rarely observed, and Shafrir and Siegel reported significantly lower performance among adults with dyslexia compared to control groups for both real words and pseudowords. In general, the use of compensatory strategies of a visual and orthographic nature appears to be poorly supported by the literature, largely due to studies identifying a visuospatial-attentional deficit in dyslexia (for a synthesis of the literature on this issue, see Chapter 4 of this book). However, and interestingly, a recent study conducted on a population of French-speaking university-level dyslexic adults (Castet et al., 2019) helps in understanding better the origin of the visuospatial-attentional deficits present in certain dyslexic readers. In this study, the authors employed a specific methodology involving a partial report task. In this task, a string of letters was presented with a target letter highlighted. The target letter was cued either before the presentation of the string (i.e., pre-cued condition) or after (i.e., post-cued condition), allowing the researchers to dissociate the effects attributable to processes involving iconic memory from those more closely related to visuospatial-attentional processing. The results show poorer performance for adults with dyslexia compared to typically developing adults only in the post-cued condition, and not in the pre-cued condition. This result suggests that the transfer of information between iconic memory and short-term visual memory is impaired in dyslexic individuals, and this transfer seems to rely partially on the attentional capacities of the readers. This finding aligns with recent work (Ktori, Cavalli, Doignon-Camus, & Colé, 2017, unpublished study), suggesting that dyslexic readers are sensitive to and utilize visual and visuographic cues in the early stages of word recognition. The consideration of certain characteristic letter traits, particularly the shape of the letters and the word envelope, appears to be more critical for readers with significant phonological deficits and may interfere (i.e., inhibit) with the lexical selection process, thus suggesting that dyslexic readers use visuographic cues in reading to compensate for their phonological difficulties. This result is similar to what research has already shown concerning the use of contextual cues as a compensatory strategy in dyslexic readers (Bruck, 1990). In fact, Maggie Bruck (1990) was one of the first to report that adults with dyslexia would systematically rely on the context in which words appear to read them. The participants were asked to read aloud sentences presented on a screen, with the final word appearing only after the penultimate word was read, and the experimenter would press a button to make the target word appear. Two types of context were presented: control sentences (always the same) with a neutral context "When I press the button, you will see the word **contempt**" and a congruent meaningful context in which target words appeared in a prose passage (e.g., "Perhaps no creature on the face of the earth has been so persistently misrepresented as the pig. The English language treats the pig with **contempt**"). Although the reading times remained significantly longer than those of the control group, dyslexic readers showed stronger facilitation effects from the contextual sentence than the two control groups (matched for chronological age and lexical age). This was observed even though the context was not particularly predictive of the words to be read (but see also Ben-Dror, Pollatsek, & Scarpati, 1991).

Corkett and Parrila (2008) focused on determining the nature of the contextual effects observed. They presented sentences that were either semantically congruent with the final word to be read, the (target word (e.g., "the wine was served from the **decanter**") or incongruent (e.g., "the politician appealed to the **decanter**"). While the authors observed a facilitation effect from semantic congruence in both groups, the inhibitory effect generated by the incongruent condition was only observed in adults with dyslexia, even when reading speed was controlled. This suggests, according to the authors, a highly interactive processing mechanism rather than an artefact of slow reading. These findings suggest a cognitive compensation that allows the development and use of reading procedures strongly assisted by the knowledge stored in memory, enabling the modulation of deficit-driven processes engaged at the lower levels of reading, such as decoding or word recognition. This would be a top-down reading process (driven by concepts). Several studies support this hypothesis, particularly those focusing on the use of oral and semantic language skills, as well as high-level (contextual and semantic) processes by dyslexic readers to compensate for reading deficits. A detailed summary of these studies, along with an introduction to theoretical models conceptualizing the dynamics of these compensation mechanisms, is presented in Chapter 3 of this book. However, although these studies provide valuable insights into the cognitive processes involved in reading success, they offer limited information on the strategies used by dyslexic students to read and understand text correctly. To address this question, studies directly focusing on reading comprehension are of particular interest. However, to our knowledge, there are very few studies that identify the processing mechanisms involved in reading comprehension in adults with dyslexia. As reported in Section 12.4 of this chapter, the study by Ransby and Lee Swanson (2003) suggests a more significant role for semantic skills and general knowledge compared to phonological and decoding skills in reading comprehension in adults (both dyslexic and non-dyslexic). The recent findings reported by Brèthes et al. (2022) support this hypothesis. This study investigated the cognitive skills underlying text reading comprehension in a sample of 54 French university students with dyslexia and 63 university students without dyslexia. The assessment was based on a battery of tests adapted for an adult population, including listening comprehension, word reading, pseudoword reading (i.e., decoding), phonemic awareness, spelling, visual span, reading span, vocabulary, non-verbal reasoning, and general knowledge. Using stepwise multiplicative linear regression, the model that best accounted for text reading comprehension included listening comprehension, general knowledge, and vocabulary. Furthermore, the presence of a significant positive interaction between general knowledge and group status suggests that general knowledge contributed more strongly to text reading comprehension in readers with dyslexia than in skilled readers. These findings indicate that certain processes involved in extended text reading comprehension in adults with dyslexia may differ from those of skilled readers. Specifically, adults with dyslexia may rely more heavily on semantic information, potentially as a compensatory mechanism, to support their understanding of written texts.

Recently, a study conducted by Lefèvre, Law, Prado, Anders, and Cavalli (2025) examined how certain cognitive and environmental factors contribute to Reading Comprehension Resiliency (RCR) in adolescents with and without dyslexia. While individuals with dyslexia typically struggle with reading comprehension due to impaired reading fluency, some show resilience and achieve strong comprehension skills despite these difficulties. This study involved 95 adolescents, including 56 with dyslexia and 39 without, with an average age of 16 years, and aimed to identify which factors support this resilience, focusing on vocabulary, listening comprehension, and socioeconomic status (SES). Participants were assessed on phonological skills, oral reading fluency, reading comprehension, listening comprehension, vocabulary skills, and socioeconomic status. Lefèvre et al. (2025) used a double mediation model to analyze how vocabulary influences listening comprehension and, in turn, affects RCR. They also examined whether SES indirectly impacts RCR through vocabulary development. The findings revealed that adolescents with dyslexia had significantly higher RCR scores, demonstrating resilience in reading comprehension despite fluency difficulties. Vocabulary and listening comprehension played a crucial role in RCR, with vocabulary influencing listening comprehension, which in turn contributed to reading comprehension resilience. Additionally, SES was indirectly linked to RCR, as adolescents from lower SES backgrounds tended to have weaker vocabulary skills, which affected their ability to compensate for reading fluency deficits. Lefèvre et al. (2025) concluded that strengthening vocabulary and listening comprehension skills can help dyslexic adolescents improve reading comprehension, even when fluency remains impaired. They emphasized the importance of considering SES in educational interventions, as early exposure to rich language environments can significantly impact reading outcomes. These findings highlight the potential of targeted language interventions to support individuals with dyslexia, particularly those from lower SES backgrounds.

On adults with dyslexia, Pedersen et al. (2016) suggest that despite difficulties in reading, reading fluency, and sometimes certain aspects of written comprehension, the academic success of university dyslexic students does not appear to be affected, and they seem to understand academic texts relatively well. However, reading comprehension remains a relatively complex activity that involves not only cognitive skills but also reading strategies. Among the reading strategies, the use of "paratextual" cues, which help readers follow the chronology of the story or text by taking into account spatiotemporal information present in the text, appears to be effective in guiding the reading comprehension of university adults with dyslexia (Cavalli, Colé, Brèthes, Lefèvre, & Lascombe, 2019). In this study, the authors compared the reading comprehension of dyslexic adults and typically developing adults on relatively long texts, using two different reading formats: paper books and e-books. The questions were presented orally, and participants' answers were also given orally. The hypothesis of this study was that reduced access to spatiotemporal cues (i.e., paratextual cues) in the e-book format would prevent dyslexic readers from using effective and compensatory reading strategies. For this, different questions evaluating various levels of reading comprehension were created and administered (e.g., literal comprehension, inferential comprehension, location of events in the text, and chronological reconstruction). The results showed that with the paper book format, dyslexic adults performed similarly to typically developing adults on the literal and inferential comprehension tasks. Additionally, dyslexic adults scored similarly or even better than typically developing adults on tasks evaluating the spatiotemporal dimensions of reading (location of events and chronological reconstruction). In contrast, with the e-book format, dyslexic adults performed worse than typically developing adults on both the literal comprehension task and the tasks evaluating the spatiotemporal dimension. These results suggest that reading in an electronic format impacts certain aspects of reading comprehension in adults with dyslexia. Furthermore, this study highlights the effectiveness of a reading strategy based on searching for paratextual cues, as dyslexic adults obtained similar or even superior performance compared to their peers on certain aspects of reading comprehension when using paper format.

In this context, an increasing number of studies aim to identify how dyslexic students manage their studies. Among these, the works of Kirby, Silvestri, Allingham, Parrila, and La Fave (2008), Pino and Mortari (2014), and Olofsson, Ahl, and Taube (2012) suggest that these students have developed study strategies that enable them to best meet academic demands. Although these strategies may be specific to each individual, the aforementioned studies show that a number of these strategies are common across a large group of students. For instance, in order to understand and retain a text, these students place particular importance on visuospatial information that structures the text, such as section headings, italicized words, or highlighted key information.

They also employ very rigorous time management strategies, including careful planning of study time and exam preparation. As a result, they dedicate considerably more time to their studies than their typically reading peers. Dyslexic students also implement learning strategies that differ from those of their typically reading peers. For example, while a typically reading student would revise a lesson by directly memorizing its content, a dyslexic student would first reorganize the lesson to bring out its logical structure before attempting to learn it (Kirby et al., 2008). However, as discussed in Chapter 9 of this book, although these strategies have been developed, their direct influence on academic performance, particularly in reading comprehension, has not been tested.

However, the examples presented suggest the involvement of metacognitive strategies in learning activities and reading tasks. More generally, the role of cognitive control in the reading activity of dyslexic adults (see Chapter 5 of this book) as well as in dyslexic children and adolescents has rarely been studied, although a number of investigations confirm its involvement in typical reading. For example, Colé, Duncan, and Blaye (2014) demonstrated in children (average age 8 years) that flexibility (a component of cognitive control) predicts performance in both text comprehension and reading of isolated words, beyond the classic influence of decoding skills (for results in adults, see Georgiou & Das, 2018).

For children, studies focusing on executive functions in developmental dyslexia report conflicting data (see the meta-analysis by Booth, Boyle, and Kelly (2010), covering 48 studies). In adults, more research is needed because, for example, Beidas, Khateb, and Breznitz (2013) observed equivalent performance on tasks assessing inhibition, flexibility, and planning when compared to their chronological age controls (in contrast with their performance on visual short-term memory, naming, visual perception, and processing speed). In contrast, Brosnan et al. (2002) reported significantly lower inhibition performance in dyslexic adults compared to their chronological age controls (see also Chapter 5 of this book). However, the involvement of these functions in reading comprehension has not been evaluated in these studies. Therefore, the role of executive functions in reading in dyslexic adults needs to be further explored.

12.6.4 Socio-Emotional Factors in Compensation

Chapter 9 of this book, along with the study by Haft et al. (2016), provides valuable insights into this topic. Persistent reading difficulties may explain why, according to the British study conducted by Carroll and Iles (2006) and the Italian study by Ghisi, Bottesi, Re, Cerea, and Mammarella (2016), dyslexic students report being more anxious than their non-dyslexic peers, with this anxiety manifesting in many other social situations. The ongoing challenges in reading lead to lower self-esteem (MacCullagh, Bosanquet, & Badcock, 2017) and a diminished sense of self-efficacy in various academic domains (Stagg, Eaton, & Sjoblom, 2018). The concept of self-efficacy, developed by Bandura (1977), is defined as "the perception individuals have of their abilities to perform a specific task." The study by Stagg et al. (2018) also highlights the motivating role of identification models provided by teachers for these students. The study by Andreassen, Jensen, and Bråten (2017) shows that the use of self-regulation strategies can impact self-efficacy and academic performance in dyslexic students but not in non-dyslexic students. Among these strategies are: note-taking, summarizing texts, highlighting or underlining text, making diagrams, listening to audiobooks, listening to recorded lectures, and text-to-speech translation. Furthermore, although both groups use these strategies, dyslexic students more systematically rely on visual (highlighting/underlining, making diagrams) and social (participating in class discussions, consulting peers, seeking help from fellow students, friends, and professors) strategies. They also perceive these strategies as particularly effective and closely tied to their self-efficacy and academic performance, which is not the case for non-dyslexic students. However, Bergey, Parrila, Laroche, and Deacon (2019) found no positive effect of study strategies on self-efficacy in first-year university dyslexic students.

Haft et al. (2016) report studies showing that individual characteristics, such as a tendency toward positive thinking in dyslexic high school students (Idan & Margalit, 2014), or family factors like family cohesion, have a positive impact on academic performance. Social support from friends also appears to play a positive role. Ahrens, DuBois, Lozano, and Richardson (2010) found that stable friendships positively influence self-esteem in dyslexic university students. However, once again, the academic performance in these studies is only a very indirect measure of reading performance.

12.6.5 Cultural Factors in Compensation

To our knowledge, there are no studies directly examining the type of compensation potentially provided by interactions with the cultural environment (although this has been considered in the models described in the previous sections). However, an article entitled "Cultural Diversity and Biological Unity" by Paulesu et al. (2001) provides interesting insights in a comparison of dyslexic university students with chronological-age matched controls reading in transparent (Italian), opaque (English), and intermediate (French) orthographies. Even though it was not specifically designed for this purpose and is subject to methodological limitations, it suggests an influence of orthographic transparency on reading abilities that persists into adulthood, both in dyslexic and non-dyslexic individuals (for a similar study with children, see, e.g., Diamanti, Goulandris, Campbell, & Protopapas, 2018). Although all dyslexic individuals, regardless of the orthographic system to which they had been exposed, read significantly more slowly than their non-dyslexic peers, the more transparent the system, the closer their performance became to that of non-dyslexic readers (Italian > French > English). Exposure to a transparent system therefore, seems to reduce the detrimental effects of dyslexia on reading. Indeed, in transparent orthographies, the correspondence between graphemes (G) and phonemes (P) is regular, which allows readers to store them more easily and thus more quickly during reading acquisition. The use of these G-P correspondences during the decoding of pseudo-words, for example, is facilitated by their high regularity compared to the inconsistent correspondences present in less transparent orthographies.

The meta-analysis by Reis et al. (2020), conducted on 178 studies comparing adults with dyslexia and matched controls, reveals that orthographic transparency has a significant impact on the manifestation of dyslexia. In adulthood, dyslexic individuals who learned to read and write in transparent orthographies exhibited overall milder deficits compared to those who learned in more opaque orthographies. Significant differences were observed in word and pseudoword reading, reading comprehension, and spelling, all of which favoured transparent orthographies.

12.7 Conclusions

The studies reviewed in this chapter have helped to identify various indicators of what is known as compensation in dyslexia at different explanatory levels (genetic, environmental, neurological, cognitive, and behavioural). It is important to note that research on compensation in the field of neurodevelopmental disorders, particularly developmental dyslexia, has made significant progress in recent years. Indeed, the emerging conceptualizations of compensation presented in this chapter now move away from the theoretical models commonly used in the field of acquired disorders, particularly in acquired language pathologies (for a review on this issue, see Cavalli & Colé, 2018). This new, more developmental perspective allows for a reconsideration of rehabilitation activities that were previously proposed (whose effectiveness remained limited in the domain of neurodevelopmental disorders) and thus opens the way to new remediation practices aimed at compensating for these disorders.

In this context, a study conducted by van Viersen, de Bree, and de Jong (2019) highlights, through a multiple-case study approach, the role of cognitive protective factors and compensatory mechanisms in a particular population of young adolescents with dyslexia and high intellectual ability (IQ ≥ 120). Indeed, the presence of highly efficient cognitive skills in these individuals (acting as strengths for the cognitive system) could facilitate the development of compensatory strategies, leading some dyslexic individuals to no longer exhibit the characteristic symptoms of dyslexia. According to the authors, comparing the strengths and weaknesses within the cognitive skill spectrum of these individuals (i.e., studying cognitive profiles) could help explain why some dyslexic individuals manage to overcome symptoms associated with dyslexia (i.e., considered in the study as resolving dyslexia) while others do not (i.e., persistent dyslexia). The authors conclude that a diagnostic and therapeutic approach to dyslexia based on risk and protective factors would provide insights not only into the specific causes of dyslexia but also into resilience and compensation in dyslexia (Cavalli et al., 2017; Haft et al., 2016), thus opening up new avenues for effective remediation.

These studies on dyslexia compensation, although limited in number, also provide valuable insights into at least three areas. The first concerns the very concept of compensation and its operationalization, particularly in the neurological, cognitive, and behavioural domains, even though many questions remain unanswered at each level, and compensations resulting from interactions between levels need to be identified. The second area concerns the theoretical framework of dyslexia, which is evolving remarkably, partly due to the inclusion of comorbidities associated with dyslexia. Thus, a deterministic framework (dyslexia as an all-or-nothing disorder) and a single-factor approach (e.g., a unique phonological deficit is the cause of dyslexia) are transitioning to a probabilistic and multifactorial conception (e.g., dyslexia results in a probabilistic manner from a set of multiple deficits, each varying in intensity). The third area, rarely explored, is that of clinical applications, particularly in the field of reading remediation for adults with dyslexia. To our knowledge, no studies have identified cognitive processing abilities that are typical or more developed in dyslexic adults to improve their word recognition or reading fluency, for example (see, in French, the study by Casalis & Colé, 2005, with dyslexic adolescents who develop and use their morphological knowledge to build a morphological word recognition strategy). However, some studies do focus on the development of compensatory reading strategies to improve oral reading fluency, focusing, for instance, on speeding up the reading rate. One such program is the Reading Acceleration Program (RAP), a computer-based program that displays sentences at an accelerated speed using a moving window. The goal of this program is to develop a compensatory reading strategy that "forces" the reading system to use direct access quickly rather than relying on slow phonological decoding, essentially "forcing" the system to use the visual-orthographic route. While the reported effects are clearly positive on the reading fluency of trained dyslexic adults (Breznitz et al., 2013), it remains unclear whether this training is based on better-preserved visual-orthographic processing or phonological processing (see Section 12.6.3 of this chapter and also Chapter 10 of this book);

Dyslexia is a persistent neurodevelopmental disorder that has significant socioeconomic repercussions into adulthood. For instance, MacDonald and Deacon (2019), in a large-scale study involving 442 adults with dyslexia from different social classes, found that only 47.5% of adults with dyslexia from working-class backgrounds were employed, significantly less that those from middle-class (70.2%) or upper-class (72.2%) backgrounds. However, individuals from all socioeconomic groups express concerns that dyslexia negatively affects their career progression, with 44% of respondents believing that dyslexia has had an impact on this progression. Nalavany, Logan, and Carawan (2018) found that the more negative the emotions and discomfort associated with dyslexia among a sample of 173 workers with dyslexia (average age 43.5 years), the lower their sense of self-efficacy and job competence, while workplace anxiety was higher, irrespective of other contextual variables such as education level or age. There are, therefore, inequalities that make the professional and everyday life of adults with dyslexia more complex (as supported by the findings reported in Chapter 5). Consequently, it is important to further explore the identification of protective factors that could facilitate their professional integration and daily living.

Recent work by Appels, van Viersen, van Erp, Hornstra, and de Bree (2024) adds to the scarce literature on this issue. Protective factors are defined as conditions or attributes that **reduce** the adverse effects of dyslexia-related risks, helping children achieve better literacy outcomes despite their challenges. Examples of such factors include strong social support, positive self-perception, adaptive learning environments, and **cognitive protective factors** like strong verbal working memory and phonological awareness. For instance, a child with dyslexia who has strong phonological awareness may better decode unfamiliar words, helping them to compensate for reading difficulties and thereby improving literacy outcomes.

The study distinguishes protective factors from promotive and skill-enhancing factors, highlighting their unique roles in literacy development. **Promotive factors** are those that foster positive literacy outcomes for all children, regardless of their risk for reading difficulties (RD). Examples of promotive factors include access to high-quality early childhood education, supportive parenting practices such as shared reading and encouraging curiosity, and positive teacher relationships that create a motivating and inclusive classroom environment. Additionally, access to rich literacy resources, such as books and digital tools, serves as a promotive factor by universally enhancing exposure to reading opportunities. While promotive factors benefit both children with RD and typically developing (TD) peers, they do not reduce the literacy gap between these groups. Instead, they consolidate literacy outcomes across the board. In contrast, protective factors specifically benefit children with RD, enabling them to achieve better-than-expected outcomes compared to their peers at lower risk for RD. These factors play a crucial role in narrowing the literacy gap between at-risk children and their TD peers. Examples of cognitive protective factors include robust executive functioning skills, such as the ability to plan and organize tasks effectively, or strong visual-spatial processing abilities that help to lessen the challenges of word recognition. Skill-enhancing factors are most effective for children with the lowest risk of RD, further improving the abilities of proficient readers. Examples of skill-enhancing factors include advanced vocabulary-building programs, exposure to complex texts, and individualized literacy instruction that challenges and extends high-achieving readers' capabilities. These factors help already proficient readers to develop even stronger literacy skills, such as advanced comprehension and critical reading abilities. However, their impact is less significant for children with RD, as they are designed to elevate performance above baseline rather than address foundational deficits.

The authors also identify the possible levels at which compensation takes place in individuals with dyslexia. Compensation can occur at the behavioural level, where individuals develop alternative strategies to address reading challenges, such as relying on context clues or memory. At the cognitive level, individuals might leverage strengths in areas like verbal working memory or visual-spatial reasoning to compensate for deficits in phonological processing. Lastly, compensation can happen at the neurobiological level, where brain plasticity allows for the recruitment of alternative neural pathways to support reading tasks. These levels highlight the complexity of dyslexia compensation and the interplay between individual strengths and external support systems. By emphasizing the distinct and complementary roles of these factors and the levels of compensation, the study underscores the importance of protective factors, including cognitive abilities like phonological awareness and executive functioning, promotive factors such as enriched educational environments, and skill-enhancing factors like advanced literacy programs. Together, these elements foster resilience, reduce disparities in literacy outcomes, and provide a deeper understanding of how children with dyslexia (and adults) adapt to and overcome challenges.

The authors' proposals suggest several directions for research that could be valuable for understanding and supporting adults with dyslexia. First, they imply the need for **longitudinal studies** that track the literacy development of adults with dyslexia over time. These studies would help identify how protective, promotive, and skill-enhancing factors evolve in adulthood and what role they play in maintaining or improving reading and writing skills over the lifespan. This research could shed light on how adults continue to adapt to their dyslexia and how their coping strategies change as they encounter new life challenges, such as changes in employment or social roles. Additionally, the authors' emphasis on **interdisciplinary research** suggests that studies involving cognitive psychology, neuroscience, education, and social sciences could be particularly beneficial for adults with dyslexia. Research in these areas could focus on how dyslexia impacts adults in various aspects of life, including work, relationships, and mental health. This approach could lead to a better understanding of the complex interplay between individual cognitive abilities, environmental factors, and social support systems that contribute to literacy outcomes for adults with dyslexia.

The authors also highlight the importance of **individual-centred research**, which would be crucial for understanding the unique coping mechanisms and strategies that different adults with dyslexia may develop. For example, some adults may rely on technology tools, while others may use compensatory strategies such as leveraging their strengths in memory or visual processing. Research could explore how these strategies vary and how they can be supported or enhanced through targeted interventions. This framework suggests that further exploration is needed into **compensatory strategies** for adults. While children with dyslexia might rely on specific educational interventions, adults may require more tailored solutions that consider their work, personal, and social contexts. Research could investigate workplace accommodations, specialized training programs, and other practical strategies that could help adults with dyslexia manage their literacy challenges effectively in real-world settings.

Neurobiological aspects of dyslexia are also worthy of exploration in adults to investigate how the brain adapts over time and how neuroplasticity might support the development of new reading strategies.

In summary, research on adults with dyslexia should focus on their unique challenges, the long-term development of compensatory mechanisms in view of protective factors, and the design of tailored interventions that consider their life context. This approach could lead to more effective strategies and support systems for adults with dyslexia, helping them to thrive in spite of their challenges.

References

Ahrens, K., DuBois, D. L., Lozano, P., & Richardson, L. P. (2010). Naturally acquired mentoring relationships and young adult outcomes among adolescents with learning disabilities. *Learning Disabilities Research & Practice, 25*(4), 207–216.

Andreassen, R., Jensen, M. S., & Bråten, I. (2017). Investigating self-regulated study strategies among postsecondary students with and without dyslexia: A diary method study. *Reading and Writing, 30*(9), 1891–1916.

Anthoni, H., et al. (2007). A locus on 2p12 containing the co-regulated MRPL19 and C2ORF3 genes is associated to dyslexia. *Human Molecular Genetics, 16*, 667–677.

Appels, S., van Viersen, S., van Erp, S., Hornstra, L., & de Bree, E. (2024). A scoping review on word-reading resilience in literacy: Evaluating empirical evidence for protective factors. *Learning and Instruction, 93*, 101969.

Bandura, A. (1977). Self-efficacy: Toward a unifying theory of behavioral change. *Psychological Review, 84*(2), 191.

Bates, T. C., Lind, P. A., Luciano, M., Montgomery, G. W., Martin, N. G., & Wright, M. J. (2010). Dyslexia and DYX1C1: Deficits in reading and spelling associated with a missense mutation. *Molecular Psychiatry, 15*(12), 1190.

Beidas, H., Khateb, A., & Breznitz, Z. (2013). The cognitive profile of adult dyslexics and its relation to their reading abilities. *Reading and Writing, 26*(9), 1487–1515.

Ben-Dror, I., Pollatsek, A., & Scarpati, S. (1991). Word identification in isolation and in context by college dyslexic students. *Brain and Language, 40*(4), 471–490.

Bergey, B. W., Parrila, R. K., Laroche, A., & Deacon, S. H. (2019). Effects of peer-led training on academic self-efficacy, study strategies, and academic performance for first-year university students with and without reading difficulties. *Contemporary Educational Psychology, 56*, 25–39.

Bishop, D. V. (2015). The interface between genetics and psychology: Lessons from developmental dyslexia. *Proceedings of the Royal Society B: Biological Sciences, 282*(1806), 20143139.

Bishop, D. V., McDonald, D., Bird, S., & Hayiou-Thomas, M. E. (2009). Children who read words accurately despite language impairment: Who are they and how do they do it? *Child Development, 80*(2), 593–605.

Bjornsdottir, G., Halldorsson, J. G., Steinberg, S., Hansdottir, I., Kristjansson, K., Stefansson, H., & Stefansson, K. (2014). The adult reading history questionnaire (ARHQ) in Icelandic: Psychometric properties and factor structure. *Journal of Learning Disabilities, 47*(6), 532–542.

Boets, B., de Beeck, H. P. O., Vandermosten, M., Scott, S. K., Gillebert, C. R., Mantini, D., & Ghesquière, P. (2013). Intact but less accessible phonetic representations in adults with dyslexia. *Science, 342*(6163), 1251–1254.

Booth, J. N., Boyle, J. M., & Kelly, S. W. (2010). Do tasks make a difference? Accounting for heterogeneity of performance of children with reading difficulties on tasks of executive function: Findings from a meta-analysis. *British Journal of Developmental Psychology, 28*(1), 133–176.

Brèthes, H., Cavalli, E., Denis-Noël, A., Melmi, J. B., El Ahmadi, A., Bianco, M., & Colé, P. (2022). Text reading fluency and text reading comprehension do not rely on the same abilities in university students with and without dyslexia. *Frontiers in Psychology, 13*, 866543.

Breznitz, Z., Shaul, S., Horowitz-Kraus, T., Sela, I., Nevat, M., & Karni, A. (2013). Enhanced reading by training with imposed time constraint in typical and dyslexic adults. *Nature Communications, 4*, 1486.

Brosnan, M., Demetre, J., Hamill, S., Robson, K., Shepherd, H., & Cody, G. (2002). Executive functioning in adults and children with developmental dyslexia. *Neuropsychologia, 40*(12), 2144–2155.

Bruck, M. (1990). Word-recognition skills of adults with childhood diagnoses of dyslexia. *Developmental Psychology, 26*(3), 439–454.

Bruck, M. (1992). Persistence of dyslexics' phonological awareness deficits. *Developmental Psychology, 28*(5), 874.

Bruck, M. (1993). Component spelling skills of college students with childhood diagnoses of dyslexia. *Learning Disability Quarterly, 16*(3), 171–184.

Callens, M., Tops, W., & Brysbaert, M. (2012). Cognitive profile of students who enter higher education with an indication of dyslexia. *PLoS One, 7*(6), e38081.

Carroll, J. M., & Iles, J. E. (2006). An assessment of anxiety levels in dyslexic students in higher education. *British Journal of Educational Psychology, 76*(3), 651–662. https://doi.org/10.1348/000709905X66233

Casalis, S., & Colé, P. (2005). L'entraînement à l'analyse morphologique chez des collégiens dyslexiques. In *Les Entretiens d'Orthophonie, Entretiens Bichat*. Paris: l'Expansion Scientifique Française.

Castet, É., Descamps, M., Denis-Noël, A., & Colé, P. (2019). Dyslexia research and the partial report task: A first step toward acknowledging iconic and visual short-term memory. *Scientific Studies of Reading*, 1–11.

Cavalli, E., Casalis, S., El Ahmadi, A., Zira, M., Poracchia-George, F., & Cole, P. (2016). Vocabulary skills are well developed in university students with dyslexia: Evidence from multiple case studies. *Research in Developmental Disabilities, 51*, 89–102.

Cavalli, E., Chanoine, V., Tan, Y., Anton, J.-L., Giordano, B. L., Pegado, F., & Ziegler, J. C. (2024). Atypical hemispheric Re-Organization of the Reading Network in high-functioning adults with dyslexia: Evidence from representational similarity analysis. *Imaging Neuroscience, 2*, 1–23.

Cavalli, E., & Colé, P. (2018). Les dyslexies chez l'adulte. In S. Casalis (Ed.), *Les dyslexies*. Elsevier Masson.

Cavalli, E., Colé. P., Brèthes, H., Lefèvre, E., Lascombe, S., & Velay, J.-L. (2019). E-book reading hinders aspects of long-text comprehension for adults with dyslexia. *Annals of Dyslexia, 69*(2), 243–259.

Cavalli, E., Colé, P., Leloup, G., Poracchia-George, F., Sprenger-Charolles, L., & El Ahmadi, A. (2018). Screening for dyslexia in French-speaking university students: An evaluation of the detection accuracy of the Alouette test. *Journal of Learning Disabilities, 51*(3), 268–282.

Cavalli, E., Duncan, L. G., Elbro, C., El Ahmadi, A., & Colé, P. (2017). Phonemic-morphemic dissociation in university students with dyslexia: An index of reading compensation? *Annals of Dyslexia, 67*(1), 63–84.

Colé, P., Cavalli, E., Duncan, L. G., Theurel, A., Gentaz, E., Sprenger-Charolles, L., & El-Ahmadi, A. (2018). What is the influence of morphological knowledge in the early stages of Reading acquisition among low SES children? A Graphical Modeling Approach. *Front. Psychol., 9*, 547.

Colé, P., Duncan, L. G., & Blaye, A. (2014). Cognitive flexibility predicts early reading skills. *Frontiers in Psychology, 5*, 565.

Corkett, J. K., & Parrila, R. (2008). Use of context in the word recognition process by adults with a significant history of reading difficulties. *Annals of Dyslexia, 58*(2), 139–161.

Cutting, L. E., & Scarborough, H. S. (2012). *Multiple bases for comprehension difficulties: The potential of cognitive and neurobiological profiling for validation of subtypes and development of assessments* (pp. 101–116). Reaching an understanding: Innovations in how we view reading assessment.

Deacon, S. H., Cook, K., & Parrila, R. (2012). Identifying high-functioning dyslexics: Is self-report of early reading problems enough? *Annals of Dyslexia, 62*(2), 120–134.

DeFries, J. C., & Fulker, D. W. (1985). Multiple regression analysis of twin data. *Behavior Genetics, 15*(5), 467–473.

DeFries, J. C., Fulker, D. W., & Olson, R. K. (2005). The Colorado learning disabilities research Center twin study. In M. Snowling & C. Hulme (Eds.), *The science of reading: A handbook* (pp. 60–77). Oxford, UK: Blackwell Publishing.

Diamanti, V., Goulandris, N., Campbell, R., & Protopapas, A. (2018). Dyslexia profiles across orthographies differing in transparency: An evaluation of theoretical predictions contrasting English and Greek. *Scientific Studies of Reading, 22*(1), 55–69.

Eckert, M. A., Berninger, V. W., Vaden, K. I., Jr., Gebregziabher, M., & Tsu, L. (2016). Gray matter features of reading disability: A combined meta-analytic and direct analysis approach. *eneuro, 3*(1), https://doi.org/10.1523/ENEURO.0103-15.2015

Elbro, C., & Arnbak, E. (1996). The role of morpheme recognition and morphological awareness in dyslexia. *Annals of Dyslexia, 46*(1), 209–240.

Faísca, L., Reis, A., & Araújo, S. (2023). Cognitive subtyping of university students with dyslexia in a semi-transparent orthography: What can weaknesses and strengths tell us about compensation? *Journal of Cultural Cognitive Science, 7*(2), 121–136.

Fischer, J., Biscaldi, M., & Hartnegg, K. (2006). Stability of dyslexic visual attention span deficits in time and after training. *Brain and Language, 97*(2), 198–210.

Fisher, S. E., & Francks, C. (2006). Genes, cognition and dyslexia: Learning to read the genome. *Trends in Cognitive Sciences, 10*(5), 250–257.

Francks, C., et al. (2004). A 77-kilobase region of chromosome 6p22.2 is associated with dyslexia in families from the United Kingdom and from the United States. *American Journal of Human Genetics*, *75*, 1046–1058.

Friend, A., DeFries, J. C., & Olson, R. K. (2008). Parental education moderates genetic influences on reading disability. *Psychological Science*, *19*(11), 1124–1130.

Frith, U., & Snowling, M. (1983). Reading for meaning and reading for sound in autistic and dyslexic children. *British Journal of Developmental Psychology*, *1*(4), 329–342.

Gayán, J., Willcutt, E. G., Fisher, S. E., Francks, C., Cardon, L. R., Olson, R. K., & DeFries, J. C. (2005). Bivariate linkage scan for reading disability and attention-deficit/hyperactivity disorder localizes pleiotropic loci. *Journal of Child Psychology and Psychiatry*, *46*(10), 1045–1056.

Georgiou, G. K., & Das, J. P. (2018). Direct and indirect effects of executive function on reading comprehension in young adults. *Journal of Research in Reading*, *41*(2), 243–258.

Ghisi, M., Bottesi, G., Re, A. M., Cerea, S., & Mammarella, I. C. (2016). Socioemotional features and resilience in Italian university students with and without dyslexia. *Frontiers in Psychology*, *7*, 478.

Gialluisi, A., Andlauer, T. F., Mirza-Schreiber, N., Moll, K., Becker, J., Hoffmann, P., & Honbolygó, F. (2019). Genome-wide association scan identifies new variants associated with a cognitive predictor of dyslexia. *Translational Psychiatry*, *9*(1), 77.

Giraud, A. L., & Ramus, F. (2013). Neurogenetics and auditory processing in developmental dyslexia. *Current Opinion in Neurobiology*, *23*(1), 37–42.

Gough, P. B., & Tunmer, W. E. (1986). Decoding, reading, and reading disability. *Remedial and Special Education*, *7*(1), 6–10.

Haft, S. L., Myers, C. A., & Hoeft, F. (2016). Socio-emotional and cognitive resilience in children with reading disabilities. *Current Opinion in Behavioral Sciences*, *10*, 133–141.

Hancock, R., Richlan, F., & Hoeft, F. (2017). Possible roles for fronto-striatal circuits in reading disorder. *Neuroscience and Biobehavioral Reviews*, *72*, 243–260.

Hatcher, J., Snowling, M. J., & Griffiths, Y. M. (2002). Cognitive assessment of dyslexic students in higher education. *British Journal of Educational Psychology*, *72*(1), 119–133.

Hebert, M., Zhang, X., & Parrila, R. (2018). Examining reading comprehension text and question answering time differences in university students with and without a history of reading difficulties. *Annals of Dyslexia*, *68*(1), 15–24.

Hillary, F. G. (2008). Neuroimaging of working memory dysfunction and the dilemma with brain reorganization hypotheses. *Journal of the International Neuropsychological Society*, *14*, 526–534.

Hoeft, F., Meyler, A., Hernandez, A., Juel, C., Taylor-Hill, H., Martindale, J. L., McMillon, G., Kolchugina, G., Black, J. M., Faizi, A., et al. (2007). Functional and morphometric brain dissociation between dyslexia and reading ability. *Proceedings of the National Academy of Sciences of the United States of America*, *104*, 4234–4239.

Horowitz-Kraus, T., & Breznitz, Z. (2014). Can reading rate acceleration improve error monitoring and cognitive abilities underlying reading in adolescents with reading difficulties and in typical readers? *Brain Research*, *1544*, 1–14.

Idan, O., & Margalit, M. (2014). Socioemotional self-perceptions, family climate, and hopeful thinking among students with learning disabilities and typically achieving students from the same classes. *Journal of Learning Disabilities*, *47*(2), 136–152.

Keenan, J. M., Betjemann, R. S., & Olson, R. K. (2008). Reading comprehension tests vary in the skills they assess: Differential dependence on decoding and oral comprehension. *Scientific Studies of Reading*, *12*(3), 281–300.

Kirby, J. R., Silvestri, R., Allingham, B. H., Parrila, R., & La Fave, C. B. (2008). Learning strategies and study approaches of postsecondary students with dyslexia. *Journal of Learning Disabilities*, *41*(1), 85–96.

Ktori, M., Cavalli, E., Doignon-Camus, N., & Colé, P. (2017, October). Visual orthographic processing in adults with dyslexia. Interactive paper (poster), European Dyslexia Association, Munich, German.

Law, J. M., Veispak, A., Vanderauwera, J., & Ghesquière, P. (2018). Morphological awareness and visual processing of derivational morphology in high-functioning adults with dyslexia: An avenue to compensation? *Applied PsychoLinguistics*, *39*(3), 483–506.

Law, J. M., Wouters, J., & Ghesquière, P. (2015). Morphological awareness and its role in compensation in adults with dyslexia. *Dyslexia*, *21*(3), 254–272.

Lazaroo, N., Bates, T., Hansell, N., Wright, M., Martin, N., & Luciano, M. (2019). Genetic structure of IQ, phonemic decoding skill, and academic achievement. *Frontiers in Genetics*, *10*, 195.

Lefèvre, E., Law, J. M., Prado, M. J., Anders, R., & Cavalli, E. (2025). Reading comprehension resiliency in adolescents with and without dyslexia relates to vocabulary, listening comprehension and socioeconomic status. *Learning & Instruction.*, *96*, 102081.

Lefly, D. L., & Pennington, B. F. (1991). Spelling errors and reading fluency in compensated adult dyslexics. *Annals of Dyslexia*, *41*(1), 141–162.

Livingston, L. A., & Happé, F. (2017). Conceptualising compensation in neurodevelopmental disorders: Reflections from autism spectrum disorder. *Neuroscience & Biobehavioral Reviews*, *80*, 729–742.

MacCullagh, L., Bosanquet, A., & Badcock, N. A. (2017). University students with dyslexia: A qualitative exploratory study of learning practices, challenges and strategies. *Dyslexia*, *23*(1), 3–23.

Macdonald, S. J., & Deacon, L. (2019). Twice upon a time: Examining the effect socio-economic status has on the experience of dyslexia in the United Kingdom. *Dyslexia*, *25*(1), 3–19.

Marchetti, R., Pinto, S., Spieser, L., Vaugoyeau, M., Cavalli, E., El Ahmadi, A., & Colé, P. (2023). Phoneme representation and articulatory impairment: Insights from adults with comorbid motor coordination disorder and dyslexia. *Brain Sciences*, *13*(2), 210.

Martin, J., Frauenfelder, U., & Colé, P. (2013). Morphological awareness in dyslexic students. *Applied PsychoLinguistics*, *35*, 1–21.

McGrath, L. M., Pennington, B. F., Shanahan, M. A., Santerre-Lemmon, L. E., Barnard, H. D., Willcutt, E. G., et al. (2011). A multiple deficit model of reading disability and attention-deficit/hyperactivity disorder: Searching for shared cognitive deficits. *Journal of Child Psychology and Psychiatry*, *52*(5), 547–557.

Meng, H., et al. (2005). DCDC2 is associated with reading disability and modulates neuronal development in the brain. *Proceedings of the National Academy of Sciences of the United States of America*, *102*, 17053–17058.

Miller-Shaul, S. (2005). The characteristics of young and adult dyslexics readers on reading and reading related cognitive tasks as compared to normal readers. *Dyslexia*, *11*(2), 132–151.

Morton, J., & Frith, U. (1993). Approche de la dyslexie développementale par la modélisation causale. *Les actes de la villette*, 263–278.

Morton, J., & Frith, U. (2001). Why we need cognition: Cause and developmental disorder. In E. Dupoux (Ed.), *Language, brain, and cognitive development: Essays in honor of Jacques Mehler* (pp. 263–278). Cambridge: MIT Press.

Nalavany, B. A., Logan, J. M., & Carawan, L. W. (2018). The relationship between emotional experience with dyslexia and work self-efficacy among adults with dyslexia. *Dyslexia*, *24*(1), 17–32.

Olofsson, Å., Ahl, A., & Taube, K. (2012). Learning and study strategies in university students with dyslexia: Implications for teaching. *Procedia-Social and Behavioral Sciences*, *47*, 1184–1193.

Parhiala, P., Torppa, M., Eklund, K., Aro, T., Poikkeus, A. M., Heikkilä, R., & Ahonen, T. (2015). Psychosocial functioning of children with and without dyslexia: A follow-up study from ages four to nine. *Dyslexia, 21*(3), 197–211.

Parrila, R., Georgiou, G., & Corkett, J. (2007). University students with a significant History of reading difficulties: What is and is not compensated? *Exceptionality Education International, 17*(2), 195–220.

Patael, S. Z., Farris, E. A., Black, J. M., Hancock, R., Gabrieli, J. D., Cutting, L. E., & Hoeft, F. (2018). Brain basis of cognitive resilience: Prefrontal cortex predicts better reading comprehension in relation to decoding. *PLoS One, 13*(6), e0198791.

Paulesu, E., Démonet, J. F., Fazio, F., McCrory, E., Chanoine, V., Brunswick, N., & Frith, U. (2001). Dyslexia: Cultural diversity and biological unity. *Science, 291*(5511), 2165–2167.

Pedersen, M. L., Hedegaard, K. L., & Elbro, C. (2016). The effects of morphological awareness training on reading and spelling in Danish students with dyslexia. *Annals of Dyslexia, 66*(3), 145–160.

Pennington, B. F. (2006). From single to multiple deficit models of developmental disorders. *Cognition, 101*(2), 385–413.

Pennington, B. F., Santerre-Lemmon, L., Rosenberg, J., MacDonald, B., Boada, R., Friend, A., & Olson, R. K. (2012). Individual prediction of dyslexia by single versus multiple deficit models. *Journal of Abnormal Psychology, 121*(1), 212.

Pennington, B. F., Van Orden, G. C., Smith, S. D., Green, P. A., & Haith, M. M. (1990). Phonological processing skills and deficits in adult dyslexics. *Child Development, 61*(6), 1753–1778.

Peterson, R. L., & Pennington, B. F. (2009). Developmental dyslexia. *The Lancet, 379*(9830), 1997–2007.

Pino, M., & Mortari, L. (2014). The inclusion of students with dyslexia in higher education: A systematic review using narrative synthesis. *Dyslexia, 20*(4), 346–369.

Pugh, K. R., Mencl, W. E., Jenner, A. R., Katz, L., Frost, S. J., Lee, J. R., Shaywitz, S. E., & Shaywitz, B. A. (2000). Functional neuroimaging studies of reading and reading disability (developmental dyslexia). *Mental Retardation and Developmental Disabilities Research Reviews, 6*, 207–213.

Ramus, F., Rosen, S., Dakin, S., Day, B., Castello, J., & White, S. (2003). Theories of developmental dyslexia: Insights from a multiple case study of dyslexic adults. *Brain, 126*, 841–865.

Ransby, M. J., & Lee Swanson, H. (2003). Reading comprehension skills of young adults with childhood diagnoses of dyslexia. *Journal of Learning Disabilities, 36*(6), 538–555.

Reis, A., Araújo, S., Morais, I. S., & Faísca, L. (2020). Reading and reading-related skills in adults with dyslexia from different orthographic systems: A review and meta-analysis. *Annals of Dyslexia, 70*(3), 339–368.

Richlan, F., Kronbichler, M., & Wimmer, H. (2011). Meta-analyzing brain dysfunctions in dyslexic children and adults. *NeuroImage, 56*(3), 1735–1742.

Richlan, F., Kronbichler, M., & Wimmer, H. (2013). Structural abnormalities in the dyslexic brain: A meta-analysis of voxel-based morphometry studies. *Human Brain Mapping, 34*(11), 3055–3065.

Sánchez-Morán, M., et al. (2018). Genetic association study of dyslexia and ADHD candidate genes in a Spanish cohort: Implications of comorbid samples. *PLoS One, 13*, e020643.

Shafrir, U., & Siegel, L. S. (1994). Preference for visual scanning strategies versus phonological rehearsal in university students with reading disabilities. *Journal of Learning Disabilities, 27*(9), 583–588.

Share, D. L., & Geva, E. (1995). Learning to read and write in a second language: Cross-linguistic contrasts and second-language learning. In M. Snowling & C.

Hulme (Eds.), *The science of reading: A handbook* (pp. 379–396). Oxford, UK: Blackwell Publishing.

Simmons, F., & Singleton, C. (2000). The reading comprehension abilities of dyslexic students in higher education. *Dyslexia, 6*(3), 178–192.

Snowling, M., Bishop, D. V. M., & Stothard, S. E. (2000). Is preschool language impairment a risk factor for dyslexia in adolescence? *The Journal of Child Psychology and Psychiatry and Allied Disciplines, 41*(5), 587–600.

Snowling, M. J. (2008). Specific disorders and broader phenotypes: The case of dyslexia. *Quarterly Journal of Experimental Psychology, 61*(1), 142–156.

Sprenger-Charolles, L., & Colé, P. (2013). *Lecture et dyslexie-2e éd.: Approche cognitive*. Dunod.

Stagg, S. D., Eaton, E., & Sjoblom, A. M. (2018). Self-efficacy in undergraduate students with dyslexia: A mixed methods investigation. *British Journal of Special Education, 45*(1), 26–42.

Stanovich, K. E. (1980). Toward an interactive-compensatory model of individual differences in the neural mechanisms underlying compensation in dyslexia 24 development of reading fluency. *Reading Research Quarterly, 16*, 32–71.

Stanovich, K. E. (1984). The interactive-compensatory model of Reading: A confluence of developmental, experimental, and Educational Psychology. *Remedial and Special Education, 5*, 11–19.

Stanovich, K. E., West, R. F., & Cunningham, A. E. (1991). Beyond phonological processes: Print exposure and orthographic processing. *Phonological Processes in Literacy: A Tribute to Isabelle Y. Liberman* (pp. 219–235). Hillsdale, NJ: Lawrence Erlbaum Associates

Swanson, H. L., & Hsieh, C. J. (2009). Reading disabilities in adults: A selective meta-analysis of the literature. *Review of Educational Research, 79*(4), 1362–1390.

Szenkovits, G., & Ramus, F. (2005). Exploring dyslexics' phonological deficit I: Lexical vs sub-lexical and input vs output processes. *Dyslexia, 11*(4), 253–268.

Tran, C., et al. (2014). Association of the ROBO1 gene with reading disabilities in a family-based analysis. *Genes, Brain and Behavior, 13*, 430–438.

Tunmer, W. E., & Chapman, J. W. (2012). The simple view of reading redux: Vocabulary knowledge and the independent components hypothesis. *Journal of Learning Disabilities, 45*, 453–466.

van Bergen, E., van der Leij, A., & de Jong, P. F. (2014). The intergenerational multiple deficit model and the case of dyslexia. *Frontiers in Human Neuroscience, 8*, 346.

van der Sluis, S., de Jong, P. F., & van der Leij, A. (2004). Inhibition and shifting in children with learning deficits in arithmetic and reading. *Journal of Experimental Child Psychology, 87*(3), 239–266.

van Viersen, S., de Bree, E. H., & de Jong, P. F. (2019). Protective factors and compensation in resolving dyslexia. *Scientific Studies of Reading, 23*(6), 461–477.

Vaughn, S., Elbaum, B., & Boardman, A. G. (2001). The social functioning of students with learning disabilities: Implications for inclusion. *Exceptionality, 9*(1–2), 47–65.

Wagner, R. K., Herrera, S. K., Spencer, M., & Quinn, J. M. (2015). Reconsidering the simple view of reading in an intriguing case of equivalent models: Commentary on Tunmer and Chapman (2012). *Journal of Learning Disabilities, 48*, 115–119.

Wallot, S., O'Brien, B. A., Haussmann, A., Kloos, H., & Lyby, M. S. (2014). The role of reading time complexity and reading speed in text comprehension. *Journal of Experimental Psychology: Learning, Memory, and Cognition, 40*(6), 1745.

White, S., Frith, U., Milne, E., Rosen, S., Swettenham, J., & Ramus, F. (2006). A double dissociation between sensorimotor impairments and reading disability: A comparison of autistic and dyslexic children. *Cognitive Neuropsychology, 23*(5), 748–761.

Willcutt, E. G., & Pennington, B. F. (2000a). Comorbidity of reading disability and attention-deficit/hyperactivity disorder: Differences by gender and subtype. *Journal of Learning Disabilities, 33*(2), 179–191.

Willcutt, E. G., & Pennington, B. F. (2000b). Psychiatric comorbidity in children and adolescents with reading disability. *The Journal of Child Psychology and Psychiatry and Allied Disciplines, 41*(8), 1039–1048.

Willcutt, E. G., Pennington, B. F., Olson, R. K., Chhabildas, N., & Hulslander, J. (2000). Neuropsychological analyses of comorbidity between reading disability and attention deficit hyperactivity disorder: In search of the common deficit. *Developmental Neuropsychology, 27*(1), 35–78.

Zhang, Y., Li, J., Tardif, T., Burmeister, M., Villafuerte, S. M., McBride-Chang, C., & Shu, H. (2012). Association of the DYX1C1 dyslexia susceptibility gene with orthography in the Chinese population. *PLoS One, 7*(9), e42969.

13
SUPPORTING STUDENTS WITH DYSLEXIA IN HIGHER EDUCATION
Predictors of Success and Inclusive Adjustments

Émilie Collette, Mariane Frenay and Marie-Anne Schelstraete

Introduction

A successful pathway in higher education is a challenge for many students. This is demonstrated by the high percentage of failures observed in France, Belgium, and the United States, particularly in the first year (failure rate of around 50%) (De Clercq et al., 2023).

Presumably, the challenge is even greater for students with learning difficulties, such as dyslexia. However, more and more students with learning disorders are present in higher education (Holmes & Silvestri, 2019; Pino & Mortari, 2014). The question of "how best to support students with dyslexia" therefore deserves attention.

In this chapter, a description of factors that may play a role in the success or failure of students with dyslexia is provided, as well as an identification of the means that could be used to support student success. In order to define the useful and relevant supports to be put in place, difficulties expressed by students with dyslexia will be considered, together with the obstacles they encounter in higher education.

The Context of Higher Education

Numerous authors have sought to identify predictors of success in higher education (Kocsis & Molnár, 2024; Neuville et al., 2013; Schneider & Preckel,

DOI: 10.4324/9781003491125-14

2017). In their review of the literature, De Clercq et al. (2023) distinguish four categories of factors, based on the classifications proposed in models of engagement:

1 **Input characteristics**: socio-economic status, gender, age, general intellectual skills, personality (including conscientiousness and openness to experience), and past performance.
2 **Social environment**: the different parties supporting the student (their peers, family, teaching staff, and the higher education institution).
3 **Motivational beliefs**: the student's motivation, the value they place on their studies, their expectations of success, their feelings of self-efficacy, and the goals they pursue in their studies.
4 **Engagement**: emotional engagement, cognitive engagement (information processing strategies), metacognitive engagement (self-regulatory strategies), and behavioural engagement (efforts), which reflect the quality of the student's investment in his or her studies.

These four categories are placed on a continuum ranging from those considered to be the most distal predictors of success (input characteristics) to the most proximal predictors (motivational beliefs and engagement). According to De Clercq et al. (2023), a sense of self-efficacy (i.e., the confidence of the learner in his or her ability to succeed), as well as behavioural engagement (student efforts) and self-regulatory strategies (planning, managing, controlling, and regulating the learning process), emerge as particularly important predictors of success.

While some factors, such as gender, age, or economic status, cannot be changed, it is possible to act on other elements, such as the social environment, motivational beliefs, or engagement. This is what prompts some higher education institutions to implement success support devices aimed at providing better support for students. Robbins et al. (2009) describe different types of interventions aimed at, for example, skills necessary for academic success (i.e., learning strategies, note-taking), self-management (i.e., management of stress and anxiety), or socialisation (integration of students).

Even if a student enjoys favourable conditions for success by being, for example, motivated, committed to their studies, and well supported, the presence of severe difficulties in reading or writing can nevertheless constitute a significant barrier to the success of that student. The question then arises as to what specific provisions can be proposed to facilitate the student's progress in higher education or their integration within this context. This question may be posed at an institutional or system-wide level and refers more broadly to the way in which these issues are considered: inclusive education, reasonable adjustments, or an integrative approach.

At present, legislation in many countries establishes benchmarks to facilitate the integration of students exhibiting a learning disorder (Moriña, 2017). The objective is to limit the impact of the difficulties experienced by students (in this case, difficulties in written language) in their curriculum. In this context, different types of support (i.e., tutoring) or adjustments (i.e., extra time during exams) are offered to students. However, for these to be effective, it is essential that they meet the needs of these students.

Difficulties Expressed by Students with Dyslexia

In order to obtain precise information concerning the specific difficulties of students with dyslexia, two complementary approaches are possible: standardised tests and self-assessment questionnaires.

The use of standardised tests enables the assessment of written language skills (via reading and spelling tasks) and various associated skills (i.e., phonological awareness, verbal memory, etc.). This assessment is critical to provide appropriate support to students. It will not be detailed here, but it is the subject of Chapter 8 of this book. It should also be noted that "ecological" simulations, such as writing tests, with or without time constraints, are interesting for giving relevant advice to students.

Self-report questionnaires are used to address difficulties that students encounter along their higher education path. While the relevance of self-assessment is often questioned (possible over-estimation or under-estimation of difficulties faced by students), studies which have employed this method with adults with the goal of identifying subjects with dyslexia through questionnaires addressing their difficulties in written language (the questions focus either on their current performance or on the history of their difficulties), point to the responsiveness, ease and speed of using the questionnaires. These assessments are successful in identifying students with dyslexia, and the results of the questionnaires are correlated with objective measures of reading (Deacon et al., 2012; Giménez et al., 2015; Snowling et al., 2012). While these studies have used questionnaires as screening tools, others have sought to identify specific difficulties experienced by students with dyslexia. In their study, Mazur-Palandre et al. (2015), for example, examined difficulties these students experienced in their university life. They observe that the most significant complaints relate to note-taking, disturbance due to noise in class, understanding written instructions during exams, written expression, and learning English (as a foreign language). These complaints, in turn, seem to be confirmed by the cognitive assessments carried out on these students.

Self-assessment is therefore a relevant method for obtaining information, and it consequently represents an interesting tool for clinicians. It is from this perspective that two questionnaires were given to students performing a diagnostic assessment at the Consultations Psychologiques Spécialisées (CPS)[1] at the Université catholique de Louvain (Belgium), each with very specific objectives: a questionnaire centred on difficulties related to academic activities and a questionnaire centred on attentional difficulties.

Questionnaire for Self-Assessment of the Difficulties Related to University Activities

The first questionnaire is a "self-assessment questionnaire on difficulties related to university activities". It consists of 30 items (see table in Appendix 13.1) for which students must state whether they encounter difficulties on a 6-point Likert scale ranging from "never" to "always" (i.e., "difficulties in taking notes in lectures", "difficulties in learning the written format of foreign languages"). Items were selected based on frequently reported difficulties from previous student anamneses or from the literature. The last two items concern the quantity of work provided and how efforts made by students may or may not be rewarded. Finally, the questionnaire concludes with an open-ended question allowing students to describe their "strengths", in other words, the strengths on which they can rely to overcome or circumvent their difficulties.

The purpose of this questionnaire is multifaceted: (1) to deepen the anamnesis; (2) to reveal weaknesses which could lead the clinician to carry out further evaluations in the case of suspected associated disorders (e.g. difficulties in oral language, dyscalculia, developmental coordination disorder, attention deficit disorder); and (3) to better understand the impact of identified disorders by the diagnostic report on their courses activities in order to suggest suitable adjustments or assistance.

This questionnaire was given to 121 students exhibiting developmental dyslexia (DD) and 50 control students (CTR) with no history of learning disabilities. The students with dyslexia were recruited following a diagnostic assessment conducted at the CPS (UCLouvain), confirming written language disorders. Nearly all of these students completed this assessment as part of the procedures for accessing adjustments during their higher education studies.[2] Students with dyslexia and control students participated in a wider study during which behavioural tests were also offered to them. Within the scope of this chapter, we will detail the results obtained by students on the Alouette test (Lefavrais, 1967, 2005), a text reading task that takes into account reading speed and precision. The text used is syntactically and grammatically correct, but poor in semantic structure, thus preventing the reader from using the context to read it. The sensitivity and specificity of this test have already been demonstrated in the literature among French-speaking adults (Cavalli et al., 2018).

Our aim was to have a clinical sample representative of students with dyslexia who were seeking help. We therefore took the opposite approach to the majority of studies by including bilingual students in our analyses (on condition that French is one of their mother languages), and students who had been schooled partly in a foreign language (on condition that the majority of schooling was conducted in French). We considered in both cases that their mastery of oral and written French would be sufficient ($N = 12$ and $N = 5$ respectively). We also included students with dyslexia for whom an associated disorder had been diagnosed in the past (attention deficit disorder, memory impairment, language development disorder, dyscalculia, developmental coordination disorder, etc.) because the comorbidity between these disorders, widely described in the literature, is a reality in clinical practice (Inserm, 2007). Only 66% of the students in our sample do not present any diagnosed associated disorder. Among the associated disorders, we note that the most frequent is attention deficit disorder (21 students with dyslexia, 17%), followed by a language development disorder (11%) and then other disorders (7% in total). Several points may be highlighted from the statistical analyses:

- Overall, students with dyslexia ($N = 121$) report difficulties ranging, on average, from "rarely" (=2) to "very often" (=5) depending on the items[3] (see table in Appendix 13.1). Students with dyslexia, therefore, seem to nuance their difficulties. Items which they complain about the most (between "often" and "very often", on average) are the items related to reading (fluency, accuracy, and comprehension), written production (spelling, organising ideas and structuring phrases in writing), foreign language learning (oral and written), the amount of work done, and the unrewarded efforts. These observations are consistent with the results of Mazur-Palandre et al. (2015), of Mortimore and Crozier (2006), and of MacCullagh et al. (2017), to whom students with dyslexia also reported difficulties with note-taking, organising essays, and expressing ideas in writing.
- Responses of students without a learning disorder ($N = 50$) are situated, on average, between "never" (=1) and "often" (=4) (see table in Appendix 13.1). The items for which control students have the most complaints (between "sometimes" and "often" on average) are those concerning general memorisation and foreign language learning (oral and written).
- Students with dyslexia are significantly different from control students for 22 of the 30 items[4] (see table in Appendix 13.1, items in grey). Among these items are numerous activities that occur very frequently in the curriculum (i.e., taking notes in class, writing summaries) as well as elements involved in studying (i.e., memorising verbal information) and assessment (i.e., understanding written instructions, responding to a multiple choice questionnaire, completing their exams within the allotted time). Items for which we did not observe any significant difference are, for example, expressing ideas orally, mastering mathematical competency in general, organising one's study, and managing spatial information.

- The questionnaire seems sensitive to the associated difficulties experienced by students with dyslexia. For example, when comparing students with dyslexia without a documented associated disorder ($N = 80$) to students with dyslexia and attention deficit disorder (ADHD) ($N = 19$), significant differences on two items of the questionnaire are observed, to the disadvantage of students with ADHD: "managing/maintaining my attention, my concentration" and "managing spatial information". Similarly, when comparing students with dyslexia without an associated disorder to students with dyslexia and developmental language disorder ($N = 10$), significant differences were reported against students with developmental language disorder on three items: spelling words, structuring written sentences, and memorising verbal information, which is consistent with the persistence of a fragility in oral language. The size difference between samples claims to be very cautious in our derived interpretations, but the results nevertheless indicate some interesting tendencies.
- Finally, not surprisingly, in the reading text test (Alouette), students with dyslexia scored significantly lower than control students in both speed and accuracy.[5] Within each subgroup (students with dyslexia and control students), reading time is positively correlated with the difficulties expressed in four items targeting reading and writing (reading quickly in a reading-aloud situation or in a silent reading situation, reading accurately, and spelling words correctly). These results are consistent with reliable and lucid self-assessment by students with dyslexia and control students, as shown previously (Deacon et al., 2012).

Even if some difficulties related to the characteristics of dyslexia, such as persistent difficulties in reading or spelling, are found among all students with dyslexia, each student has his or her own strengths and weaknesses. Thus, clinically, problems reported by students with dyslexia are not always identical. The resulting assistance must therefore be adapted to each profile. In order to take into account the inter-individual variability of this population, we have conducted cluster analyses, the objective of which is to distinguish groups of individuals with similar profiles. These analyses were carried out on the entire group of 171 students with or without learning difficulties and revealed four distinct groups, presented succinctly in Table 13.1.

These analyses therefore indicate that the questionnaire allows for distinguishing students with dyslexia from those without learning disorders, since the vast majority (92%) of the latter are assembled in the group reporting the fewest problems. Within the group of students with dyslexia, we note different profiles, with some students making particularly marked complaints about methodological and organisational issues, as well as issues related to mathematical competence and the understanding of course concepts.

TABLE 13.1 Description of four groups of students identified in the self-evaluation questionnaire regarding difficulties related to university activities

Groups identified	Number of control students (N = 50)	Number of students with dyslexia (N = 121)	Characteristics
Group 1	46	9	- Fewer complaints than the average for the majority of items (24 out of 30 items), especially the amount of work accomplished, spelling, reading (particularly comprehension of instructions and texts), learning foreign languages, memorising verbal information, etc.
Group 2	4	28	- More complaints about memorisation, multiplication tables, mathematical skills, and understanding of concepts. - Fewer complaints for organisation, time management, note-taking.
Group 3	0	49	- More complaints about spelling, reading, learning foreign languages, and memorising verbal information. - Fewer complaints about oral comprehension and expression, understanding of concepts, and mathematical skills.
Group 4	0	35	- More complaints for any item, particularly concentration, planning, organisation, note-taking, comprehension of oral presentations, and complex written instructions.

The questionnaire concludes with an open-ended question: "What are my strengths? Describe the strengths you can rely on to overcome/circumvent your difficulties." The elements cited by students are therefore those that come to mind spontaneously after filling in 30 items in the questionnaire referring to the difficulties encountered.

Some students with or without dyslexia did not answer this question (18% and 12% respectively). Strengths pointed out by students were classified according to the four categories of engagement models detailed above. It is interesting to note that elements referencing each of these categories were found in the responses of both groups of students (with or without dyslexia). Concerning input characteristics, a number of students refer to personal characteristics by emphasising specific skills (i.e., in mathematics) or some aspects of their personality (i.e., optimistic, creative, sociable, resourceful). In relation to the social environment, some students describe the support provided by their entourage or by professionals, for example. Motivational beliefs (i.e., motivation, interest, willingness to learn, "I am capable") are frequently cited by students. However, it is engagement that is the most often emphasised strength by the students, whether or not they have learning difficulties.

In terms of engagement, four sub-categories were distinguished: emotions and affects (e.g. calmness vs. anxiety), information processing strategies (the different learning strategies implemented by the student), self-regulation (e.g. organisation, planning, and time management), and behavioural engagement (e.g. the efforts made, participation in courses, study, etc.). Again, we find responses from students with and without learning difficulties, highlighting each of these sub-categories. Note, however, that control students are more likely to cite their good information processing strategies (i.e., in-depth understanding, synthesis skills, visual and/or auditory learning strategies) and self-regulation. Students with dyslexia more often refer to behavioural engagement than students without a learning disorder: the amount of work, effort, and perseverance. This is consistent with observations from other studies in which adults with dyslexia describe themselves as persevering and responsible (Hellendoorn & Ruijssenaars, 2000). Behavioural engagement, like self-regulatory strategies, is strongly related to success (De Clercq et al., 2023; Dupont et al., 2015).

In conclusion, students seem to be able to correctly identify their difficulties, and their self-assessments appear to be reliable. Students with dyslexia differ significantly from students without learning disabilities on the majority of the items, but our results emphasise the importance of adapting the support offered to each student according to their associated disorders, of course, but also according to their individual profile. For example, planning and organisation seem to be a major difficulty for some students, while others consider this to be one of their strengths. Some students with dyslexia report severe difficulties in expressing their ideas in writing or in reading (accuracy, speed, and comprehension). For these students, the implementation of computer-based software could be particularly useful (see Section 0). Finally, what stands out particularly for students with dyslexia is the amount of work required to achieve the same results as other students.

Questionnaire for Self-Assessment of Attention in Different Situations

The second questionnaire is a "questionnaire for self-assessment of attention in different situations" (see table in Appendix 13.2). It was created following recurring complaints from students with dyslexia who showed difficulties in controlling and maintaining their attention. This complaint has already been reported in previous publications (Mortimore & Crozier, 2006). However, despite the relatively high comorbidity between dyslexia and attention deficit disorder (Inserm, 2007), students do not systematically present an associated attentional disorder. It therefore seemed essential to clarify this complaint by identifying the situations in which students found themselves in difficulty. The items in this questionnaire stem largely from the Attention Self-Assessment Questionnaire (QAA; Coyette et al., 1999), which we have adapted and completed since it was not created for the same purpose nor for our population. The point of this questionnaire is to present the same items several times but in different life situations (e.g. "When I read, I am distracted by outside noise and/or the comings and goings around me" vs. "During conversations/meetings, I am distracted [...]" vs. "When I engage in an activity, I am distracted [...]"). We have also translated and adapted some items from two other existing attentional questionnaires: the Adult ADHD Self-report Scale - ASRS-V1.1 (Kessler et al., 2005) and the Brown attention deficit disorder scales (Brown, 1996). Finally, we have added a number of items, notably related to the context of reading and writing (e.g. "Reading and understanding a text requires a lot of energy and concentration"). All in all, this questionnaire consists of 50 items (see table in Appendix 13.2).[6]

The aims of this questionnaire are: (1) to have in-depth insight into attentional complaints related to situations requiring reading and written production; and (2) to differentiate between "global" attentional difficulties, present in all situations of daily life, and "targeted" attentional difficulties relating to written material, which may be the result of consecutive cognitive overload due to a lack of automated reading procedures.

We offered this questionnaire to 121 students with dyslexia (including 21 students with attention deficit disorder) and 50 control students without a learning disorder.[7] The recruitment criteria were the same as in the first questionnaire. Statistical analyses revealed several points:

- Students without learning disabilities ($N = 50$) and students with dyslexia and no associated ADHD ($N = 100$) differ significantly on the general item ("Do you have attention difficulties in everyday life?") and on all items relating to attention difficulties in reading and writing situations (e.g. "When I read, I gradually forget the information I read") (see table in Appendix 13.2, shaded items). Among the other items with a significant difference, we note some items related to the performance of tasks (i.e., forgetting instructions or some elements of the instructions; work that is not of consistent quality) or other items, such as getting fatigued when it is necessary to concentrate over a long period of time, etc.

- Students with dyslexia without associated ADHD ($N = 100$) also differ significantly from students with dyslexia and ADHD on the general item. Of the 10 items related to written language, only two items distinguish them from students with dyslexia and ADHD (having a wandering mind or a "blank" in reading situations). This is consistent with the fact that students with dyslexia without ADHD also report difficulties with items related to written language. Furthermore, as expected, students with dyslexia with and without ADHD are distinguished on many other items related to conversational situations, activities, distraction, fatigue, etc., to the disadvantage of students with ADHD (see table in Appendix 13.2, shaded items).
- Finally, among students with dyslexia ($N = 121$), reading time on the Alouette is positively correlated with the scores obtained on the items, "even if I am in a quiet place, it takes me a long time to read a text", "reading and understanding a text requires a lot of energy and concentration", and "when I read, I do not record the meaning of what I read", but not with the scores on the other items of the questionnaire. Moreover, the number of reading errors is positively correlated with the score on the item, "when I read, I skip words/I read one word instead of another". These results are again in line with accurate self-evaluation on the part of students with dyslexia.

In order to identify if different profiles emerged, cluster analyses were again conducted (without taking into account groups that had been focused on for the first questionnaire). This time, these analyses indicate the presence of five profiles (described in Table 13.2 below) varying in relation to two aspects in particular: the presence or absence of overall attentional difficulties and the presence or absence of particularly pronounced difficulties for items related to written language.

The questionnaire, therefore, reveals attentional items linked to situations requiring written language processing as being dissociated from items referring to other situations in our population. A portion of students with dyslexia and no associated attentional disorder (41%) present a similar profile to students without learning disabilities, indicating that they do not have any particular attentional problems, even in situations of reading or writing production (Groups 1 and 2). However, almost half of students with dyslexia (47%) present particularly pronounced difficulties when faced with written material (groups 3 and 4). For these students, attentional problems could be the result of cognitive overload due to persistent difficulties in written language. The lack of automation of low-level processes would put these students in a dual-task situation, with fewer resources available for the high-level processes necessary to complete the task (reasoning, comprehension, etc.).

Finally, nearly 60% of the students with an associated attention deficit disorder are found in the group with particularly pronounced complaints across

TABLE 13.2 Description of the five groups of students identified in the self-assessment questionnaire of attention in different situations

Groups identified	Number of control students (N = 50)	Number of students with dyslexia without ADHD (N = 100)	Number of students with dyslexia with ADHD (N = 21)	Characteristics
Groups 1 and 2	49	41	4	- Fewer complaints than the average for the questionnaire as a whole (slightly more complaints for Group 2 than for Group 1).
Groups 3 and 4	1	47	6	- More complaints for items related to written language. - For other items: Groups 3 and 4 are similar to Groups 1 and 2 respectively.
Group 5	0	12	11	- More complaints on the questionnaire as a whole.

the entire attentional questionnaire (Group 5). The attentional competence of the 12 students with dyslexia and without a documented attention deficit disorder present in this same group is uncertain. An attentional and executive function evaluation would be of interest in this case. Concerning the 4 students who have been diagnosed with attentional disorders but who are among the students with the fewest complaints, it can be hypothesised that they have managed to compensate for their difficulties over time.

Finally, it should be noted that some items in the questionnaire seem less sensitive (e.g. procrastination, leaving a room without the object sought).

In conclusion, the questionnaire for self-evaluation of attentiveness in different situations seems relevant for use with students with dyslexia reporting attentional problems during the anamnesis. It allows us to distinguish between complaints related to written language and more general complaints, which may lead to proposing a more in-depth attentional and executive function assessment. In the case of attentional complaints focused primarily on written language, assistance and adaptations could be offered according to the issues that emerge: for example, moving into a quiet, uncluttered environment in the case of distractibility, breaking up reading time and using attentional reminder strategies if the student tends to have a wandering mind, using comprehension verification and self-questioning strategies if the student feels that they are not memorising or are forgetting information as they go along. A further suggestion may be the implementation of text-to-speech software for the student to focus on the content without having to read it himself or herself, or to use voice dictation software to avoid the risk of forgetting words and to allow the student to concentrate more on the content in a written production situation (see Section 0).

Monitoring, Adaptations, and Adjustments

As we have just seen, the persistence of difficulties in written language has a direct and indirect impact on students' pathways through higher education: a direct impact on reading (i.e., reading speed and accuracy) and written production activities (i.e., spelling), and an indirect impact on all the more complex tasks involving written material such as note-taking, learning lectures, writing assignments, written examinations, etc.

The challenge is therefore to limit this impact as much as possible. To do this, action can be taken at several levels: targeted improvement of weak skills (i.e., written language), but equally, compensating for and circumventing existing difficulties.

Targeted Support for Written Language

The background of each student is different: some have already benefited from speech and language therapy throughout their academic career, others have had a much more limited monitoring over time, and others still have never benefited from any type of intervention. Whatever the background of the student, if he or she is a participant, it could be worthwhile to set up monitoring during their university courses. In fact, adults can still improve their reading and spelling abilities: written language support for adults presents a range of advantages (Collette & Schelstraete, 2015). We will not, however, discuss this further (see Chapter 10 of this book).

Improving Learning and Self-Regulation Strategies

Self-regulation and learning strategies are predictors of success at university in the general population (Dupont et al., 2015).

Self-regulation refers to strategies deployed by the student to plan, manage, regulate, and control his or her learning, notably setting objectives, managing time, evaluating progress, managing sources of distraction, controlling the effectiveness of learning strategies, etc. (Pintrich, 2000). Processing strategies refer to anything that is implemented by the student to process information for the purpose of learning: for example, restructuring courses, connecting information together, making syntheses, etc. (Pintrich, 2000).

Some students with dyslexia have, over time, been able to develop effective learning strategies (MacCullagh et al., 2017; Richardson, 2021) either solely by virtue of their own expertise or with the help of a professional. For example, Kirby et al. (2008) gave questionnaires about learning strategies to both students with dyslexia and students with typical reading. Students with dyslexia make fewer references than typically reading students to the use of strategies, such as identifying key ideas and test-taking strategies. In contrast, students with dyslexia report greater use of time management strategies, use of studying aids that help them to learn or memorise information (i.e., title, italics), and in-depth processing strategies (i.e., understanding underlying concepts, being critical, making connections, etc.). The authors interpret these results as reflecting the means by which students with dyslexia compensate for their reading difficulties. However, as previously discussed, some students with dyslexia report significant problems at this level: problems with general organisation and time management are among the difficulties often reported by students with dyslexia (Mortimore & Crozier, 2006).

Several players can intervene to improve these different strategies: sometimes the support offered by institutions is aimed at all students (Robbins et al., 2009) and has an impact on performance at the end of the year (Hofer & Yu, 2003), but in this case, the support provided is not specific to the dyslexia profile. Specific help can also be provided by therapists or tutors trained in the field of dyslexia. We refer the reader interested in information about learning strategies and metacognition to Chapter 9 of this book.

Learning strategies must be adapted according to the difficulties and content of each course. The next section briefly discusses foreign language learning in relation to dyslexia. Indeed, foreign language learning has been identified in our questionnaires and in the literature as particularly problematic for students with dyslexia (Crombie, 2000; Downey et al., 2000; Mazur-Palandre et al., 2015). However, language courses are mandatory in many fields of study, and mastery of a foreign language is a necessity for numerous professions.

The Particular Case of Learning Foreign Languages

The question of how best to teach a foreign language is an important issue. Studying strategies need to be adapted according to the difficulties of students with dyslexia. Various approaches have been proposed (e.g. Crombie, 2000; Ganschow & Sparks, 2000; von Davier, 2012), many of which have already been put into practice by educators. These approaches, far from being an exhaustive list, target such matters as learning content, methods of presenting materials, studying strategies, and adjustments.

Concerning *learning content*, the recommendation is, for example, taking explicit training on the phonology and spelling of foreign languages with an emphasis on regularities, incorporating specific training of sound differentiation, and developing knowledge of the morphology of the language in order to overcome the phonological difficulties of students with dyslexia. Concerning the *methods of presenting material*, the authors advise the use of visual clues (images, colour coding, etc.) and gestures to encourage memorisation, as well as the use of multi-sensory techniques (listening, seeing, speaking, writing, associating a movement). In the same vein, they highlight the value of presenting videos with subtitles. They also propose slowing down the speed of presentation for speech as a first step. In terms of *study strategies*, students should discover their own way of learning (i.e., the use of mnemonics that are more visual or more auditory in nature). They suggest the use of vocabulary cards that associate the written word with a picture (with audio support for pronunciation, if possible). They insist on in-depth learning of the spelling of a new word (look, say, hide, write, and check), promote the use of summary sheets, tables, and suggest that teachers transmit the vocabulary lists via a computerised file so that students can classify them as they wish (by the family, by rules, etc.). Finally, concerning *adjustments*, the use of software to assist reading or written production, which we will discuss in the next section, can be very useful, as can be the use of a monolingual dictionary, the verification of the comprehension of instructions, and written and oral evaluation during exams.

While these different approaches can be useful for students with dyslexia, several of them could also be useful for students without learning difficulties. Indeed, learning a foreign language was one of the most frequently reported difficulties by control students in our questionnaire. This is in line with the notion of "universal design for learning," which advocates a flexible learning environment that gives all individuals the same learning opportunities by providing methods, materials, and assessments that are adequate for all by adapting to the needs of each individual (Reid et al., 2013). We will return to this in the next section.

Adjustments

Introduction

As previously discussed, students with dyslexia report difficulties in a variety of tasks inherent in the university curriculum, such as note-taking and reading scientific articles (MacCullagh et al., 2017). These difficulties also re-emerge during assessment, for example, in understanding written instructions (Mazur-Palandre et al., 2015) or in the drafting of written responses (Mortimore & Crozier, 2006).

In this context, legislation in many countries imposes an obligation on institutions to provide adjustments to facilitate access to higher education (Moriña, 2017; Moriña et al., 2015). The legal framework differs from country to country and, depending on the flexibility of existing regulations, the types of adjustments and the ease with which they are implemented vary from institution to institution, and sometimes even from teacher to teacher (Lindstrom, 2007).

In the context of assessment, the purpose of reasonable adjustments is not to modify the content of what is being evaluated but to limit the impact of factors related to dyslexia (or another disorder) that interfere with assessment. However, many people are legitimately concerned about the issue of "equity", arguing that accommodating students with special needs may give them an advantage by "simplifying their lives". Indeed, some adjustments granted to students with specific needs could be useful for all students (Holmes & Silvestri, 2019). For this reason, some authors consider that a proposed adjustment for a disorder should only benefit students with that disorder (Fletcher et al., 2006). In this case, only adjustments that specifically help a particular disorder (i.e., in the case of dyslexia, reading proper names aloud or breaking up a written assessment into two sessions) would be applied, in contrast to adjustments that could potentially benefit all students (i.e., providing extra time). Other authors reply that education needs to be adapted to all students' needs (Tremblay & Loiselle, 2016). Since students with learning disabilities are not the only ones who might benefit from adjustments and to avoid discrimination based on special status, adjustments should be offered to meet the needs of all learners, recognising that each learner has his or her own style of learning, preferences, and needs (Quinlan et al., 2012). Education policies are evolving, but we are still a long way from a universal design for learning. However, some assistance, potentially beneficial to all students, can be relatively easily implemented by teachers and/or institutions (i.e., providing course materials in advance, reading written examination instructions aloud, and providing access to spell-checking software for drafting assignments). In addition, apart from the "officially" accepted institutional adjustments for examinations and assignments, there are a number of other tools that could be used or implemented on a daily basis by students with dyslexia.

Far from being an exhaustive list, we will describe some of the classic adjustments for students with dyslexia (Björklund, 2011; Fletcher et al., 2006; Fuller et al., 2004; Holmes & Silvestri, 2012, 2019; Lindstrom, 2007; MacCullagh et al., 2017; Mortimore & Crozier, 2006; Pino & Mortari, 2014). Note, however, that very few empirical studies evaluate the effectiveness of these adjustments (Holmes & Silvestri, 2019; Lindstrom, 2007). Moreover, the majority of studies focus on students exhibiting a learning disability, broadly defined, rather than a specific reading disability.

After quickly listing a series of adjustments that can be beneficial for both lectures and assignments, we will focus on the adjustments offered for exams and on technological aids.

Concerning lectures, different types of adjustments are often recommended: systematic presentation of new terms in writing in addition to oral presentation; making lecture notes available (by the teacher or by other students enrolled in the course) or an audio or video recording of the lectures (or authorising recording by the student); dissemination of planned documents and other materials in advance in a digital format (useful for technological aids); and when possible, access to the audio version of books (sometimes made available to students with visual impairment). For assignments, there are also a number of different adjustments, such as extra time or flexibility in accommodating spelling and grammar. In addition, support is sometimes offered for the organisation and planning of work, or for the improvement of writing skills. Such support can be implemented in the form of individual or group tutoring, supervised by specialised tutors. Tutoring generally targets the improvement of specific skills or a particular course.

Adjustments During Examinations

The granting of extra time during assessments is undoubtedly one of the most frequent adjustments, the idea being to make up for the slowness of reading. However, there is no consensus on the length of extra time (e.g. 25%, 33%, 50%, 100%). In a study conducted with students with learning disabilities (and therefore not only with students with dyslexia), Holmes and Silvestri (2019) observed that a number of institutions provided 50% extra time, but that the majority of students (approximately 70%) did not use this additional time at all. Moreover, only a minority (less than 20%) used more than 25% supplemental time. This then raises the question of the usefulness of this adjustment, which is very frequently offered, for some students with learning disabilities. A case-by-case consideration of relevant adjustments, therefore, seems necessary. In addition to extra time, it may also be useful to provide students with time management guidelines. To avoid fatigue, one possibility is also to split the examination by taking breaks.

Another current adjustment is the oral presentation of written material: reading aloud the instructions or some passages of the exams, or providing an audio recording of them. In addition, it is preferable to articulate the questions clearly, using short sentences and emphasising the various steps to be taken. Another option is for students to record their responses for the exam or to dictate their answers to a third party rather than writing them down themselves. If students write the response themselves, a dictionary of spelling can be made available. Both for reading the questions and for producing the responses, the use of software to assist reading or writing can be useful, as will be discussed in the next section. In some cases, the instructor agrees to orally question the student immediately after the written exam or to replace the written evaluation with an oral evaluation.

Some examinations take place in separate locations, either to benefit from a quiet place without distractions or a location allowing the use of assistive software, or simply for ease of organisation, as in the case, for example, of additional time.

A specific format can be adopted for written exams by adapting the font (e.g. Arial), the font size (e.g. size 14), the line spacing (e.g. 1.5), the colour of the paper, or the printing format (using only one side of the page).

Finally, some arrangements are simple to put in place, such as using highlighters to identify key words in the instructions, a reading window to make reading easier, a stopwatch to manage your time, a calculator if numerous operations need to be performed, earplugs or headphones to be less disturbed by ambient noise, etc.

Among these adjustments, some have no impact on the instructor's grading criteria (i.e., having a calculator, being in a separate room, etc.). In contrast, modifying the format of the print or grading spelling separately, for example, in one way or another, leads to the identification of the student and prevents "anonymous" grading. In addition, some adjustments alter the mode of evaluation (in the case of oral evaluation instead of written evaluation, for example). It is therefore essential that instructors can be trained and informed about these challenges, bearing in mind the competences targeted by the assessments.

Technological Aids

The objective of technological aids is to assist, increase, or improve the functional abilities of individuals. In the case of dyslexia, for example, this means relieving the activity of reading or writing in order to liberate resources that are then available for other types of processing, such as detailed comprehension. According to Holmes and Silvestri (2012), assistive technologies can be considered (1) as a cognitive prosthesis, which replaces or circumvents an absent or deficient skill, as in the case of software that reads in place of an individual, or (2) a cognitive partner, which supports the learning process, as in the case of software aimed at improving a particular skill. In the context of adjustments, most interest is focused on the cognitive prosthetic approach.

Technological assistance can be classified into different categories. Draffan et al. (2007) distinguish between computer-related hardware and software. In each case, they differentiate the technology whose primary purpose is not specifically targeted towards people with specific needs, from assistive technology whose primary purpose is to be an aid, even though these assistive technologies can be used by everyone.

- **Computer hardware and general electronic equipment**: computers, tablets, scanners, etc. They constitute the basic equipment used by the general population.
- **Specific computer hardware**: recorders, portable spell checkers (which can be used to check handwritten work, to provide definitions, and as a thesaurus,

for example), pens which scan the text and transfer it to the computer, reading pens which pronounce and define words, etc.
- **General-purpose software**: standard software (like Microsoft Word®) but also voice recognition software (like Dragon Naturally Speaking®), which allows students to "dictate" a text that gradually appears on the computer screen. This type of software adapts itself to the speech of the person using it and becomes more and more accurate as it is used. It can be beneficial for students with a good level of oral language but difficulties in written language (Holmes & Silvestri, 2012).
- **Software and applications for specific purposes**: there are a number of different software packages that can specifically support students with learning disabilities (Draffan et al., 2007; Holmes & Silvestri, 2012). Among the reading assistance tools are text-to-speech software programs that convert scanned text into speech, which may be of interest to students with decoding difficulties but without speech comprehension difficulties (e.g. Sprint®, Kurzweil 3000®). These software programs can read files that have been imported or downloaded from the Internet. It is possible to define a whole range of parameters (e.g. language, voice, speed) and to choose whether you want only a passage or the whole text to be read. To support the production of written work, word banks and word prediction software are available to aid students in selecting and writing the right word on the basis of criteria such as syntax, spelling, frequency, etc. (e.g. Skippy®, Text Help®). As soon as the first letters of the word are typed, the software suggests a series of words. The spell checkers help to identify and correct spelling and grammar errors (e.g. Antidote®, Médialexie®, Kurzweil 3000®). There also exist standard dictionaries with voice output or software that enables the creation of mental maps (mind mapping) to facilitate the organisation of information. Mind maps permit the visual presentation of ideas or information in a schematic form and can be used for note-taking, brainstorming, revision, planning reports and essays (e.g. Xmind®, Inspiration®). These latter tools are of use, among others, for students with a weak working memory in that they enable all of the information to be kept available (Holmes & Silvestri, 2012). The software programs most widely used by students exhibiting learning disabilities are those for speech synthesis, speech recognition, word prediction, and graphic organizers (Holmes & Silvestri, 2012). In addition, there are also a growing number of applications and software available on the Internet, which offer a wide range of functions, from reading aloud online websites and modification of web page settings (font size and colour, for example), to activity planning and the creation of checklists (so as not to forget different activities or steps), to learning aids such as "flash cards" (cards containing a word or an image), etc. (Holmes & Silvestri, 2012; Reid et al., 2013).

Holmes and Silvestri (2012) are interested in the digital tools offered to students with learning disorders and, in particular, in the effectiveness of these aids, which has rarely been investigated until now. In their review of research, they report mixed results concerning text-to-speech software: this software improves the comprehension of students with the most severe reading disorders but interferes with comprehension for students with less difficulty. This could be explained by an overload in working memory created by the continuous flow of speech from the software. It would seem that if only one word or passage is selected, the disruptive effect of the continuous reading of spoken text on the working memory processes linked to reading comprehension is avoided. Furthermore, while speech synthesis improves reading comprehension for adults with a specific phonological processing deficit, it would be a hindrance for adults with another profile (better phonological processing). The same software, when synchronised with the text that appears highlighted on the screen, can be useful for proofreading as it enables students with learning disorders to identify a greater number of errors in their writing compared to those without this assistance. Outside of speech synthesis software, the authors lament the fact that there is very little published work on the effectiveness of digital tools, but studies on the abandonment of technological aid (and therefore its lack of effectiveness) nevertheless provide some interesting information. According to Holmes and Silvestri, several reasons for abandonment are identified in studies targeting learning disabilities: the objective is not achieved (does not improve university tasks, does not meet academic needs/requirements), implementation is too tedious (requires too much assistance from another person, too difficult to use, requires a long or complicated series of commands, lack of training and support, and therefore no benefit from the technology) or obstacles arise (too difficult or costly to repair, not always reliable).

Numerous digital tools that can help students with dyslexia do exist. However, there are several elements that seem important to keep in mind. *First*, the cost of the different software packages has not been discussed here. Prices vary considerably between the most expensive software and that which is available free of charge, either in whole or in part. In some countries, if students with dyslexia receive some digital tools for free (as a part of disability allowance), this is not the case in numerous countries. Cost can therefore be a significant barrier for students. *Second*, it is very important to master the digital tools and to use them regularly and correctly in order for them to be effective and to avoid the risk of abandonment (Björklund, 2011). Inadequate technology can become an obstacle to learning. Therefore, one should not increase the number of tools without evaluating the value of each of them for the student. It is not enough to simply offer a particular software to a student, as a follow-up for selection and training must be conducted, either by a person specialised in dyslexia linked to the student's institution (but this requires resources and qualified staff, and many institutions lack the technical and human resources) or by an external therapist (which represents an additional cost for the student). *Third*, there are still too few studies specifically evaluating the effectiveness of these different tools for students with dyslexia. Some studies are rather positive: for example, in a study conducted in England (Draffan et al., 2007), students with dyslexia received a recording device, text-to-speech software, and a mind-mapping tool in addition to a standard computer. Most students reported being satisfied or very satisfied with the technological aid provided. However, the usefulness and effectiveness of the digital tools are clearly in need of qualification in some cases (Holmes & Silvestri, 2012; Perelmutter et al., 2017). It is therefore important to continue researching in this area, taking into account the feedback from students with dyslexia and using objective measures indicating the effectiveness or ineffectiveness of these different tools.

To conclude, it is worth noting that one of the advantages of using technological aid is that, in most cases, it integrates well into an inclusive perspective. Indeed, at present, almost all students have this technology at their disposal (Björklund, 2011); the use of a computer or a tablet, for example, will not be pointed to as a marker of difference but will, on the contrary, pass unnoticed fairly easily. The stigma sometimes felt by some students with dyslexia may indeed, in some instances, be a constraint on their request for adjustments and/or integration.

Support, Adjustments, and Success: What Do Students Think?

While different types of aids, adaptations, and adjustments seem to be beneficial for students with dyslexia, it is particularly enlightening to have their opinions on the utility and actual implementation of these services. With this perspective in mind, a survey was carried out among students with dyslexia who had benefited from a written language assessment at the CPS (UCLouvain). The objective of this survey was to have an overview of their experience by asking them to report on the support available to them, the usefulness of aids, and the benefits of the adjustments. Forty students with dyslexia responded to the survey, including 11 men and 29 women, all of whom were enrolled in higher education (14 in the 1st year, 10 in the 2nd year, 6 in the 3rd year, 3 in the 4th year, and 7 in the 5th year) and had already taken at least one session of exams. It should be noted that 30% of these students have a diagnosed associated disorder (attention deficit disorder, developmental coordination disorder, or dyscalculia).

The Support of Relatives, Peers, and the Educational Team

Support is an important issue because, in the general population, how the student perceives support is seen as a predictor of their success at university, their persistence, and their self-efficacy (Dupont et al., 2015). Similarly, being supported and maintaining good relationships with family, peers, friends, and teaching staff is a protective factor in dyslexia (Haft et al., 2016). The majority of students with dyslexia surveyed feel supported by their family (90%), and a large proportion can also count on the support of friends (85%). This is positive as parental support seems to be a predictor of the adaptation and well-being of adults with dyslexia (Hellendoorn & Ruijssenaars, 2000).

We note, however, more nuanced results in relation to the support of peers (42.5%) and teaching staff (37.5%). In studies conducted among students without learning difficulties, the perceived support of teachers is associated with the success of students, due to its effects on their learning strategies and engagement. Peer assistance and support behaviours, such as sharing lecture notes, communicating information, giving encouragement, or incentivising different types of activities, are also correlated with success, particularly through their impact on motivation. Furthermore, there is a relation between student performance results and feelings of rejection or discrimination experienced in everyday life, especially among minorities (Dupont et al., 2015). In our survey sample of students with dyslexia, almost all of the students feel able to talk about their difficulties in their surroundings (92.5%), and the results are quite positive in terms of their feeling of integration (only 15% answer "not at all" or "mostly not"). The results are more mixed, however, regarding the feeling of being "judged", "discriminated against", with 32.5% of students with dyslexia answering in the affirmative ("mostly yes" or "absolutely"). Some students with dyslexia report quite strong remarks coming from other students who consider the adjustments to be favouritism, who suspect them of faking their difficulties in order to take advantage of the aid, or those who refuse to work with a student with dyslexia in group work.

Raising awareness and providing information to peers and teachers are therefore critical to reduce negative behaviours and attitudes, which are often due to a lack of knowledge about dyslexia (Pino & Mortari, 2014). Among the obstacles to success identified by students with a disability, teaching staff attitude is an important element (Moriña et al., 2015): authors observe that experience reported by students on this subject varies from student to student (Fuller et al., 2004). Some have had very positive contact with open-minded teachers (Pino & Mortari, 2014), but this is not the case for all students. This is consistent with Morina's reflections (2017) on "invisible" disabilities in which students feel that teaching staff and other students question the validity of the disability. Students have an obligation to provide documentation of their disorder, which makes them feel less legitimate. And because they desire to be treated "normally" or are afraid of being judged or stigmatised, some prefer not to disclose their difficulties (Mortimore & Crozier, 2006).

Support from Professionals

When students are asked what assistance or support they benefited from or received during their course of higher education (speech therapists, neuropsychologists, educators, psychologists, etc.), almost half (42.5%) say that they have not received any particular support apart from the adjustments they have been granted. Only 17.5% received speech therapy and information about dyslexia at university. The same percentage had been helped by a tutor or a relative (other students or family members) for a particular course. Slightly more students (22.5%) received help concerning their study skills. Finally, 5% of the students received a follow-up for emotional management.

The proportions of students who have received specific support are thus low.[8] Nevertheless, students seem to be requesting it because when they are asked about what they would have liked to have benefited from, all these aids are mentioned (information on dyslexia, methodological support, emotion management, etc.). Support and guidance adapted to the profile of each student could therefore be beneficial, especially to encourage a means of compensation for these students. However, the time needed for these follow-ups and the financial aspects certainly play a role in their implementation.

Reasonable Adjustments

In relation to the adjustments offered to the 40 students with dyslexia who responded to our survey, only one student had not applied for any adjustments because he did not feel the need for them. All of the other students were given extra time in exams (one-third additional time), making this the most common adjustment among these students. Only two students reported that they did not consistently need it. In second place was: taking the exam in a separate (smaller and quieter) room. Next adjustments were: the adapted format of the written exams, the availability of a spelling dictionary, the possibility of an oral exam (either after or in place of the written exam), access to a computer with spell-checking software, tolerance for spelling errors in the marking of the exam, extra time for submitting assignments, adjustments for language classes, and having access to course materials in advance.

As far as the implementation of these adjustments is concerned, the vast majority of students are rather positive. They say that their experience of the process went well and that they feel well supported. The implementation was, according to them, natural and rapid. They felt that the institution was involved and that the contact personnel (student support service) were adequate. They spoke of real relief and a significant reduction in stress.

While most students are satisfied with the adjustments provided, some report that they were initially granted "typical" adjustments that were either not helpful (e.g. separate room, spelling dictionary) or disruptive to them (e.g.

adapted format). Only later did they benefit from truly adapted adjustments. This therefore demonstrates the value of a rigorous process of analysing needs and selection of relevant adjustments according to the difficulties of each student (cognitive and linguistic profile), the task to be performed, and the context (Lindstrom, 2007).

Among adjustments that students surveyed did not obtain/request but would have appreciated were the following: reading aloud of the instructions by the teacher, more assistance in understanding the questions (and clearer instructions with important items in bold), more adaptations for language lessons, having 50% more time instead of 33%, having the chance to listen to the texts to be covered (MP3 player, for example), being able to speak out loud during the exams, availability of a computer with software to help with reading and writing during the exam, availability of complete course notes from the teachers and a recording of the lessons.

It should nevertheless be borne in mind that students mention adjustments that they think would be useful to them. On the one hand, they may not have envisioned some adjustments that could be effective, and on the other, it is possible that they may feel that a particular adjustment could be beneficial to them without this actually being the case (Holmes & Silvestri, 2019).

Finally, note that only four students say they use reading or writing assistive software on a daily basis. One might pose the question as to whether these tools are not useful for the other students, or whether they did not have access to them (no information on this subject, financial aspects, etc.).

The University Pathway: Expectations of Success, Obstacles, and Interest in Education

Several questions in the survey refer to students' expectations of success (meaning their expectations of their future performance) and their perception of the task value. These two aspects are considered to be positively associated and predictive of success in higher education in the general population (Expectation-value model; Eccles & Wigfield, 2002).

To the question, "Do you think you will be able to succeed in your studies?", only two students answered negatively. However, more than half of the students say they feel able to do so, but on the condition that they can be provided with adjustments or support. This can be linked to students' sense of self-efficacy and thus their confidence in their ability to succeed. However, it is known that students with a higher sense of self-efficacy persist more, use more in-depth studying and self-regulatory strategies, become more committed, and achieve higher performance levels (Dupont et al., 2015).

When asked to identify the barriers to success, the responses of the students with dyslexia summarise quite well the points that were discussed previously: the need to read (books, articles, etc.) and write (notably assignments), their slowness and the amount of work required, the need to memorise things, fatigue, their difficulties in concentrating, their lack of efficiency and organisation, and stress. Yet many of them say that they are able to overcome them, particularly through consistent and substantial work, efficient organisation, and good learning strategies (which some still need to improve). This is consistent with what we observed when analysing the self-assessment questionnaire on difficulties related to university activities.

The obstacles which each student confronts during their higher education career depend not only on the support, methods, and learning objectives, but also on the modes of assessment in each field of study (and in each course). This is why some students choose their field of study taking into account their own difficulties (e.g. fields in which learning and evaluation require little written work or which involve practical elements, or which rely on technologies that allow the use of software) (Fuller et al., 2004). Note, however, that our sample includes students from all backgrounds (humanities, science and technology, health sciences, paramedical fields, etc.). The obstacles that will arise (and the relevant adjustments) will therefore be different for each of them.

Finally, two questions address the perception of the interest and usefulness of the courses, both of which touch on the concept of the task value. Almost all students with dyslexia are affirmative about their interest in their courses and the usefulness of the courses for their future profession. This is rather positive, especially when considering that having a positive perception of the task is also an important predictor of success (Dupont et al., 2015).

In conclusion, the students with dyslexia who were interviewed seemed to be interested in their studies and, even if they identified some obstacles to their success, they felt able to overcome them, particularly thanks to the strategies they put in place, the adjustments, and the targeted support they benefited from.

Conclusion and Perspectives

There is no single and best way to help students with dyslexia for the simple reason that there is no single and the same student profile. The assistance provided will therefore depend on the difficulties identified by behavioural tests, on the one hand, and on confronting these difficulties, the perceived difficulties, and the expectations of higher education, on the other hand. In order to better identify the needs of students with dyslexia, it may be useful to administer questionnaires focused on university activities, since their self-evaluation seems to be fairly reliable and lucid, illuminating their strengths and revealing their needs.

Various types of assistance can be provided during their journey, particularly by specialists (written language support, methodological aid, psychological support, etc.), but their cost and the time needed to set them up are points not to be overlooked.

Support from family, friends, peers, teaching staff, and the institution is likewise very important. While students generally feel well supported by their family and friends, it is essential to continue to raise awareness among faculty and other students. The support implemented by the institutions depends, among other things, on legislation, possible subsidies, available resources, and the willingness of the different parties involved. The students in our survey show general satisfaction with the assistance they receive, but there is much to be gained by further developing guidance offered by institutions for all students (thus promoting predictors of success), and also by offering assistance targeted according to students' difficulties (e.g. adapted learning strategies).

Students with dyslexia attribute their success in particular to the efforts they make (MacCullagh et al., 2017). Many of them seem determined and resourceful in compensating for their difficulties (Lindstrom, 2007). It is without doubt one of the elements that enables some of them to overcome obstacles and succeed in their studies. Adjustments appear to be a valuable aid for numerous students, and half of the students we surveyed indicate that they feel capable of succeeding, provided they continue to be able to benefit from them. However, these adjustments vary from one institution to another, and sometimes even from one teacher to another, so more reflection on this issue must follow. Furthermore, it is essential to continue to develop research in this area, as we still lack data on the relevance and effectiveness of the various proposed adjustments.

Reasonable adjustments are found at the heart of a debate mixing the notions of equality, equity, integration, and inclusion. Some authors advocate a universal conception of education (Tremblay & Loiselle, 2016) that gives all individuals the same learning opportunities (Reid et al., 2013). Although we are far from a totally inclusive education system, pedagogical approaches are gradually evolving, and the support implemented has the merit of permitting students with dyslexia to pursue their studies under better conditions of learning and assessment. Note that many of the obstacles identified by students with special needs in previous studies have nothing to do with their specific disorders (e.g. rigid teaching methods, distant relationship between teacher and student) and also affect other students (Moriña et al., 2015). While some modifications require significant changes, there are other modifications that seem relatively easy to implement and could benefit all students.

To conclude, let us emphasise the importance of the roles of all of the players who interact with students with dyslexia (speech therapists, neuropsychologists, psychologists, educators, tutors, support service staff, teaching staff, etc.). These different contributors are regularly brought together to discuss the choice of studies, professional orientation, follow-up, and adjustments to propose to the students. It is therefore critical that they are properly informed in order to best help all students to overcome the challenge that is the successful completion of a pathway in higher education.

Appendices

Appendix 13.1

TABLE A13.1 Average per group (students with dyslexia (DD) and controls (CTR)) for the answers to each item of the self-assessment questionnaire about difficulties related to university activities (Likert scale from 1 to 6)

	Questionnaire items for the self-assessment of difficulties related to university activities	Average DD (N = 121)	Average CTR (N = 50)
N°	I experience **difficulties** in the following activities:		
1	Taking notes in lectures.	3.64	2.70
2	Organising/expressing my ideas in my dissertations/written productions.	4.11	2.44
3	Producing summaries, abstracts.	3.56	2.52
4	Understanding and integrating the theoretical concepts of the courses.	3.19	2.84
5	Expressing my ideas orally.	3.17	2.88
6	Understanding an oral presentation in detail.	2.86	2.37
7	Reading quickly in a reading ALOUD situation (slow reading).	4.36	2.08
8	Fast reading in a SILENT reading situation (slow reading).	3.87	1.74
9	Reading accurately (errors and/or tendency to invent, to read one word for another, etc.).	4.39	2.28
10	Understanding what I am reading (e.g. needing to read several times to understand the meaning of a text, difficulty in understanding a university-level text in detail, difficulty in retaining all the information read)	4.21	2.78
11	Understanding complex written instructions/statements (e.g. exam questions).	3.91	2.38
12	Answering an MCQ (multiple choice questionnaire).	3.30	2.28
13	Spelling words correctly (basic spelling).	4.70	2.26
14	Applying basic grammar rules in spelling.	4.55	2.36
15	Structuring my written sentences correctly (errors related to syntax, writing style, wording).	4.10	2.24
16	Writing letters legibly (poorly legible handwriting).	2.53	2.52
17	Memorising in a general way (e.g. too much work needed to memorise a course).	3.47	3.06
18	Memorising verbal information (proper names, vocabulary, etc.).	3.81	2.80
19	Remembering and recalling the multiplication tables (arithmetic facts).	2.85	2.46

(Continued)

TABLE A13.1 (Continued)

Questionnaire items for the self-assessment of difficulties related to university activities		Average DD (N = 121)	Average CTR (N = 50)
20	Mastering mathematical skills in general (e.g. reasoning, logic).	2.74	2.62
21	Learning foreign languages ORALLY.	4.45	3.24
22	Learning the WRITTEN format of foreign languages	4.77	3.00
23	Organising my study, my work.	3.08	2.86
24	Managing/maintaining my attention, my concentration.	3.81	2.80
25	Managing my time (agenda, activities, studies).	3.23	2.86
26	Finishing my exams, I work on time.	3.42	2.42
27	Managing spatial information (understanding and representing space, manipulating graphs, charts, tables, etc.)	2.41	2.48
28	Coordinating my movements to carry out complex motor sequences.	2.43	2.62
29	I have to work harder than other students to achieve the same result.	4.76	2.56
30	I have the impression that my efforts are not rewarded (e.g. results that are not up to par).	4.05	2.62

Note: Shaded scores indicate a significant difference ($p < .05$) between the two groups.

Appendix 13.2

TABLE A13.2 Average per group (students with dyslexia (DD) with or without associated attention deficit disorder (ADHD) and control students (CTR)) for the answers to each item of the self-assessment questionnaire about attentional difficulties in different situations (Likert scale from 1 to 6)

Code items	Questionnaire items for the self-assessment of attentional difficulties in different situations	Average DD with ADHD (N = 21)	Average DD w/o ADHD (N = 100)	Average CTR (N = 50)
	In DAILY LIFE:			
G1	Do you think you have attention difficulties in everyday life?	4.05	3.01	2.36
	In a READING situation (silent, quiet reading):			
L1	During reading, I lose track because I am distracted by outside noise and/or the comings and goings around me.	4.33	3.78	2.86

(*Continued*)

TABLE A13.2 (Continued)

Code items	Questionnaire items for the self-assessment of attentional difficulties in different situations	Average DD with ADHD (N = 21)	Average DD w/o ADHD (N = 100)	Average CTR (N = 50)
L2	When I read, I lose track because my mind wanders and I can't stop thinking about something else.	4.38	3.58	2.98
L3	When I read, I lose the thread because I have like a "hole", a "blank", an empty head.	3.05	2.30	1.76
L4	When I read, I do not "register" the meaning of what I read.	3.38	3.47	2.48
L5	As I read, I gradually forget the information I have read.	3.29	3.13	2.20
L6	Even if I am in a quiet place, it takes me a long time to read a text.	3.81	4.03	1.96
L7	Reading and understanding a text requires a lot of energy and concentration.	4.48	4.21	2.16
L8	When I read, I skip words/I read one word instead of another.	4.05	3.94	1.88
	In a WRITING situation:			
E1	I forget letters and words as I write.	3.43	3.44	2.08
E2	When I write, I find it difficult to pay attention to content and at the same time to spelling and style.	4.71	4.66	2.12
	In a CONVERSATION situation (with two or more people)/MEETINGS:			
C1	During conversations/meetings, I lose track because I am distracted by outside noise and/or the comings and goings around me.	3.38	2.61	2.12
C2	During conversations/meetings, I lose track because my mind wanders and I can't stop thinking about something else.	3.29	2.73	2.66
C3	During conversations/meetings, I lose the thread because I have like a "hole", a "blank", an empty head	2.62	1.88	1.56

(*Continued*)

TABLE A13.2 (Continued)

Code items	Questionnaire items for the self-assessment of attentional difficulties in different situations	Average DD with ADHD (N = 21)	Average DD w/o ADHD (N = 100)	Average CTR (N = 50)
C4	During conversations/meetings, I don't always "register" what is said; I forget some information as I go along.	3.38	2.48	2.24
C5	During conversations/meetings, people point out to me that I change the subject (I go off on a tangent).	3.43	2.46	2.20
<u>C6</u>	In conversations/meetings, I tend to finish other people's sentences before they can do so.	2.71	2.48	2.60
C7	Listening and understanding a conversation/meeting requires a lot of energy and concentration.	3.43	2.47	1.78
	When I watch a film on the TELEVISION:			
T1	When I watch a film, I lose track because I am distracted by outside noise and/or the comings and goings around me.	2.19	1.94	2.04
T2	When I watch a film, I lose track because my mind wanders and I can't stop thinking about something else.	2.38	2.06	2.12
T3	When I watch a film, I lose the thread because I have like a "hole", a "blank", an empty head.	1.86	1.38	1.30
T4	When I watch a film, I don't always "register" everything; I forget some information as I go along.	2.38	1.79	2.06
	When I carry out an ACTIVITY, a TASK, or an ASSIGNMENT alone:			
A1	When I am conducting an activity, I am easily distracted by outside noise and/or the comings and goings around me.	4.38	2.93	2.54

(*Continued*)

TABLE A13.2 (Continued)

Code items	Questionnaire items for the self-assessment of attentional difficulties in different situations	Average DD with ADHD (N = 21)	Average DD w/o ADHD (N = 100)	Average CTR (N = 50)
A2	When I carry out a simple, repetitive, and monotonous activity over a long period of time, I make careless mistakes.	4.35	3.43	3.08
A3	When I carry out an activity and I am interrupted by something unexpected, I forget to come back to finish it.	3.14	2.67	2.62
A4	When I carry out an activity that involves several steps, I omit one.	3.24	2.63	2.16
A5	When I carry out an activity that requires organisation, I find it difficult to set priorities.	2.90	2.87	2.34
A6	I find it difficult to carry out several activities at the same time.	4.00	3.03	2.72
A7	When I carry out an activity, I make mistakes if people talk to me at the same time.	3.71	3.34	3.04
A8	When I run a project, I find it difficult to finalise it once the bulk of the work has been done.	3.19	2.67	2.78
A9	I tend to postpone or avoid tasks that require concentration.	3.60	3.22	2.94
A10	When I have to do a task, I feel hyperactive, like an electric battery.	3.29	2.45	2.34
A11	When I have to perform a task, I forget the instructions or some elements of the instructions.	3.52	3.30	2.34
A12	I produce work that is not of consistent quality, and my work performance is quite varied.	3.29	3.00	2.48
	DISTRACTION:			
D1	I forget where I have just placed an object a few moments before.	4.05	3.14	3.18
D2	I enter a room without knowing what I came to do there.	3.81	3.14	3.06

(Continued)

TABLE A13.2 (Continued)

Code items	Questionnaire items for the self-assessment of attentional difficulties in different situations	Average DD with ADHD (N = 21)	Average DD w/o ADHD (N = 100)	Average CTR (N = 50)
D3	I go into a room to take or do something and come out having taken or done something else.	3.62	3.11	3.14
D4	When I leave the house, I forget to turn off the lights or lock the door.	2.29	1.85	1.72
<u>D5</u>	I have difficulty remembering my appointments.	3.43	2.45	1.96
D6	My entourage considers me to have my "head in the clouds".	3.67	2.59	2.42
D7	I am considered "a dreamer", "to be lost in thought".	3.67	2.55	2.14
D8	As a child, I tended to daydream at school rather than follow classes.	4.24	3.17	2.36
	MISCELLANEOUS:			
S1	I feel tired during the day, even after a good night's sleep.	4.14	3.60	3.54
S2	I get tired when I have to concentrate for a long period of time.	4.52	4.05	3.24
<u>S3</u>	I get "fidgety"; I move my feet and hands when I have to sit for a long period of time.	4.62	3.67	2.82
S4	In general, I feel nervous, agitated, and impatient.	4.14	2.78	2.28
<u>S5</u>	I find it difficult to wait my turn when I am in a situation that requires me to take turns to intervene.	3.52	2.20	2.44
S6	I tend to bother others when they are busy.	2.857	2.185	2.14
S7	I am irritable, with bouts of sudden aggressiveness.	2.81	2.04	1.80
S8	I get discouraged easily.	3.19	2.74	2.54

Note: The shaded scores in the column for the DD students with ADHD or in the column for the CTR students indicate a significant difference ($p < .05$) between these groups and the students with dyslexia without ADHD.

Codes for items adapted from the QAA are shown in bold, those for translated and/or adapted items from the ASRS-V1.1 are underlined, and those for translated and/or adapted items from the Brown questionnaire are italicised.

Notes

1. In this chapter, we will regularly refer to the Consultations Psychologiques Spécialisées (CPS), a centre for the screening and follow-up of dyslexic students, which is part of the Psychological Sciences Research Institute at the Université catholique de Louvain (UCLouvain, Belgium), and to the 'PEPS' project (Project for Students with Specific Profiles) which has been set up at UCLouvain, specifically to promote the integration of students with learning difficulties.
2. Studies comparing students diagnosed with dyslexia and students reporting reading acquisition difficulties without a diagnosis suggest that they are the same underlying population but with different adaptive strategies (Deacon et al., 2012). Similarly, it can be assumed that the profile of students who do or do not take steps to benefit from accommodations is not quite the same (i.e., more or less effective compensatory strategies, presence or absence of an associated disorder, etc.).
3. The levels "never", "rarely", "sometimes", "often", "very often" and "always" have been recoded into a scale from 1 to 6 for statistical analysis.
4. In our analyses, we use a significance threshold of $p < .05$ (non-parametric test for two independent samples: Mann-Whitney test).
5. The efficiency score was also calculated on the basis of the speed and accuracy of reading on the Alouette. The scores for students with dyslexia (mean 342.01; SD 74.81) and control students (mean 541.77; SD 94.78) correspond to the results obtained by Cavalli et al. (2018) and to the threshold efficiency score (402.26) that emerged in their study as distinguishing between students with and without reading difficulties.
6. Codes for items adapted from the QAA are shown in bold, those for translated and/or adapted items from the ASRS-V1.1 are underlined, and those for translated and/or adapted items from the Brown questionnaire are italicized.
7. The samples of students with dyslexia and controls for the two questionnaires differed by only four students (2 students did not complete the Academic Difficulty Questionnaire and 2 students did not complete the Attention Questionnaire).
8. It should be remembered that 14 of the 40 students surveyed are in their first year in higher education, so this is a relatively short period of time and perhaps partly explains the small amount of support/follow-up that has been implemented.

References

Björklund, M. (2011). Dyslexic students: Success factors for support in a learning environment. *The Journal of Academic Librarianship, 37*(5), 423–429. https://doi.org/10.1016/j.acalib.2011.06.006

Brown, T. E. (1996). *Brown attention deficit disorder scales for adolescents and adults*. The Psychological Corporation.

Cavalli, E., Colé, P., Leloup, G., Poracchia-George, F., Sprenger-Charolles, L., & El Ahmadi, A. (2018). Screening for dyslexia in French-speaking university students: An evaluation of the detection accuracy of the Alouette test. *Journal of Learning Disabilities, 51*(3), 268–282. https://doi.org/10.1177/0022219417704637

Collette, E., & Schelstraete, M.-A. (2015). Rééducation de l'orthographe dans le cas D'une dyslexie développementale: Etude de cas clinique chez un étudiant. *Rééducation orthophonique, 261*, 91–109.

Coyette, F., Arno, P., Leclercq, M., Seron, X., & Van der Linden, M. (1999). *Questionnaire d'auto-évaluation de l'attention (QAA): Élaboration de normes à partir D'une population de 220 sujets adultes*. Centre de Revalidation Neuropsychologique des Cliniques Universitaires Saint-Luc.

Crombie, M. A. (2000). Dyslexia and the learning of a foreign language in school: Where are we going? *Dyslexia*, *6*, 112–123. https://doi.org/10.1002/(SICI)1099-0909(200004/06)6:2<112::AID-DYS151>3.0.CO;2-D

De Clercq, M., Roland, N., Dangoisse, F., & Frenay, M. (2023). *La transition vers l'enseignement supérieur*. Peter Lang.

Deacon, S. H., Cook, K., & Parrila, R. (2012). Identifying high-functioning dyslexics: Is self-report of early reading problems enough? *Annals of Dyslexia*, *62*, 120–134. https://doi.org/10.1007/s11881-012-0068-2

Downey, D. M., Snyder, L. E., & Hill, B. (2000). College students with dyslexia: Persistent linguistic deficits and foreign language learning. *Dyslexia*, *6*, 101–111. https://doi.org/10.1002/(SICI)1099-0909(200004/06)6:2%3C101::AID-DYS154%3E3.0.CO;2-8

Draffan, E. A., Evans, D. G., & Blenkhorn, P. (2007). Use of assistive technology by students with dyslexia in post-secondary education. *Disability and Rehabilitation: Assistive Technology*, *2*(2), 105–116. https://doi.org/10.1080/17483100601178492

Dupont, S., De Clercq, M., & Galand, B. (2015). Les prédicteurs de la réussite dans l'enseignement supérieur. *Revue française de pédagogie*, *191*, 105–136. https://doi.org/10.4000/rfp.4770

Eccles, J. S., & Wigfield, A. (2002). Motivational beliefs, values, and goals. *Annual Review of Psychology*, *53*, 109–132.

Fletcher, J. M., Francis, D. J., Boudousquie, A., Copeland, K., Young, V., Kalinowski, S., & Vaughn, S. (2006). Effects of accommodations on high-stakes testing for students with Reading disabilities. *Exceptional Children*, *72*(2), 136–150. https://doi.org/10.1177/001440290607200201

Fuller, M., Healey, M., Bradley, A., & Hall, T. (2004). Barriers to learning: A systematic study of the experience of disabled students in one university. *Studies in Higher Education*, *29*(3), 303–318. https://doi.org/10.1080/03075070410001682592

Ganschow, L., & Sparks, R. (2000). Reflections on foreign language study for students with language learning problems: Research, issues and challenges. *Dyslexia*, *6*, 87–100. https://doi.org/10.1002/(SICI)1099-0909(200004/06)6:2<87::AID-DYS153>3.0.CO;2-H

Giménez, A., Luque, J. L., López-Zamora, M., & Fernández-Navas, M. (2015). A self-report of reading disabilities for adults: ATLAS. *Anales de psicología*, *31*(1), 109–119.

Haft, S. L., Myers, C. A., & Hoeft, F. (2016). Socio-emotional and cognitive resilience in children with reading disabilities. *Current Opinion in Behavioral Sciences*, *10*, 133–141. https://doi.org/10.1016/j.cobeha.2016.06.005

Hellendoorn, J., & Ruijssenaars, W. (2000). Personal experiences and adjustment of Dutch adults with dyslexia. *Remedial and Special Education*, *21*(4), 227–239. https://doi.org/10.1177/074193250002100405

Hofer, B. K., & Yu, S. L. (2003). Teaching self-regulated learning through a "learning to learn" course. *Teaching of Psychology*, *30*(1), 30–33. https://doi.org/10.1207/S15328023TOP3001_05

Holmes, A., & Silvestri, R. (2012). Assistive technology use by students with LD in postsecondary education : A case of application before investigation? *Canadian Journal of School Psychology*, *27*(1), 81–97. https://doi.org/10.1177/0829573512437018

Holmes, A., & Silvestri, R. (2019). Extra time or unused time? What data from a college testing Center tells us about 50% extra time as an accommodation for students with learning disabilities. *Psychological Injury and Law*, *12*, 7–16. https://doi.org/10.1007/s12207-019-09339-9

Inserm. (2007). *Expertise collective : Dyslexie, dysorthographie, dyscalculie : Bilan des données scientifiques*. Inserm.

Kessler, R. C., Adler, L., Ames, M., Demler, O., Faraone, S., Hiripi, E., Howes, M. J., Jin, R., Scecnik, K., Spencer, T., Ustun, T. B., & Walters, E. (2005). The World Health Organization adult ADHD self-report scale (ASRS): A short screening scale for use in the general population. *Psychological Medicine*, *35*, 245–256. https://doi.org/10.1017/S0033291704002892

Kirby, J. R., Silvestri, R., Allingham, B. H., Parrila, R., & La Fave, C. B. (2008). Learning strategies and study approaches of postsecondary students with dyslexia. *Journal of Learning Disabilities*, *41*(1), 85–96. https://doi.org/10.1177/0022219407311040

Kocsis, Á., & Molnár, G. (2024). Factors influencing academic performance and dropout rates in higher education. *Oxford Review of Education*, 1–19. https://doi.org/10.1080/03054985.2024.2316616

Lefavrais, P. (1967). *Test de l'Alouette*. Les éditions du centre de psychologie appliquée.

Lefavrais, P. (2005). *Alouette-R*. Les éditions du centre de psychologie appliquée.

Lindstrom, J. H. (2007). Determining appropriate accommodations for postsecondary students with Reading and written expression disorders. *Learning Disabilities Research & Practice*, *22*(4), 229–236. https://doi.org/10.1111/j.1540-5826.2007.00251.x

MacCullagh, L., Bosanquet, A., & Badcock, N. (2017). University students with dyslexia: A qualitative exploratory study of learning practices, challenges and strategies. *Dyslexia*, *23*, 3–23. https://doi.org/10.1002/dys.1544

Mazur-Palandre, A., Abadie, R., & Bedoin, N. (2015). Étudiants dyslexiques à l'Université : Spécificité des difficultés ressenties et évaluation des déficits. *Développements (Revue interdisciplinaire du développement cognitif normal et pathologique)*, *18*(19), 139–177.

Moriña, A. (2017). Inclusive education in higher education : Challenges and opportunities. *European Journal of Special Needs Education*, *32*(1), 3–17. https://doi.org/10.1080/08856257.2016.1254964

Moriña, A., Cortés-Vega, M. D., & Molina, V. M. (2015). What if we could imagine the ideal faculty? Proposals for improvement by university students with disabilities. *Teaching and Teacher Education*, *52*, 91–98. https://doi.org/10.1016/j.tate.2015.09.008

Mortimore, T., & Crozier, W. R. (2006). Dyslexia and difficulties with study skills in higher education. *Studies in Higher Education*, *31*(2), 235–251. https://doi.org/10.1080/03075070600572173

Neuville, S., Frenay, M., Noël, B., & Wertz, V. (2013). *Persévérer et réussir à l'université*. Presses universitaires de Louvain.

Perelmutter, B., McGregor, K. K., & Gordon, K. R. (2017). Assistive technology interventions for adolescents and adults with learning disabilities: An evidence-based systematic review and meta-analysis. *Computers & Education*, *114*, 139–163. https://doi.org/10.1016/j.compedu.2017.06.005

Pino, M., & Mortari, L. (2014). The inclusion of students with dyslexia in higher education: A systematic review using narrative synthesis. *Dyslexia*, *20*(4), 346–369. https://doi.org/10.1002/dys.1484

Pintrich, P. R. (2000). Multiple goals, multiple pathways: The role of goal orientation in learning and achievement. *Journal of Educational Psychology*, *92*(3), 544–555. https://doi.org/10.1037/0022-0663.92.3.544

Quinlan, M. M., Bates, B. R., & Angell, M. E. (2012). 'What can I do to help?': Postsecondary students with learning disabilities' perceptions of instructors' classroom accommodations. *Journal of Research in Special Educational Needs*, *12*(4), 224–233. https://doi.org/10.1111/j.1471-3802.2011.01225.x

Reid, G., Strnadová, I., & Cumming, T. (2013). Expanding horizons for students with dyslexia in the 21st century: Universal design and mobile technology. *Journal of Research in Special Educational Needs*, *13*(3), 175–181. https://doi.org/10.1111/1471-3802.12013

Richardson, G. (2021). Dyslexia in higher education. *Educational Research and Reviews*, *16*(4), 125–135.

Robbins, S. B., Le, H., Oh, I.-S., & Button, C. (2009). Intervention effects on college performance and retention as mediated by motivational, emotional, and social control factors: Integrated meta-analytic path analyses. *Journal of Applied Psychology*, *94*(5), 1163–1184. https://doi.org/10.1037/a0015738

Schneider, M., & Preckel, F. (2017). Variables associated with achievement in higher education: A systematic review of meta-analyses. *Psychological Bulletin*, *143*(6), 565–600. https://doi.org/10.1037/bul0000098

Snowling, M., Dawes, P., Nash, H., & Hulme, C. (2012). Validity of a protocol for adult self-report of dyslexia and related difficulties. *Dyslexia*, *18*, 1–15. https://doi.org/10.1002/dys.1432

Tremblay, S., & Loiselle, C. (2016). Handicap, éducation et inclusion : Perspective sociologique. *Education et francophonie*, *44*(1), 9–23. https://doi.org/10.7202/1036170ar

von Davier, R. (2012). Une pédagogie adaptée – Suggestions pour les écoles genevoises. *Babylonia*, *3*, 52–56.

INDEX

Pages in **bold** refer to tables.

academic accommodations 208–210, 337–339
academic achievement 24–26, 31–33, 344–346
academic resilience *see* resilience
access to higher education 7–8, 31–33
adult dyslexia 1–7, 9–16, 22–40, 65–104, 287–290
adult literacy 23–24
alphabetic orthographies 3, 5, 72–73
American Psychiatric Association *see* Diagnostic and Statistical Manual of Mental Disorders (DSM-5)
anxiety 6, 14, 346–348
auditory hypothesis 2–3
automaticity: in reading 130–132; theoretical accounts 131–133

behavioural markers of dyslexia 4, 34–35
Bergey, B. W. 219–232
Bonnefond, A. 105–128
brain networks: functional connectivity 186–189; reading-related networks 180–184
brain plasticity *see* neuroplasticity
Brysbaert, M. 205–218

Carroll, J. 5–6
Catts, H. W. 5–6, 287–289
Cavalli, E. 1–16, 65–104, 298–336

cerebellar hypothesis 3, 133–135
clinical practice: in adulthood 8–10; implications for higher education 340–343
cognitive profiles 26–29, 33–35, 71–74
cognitive remediation: effects on reading **245–248**, 249–250; neural changes associated with 250–254
Colé, P. 1–16, 298–336
Collette, É. 337–360
comorbidity: attention deficit hyperactivity disorder (ADHD) 4, 14, 28–30; developmental language disorder 4, 29; dyscalculia 4, 28–29
compensatory mechanisms 6–7, 13–16, 31–33, 90–94, 298–336; neural correlates 302–305; strategic compensation 312–318
comprehension skills *see* reading comprehension
Costanzo, F. 243–286
Cutting, L. E. 12–13

Deacon, S. H. 219–232
decoding: deficits in adulthood 24–26, 30; relationship with oral language 70–72
definition of dyslexia: current debates 287–290; DSM-5 framework 4–5; historical perspectives 1–3

developmental dyslexia: persistence across the lifespan 3–4; risk and protective factors 5–7
diagnosis: in adulthood 205–210; in higher education 205–210; limitations of exclusionary criteria 3–5
Diagnostic and Statistical Manual of Mental Disorders (DSM-5) 4–5, 287–289
disability services: in higher education 8–9, 210–212
Doignon-Camus, N. 105–128
Duncan, L. G. 1–16, 298–336
dyscalculia see comorbidity

educational attainment 7–8, 25–26, 37–38
emotional resilience 6–7, 15–16
employment outcomes 25–26, 336–337
exclusionary criteria: limitations of 3–5; role in diagnosis 3–4
executive functions 6, 29–30, 34, 129–152; deficits in adults with dyslexia 130–134; relationship with reading comprehension 140–143; role in academic functioning 136–139

fMRI studies 180–184, **248**, 249–252
Frenay, M. 337–360
functional connectivity see brain networks

genetic factors: in dyslexia 298–301; interaction with environment 300–302
Gordon, R. 153–178
Goswami, U. 2–3, 5
growth mindset 6

higher education: access for adults with dyslexia 7–8, 31–33; inclusive practices 337–339; learning demands 32–33; support services 8–9, 210–212
Hoeft, F. 302–305

identity development 6–7, 336–337
inclusionary criteria: definition and scope 5–6; probabilistic perspective 5–7
inclusive pedagogy 337–339
International Dyslexia Association (IDA) 1–2, 5
intervention: in adulthood 243–250; neural effects of **248**, 249–252
IQ discrepancy model see exclusionary criteria

language comprehension: components of 76–79; role in academic reading 88–91
language transparency 6, 72–73
Law, J. M. 65–104
learning disabilities: in adulthood 23–25; definition of 22–23
learning strategies 219–232; metacognitive components 224–228; strategic adaptation 229–232
lexical knowledge 73–75
listening comprehension 76–78
longitudinal studies 24–26

magnocellular deficit theory 2–3, 133–135
memory 153–178; long-term memory 166–170; prospective memory 170–173; short-term memory 155–158; working memory 158–166
Menghini, D. 243–286
metacognition 6–7, 219–232
morphological awareness: contribution to reading comprehension 80–83; preserved skills in adulthood 83–84
motivation 32–33, 231–232
multiple deficit model 5–6

neural plasticity see neuroplasticity
neurodevelopmental disorders 2, 4–5, 28–30
neuroimaging research 179–204; EEG studies 190–194; fMRI studies 180–184; MEG studies 194–197
neuroplasticity 6, 15–16, **248**, 249–252; adaptive changes in adulthood 250–254
nonword reading 24–26

oral language skills **66–67**, 68–75, 88–94; as compensatory resources 89–94; interaction with decoding 70–72
orthographic processing 2–3, 105–128

Parrila, R. 219–232
Pennington, B. F. 5–6
phonological awareness 3, 41–44
phonological deficit hypothesis 2–5
phonological processing 1–5, 41–64; deficits in adulthood 44–48; interaction with oral language 70–72
processing speed 27–28, 30
protective factors 6–7
psychosocial outcomes: anxiety and depression 6, 14; self-esteem 6–7

Ramus, F. 287–297
reading comprehension 7, 12–13, 78–91; predictors in adulthood 81–85; time-unconstrained conditions 92–94
reading fluency 5–6, 30, 44–48
reading instruction quality 5
resilience 6–7, 15–16, 336–337
Richlan, F. 179–204
risk factors 5–7

Schelstraete, M.-A. 337–360
Schraeyen, K. 41–64
screening: in adulthood 205–210; in higher education 205–210
self-esteem 6–7
semantic processing: role in reading comprehension 73–76
Smith-Spark, J. H. 129–178
Snowling, M. J. 5–6
socio-emotional outcomes 26–27, 336–337
specific learning disorders 4–5
strategic compensation *see* compensatory mechanisms

support services *see* disability services
Swanson, H. L. 22–40
syntax: complexity effects 77–79

Tops, W. 205–218
Tunmer, W. E. 3–4

university students with dyslexia 31–33, 36–38, 336–339

Vanderauwera, J. 41–64
Vandermosten, M. 41–64
Vicari, S. 243–286
visual processing deficits 105–108
visuo-attentional span 2–3, 105–108
vocabulary knowledge: breadth and depth 73–75

working memory 29–31, 158–166; role in reading comprehension 31–32

Ziegler, J. C. 2–4, 6